Introduction to Vocational Rehabilitation

This text provides an overview of vocational rehabilitation (VR) practice, making it the perfect companion for students and practitioners with an interest in supporting people back to work and improving their sense of health and well-being.

The book is divided into three parts: the first covers the policy context of VR in the UK, defining VR, outlining the development of national standards in the sector, and looking at issues such as the economy and worklessness, and the legal background to the employment of disabled people. The second part examines models of VR practice and relevant standards. It explores the nature of developing services in the public and private sectors, illustrated by case studies from a range of disciplinary backgrounds. The final part presents a detailed introduction to the knowledge and skills required to provide a VR service, including consideration of the multidisciplinary processes and stages involved.

Introduction to Vocational Rehabilitation includes numerous case studies and a dedicated chapter of issues and questions to aid reflection. Comprehensive and evidence-based, this is the first multidisciplinary textbook for students and practitioners from a range of backgrounds, including occupational therapy and health, physiotherapy, human resources, nursing, social work and health psychology.

Clive Langman has held senior vocational rehabilitation positions in the public and private sectors. He is a visiting lecturer at City University, UK, and, as a member of the Vocational Rehabilitation Association's Professional Development Committee, is involved in training and standards development.

Introduction to Vocational Rehabilitation

Policies, practices and skills

Clive Langman

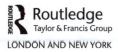

LONDON AND NEW YORK

First published 2012
by Routledge
2 Park Square, Milton Park, Abingdon, Oxon OX14 4RN

Simultaneously published in the USA and Canada
by Routledge
711 Third Avenue, New York, NY 10017

Routledge is an imprint of the Taylor & Francis Group, an informa business

British Library Cataloguing in Publication Data
A catalogue record for this book is available from the British Library

Library of Congress Cataloging in Publication Data
Langman, Clive.
  Introduction to vocational rehabilitation : policies, practices and
  skills/by Clive Langman.
     p. cm.
  1. Vocational rehabilitation – Great Britain.   I. Title.
  HD7256.G7L36 2011
  362'.0425—dc22   2011009653

ISBN: 978–0–415–60305–8 (hbk)
ISBN: 978–0–415–60306–5 (pbk)
ISBN: 978–0–203–80442–1 (ebk)

Typeset in Times
by Florence Production Ltd, Stoodleigh, Devon

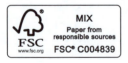

MIX
Paper from
responsible sources
FSC
www.fsc.org   FSC® C004839

Printed and bound in Great Britain by
TJ International Ltd, Padstow, Cornwall

A great number of demographic, psychological, social, medical, rehabilitation-related, workplace-related and benefit-system-related factors are associated with return to work. The different types of risk factors are associated in many ways. People with greater chances of job return after vocational rehabilitation are younger, native, highly educated, have a steady job and high income, are married and have stable social networks, are self-confident, happy with life, not depressed, have low level of disease severity and no pain, high work seniority, long working history and an employer that cares and wishes them back to the workplace. Unfortunately people with the above profile are seldom found amongst the long-term sick.

(Selander *et al.*, 2002)

Contents

Acknowledgements

Gratitude is expressed to the following individuals or organisations for their guidance and/or for permission to reproduce materials: Anne Chamberlain, Academic Department of Rehabilitation Medicine, University of Leeds; Helen Benson and Wendy Lerums, Access to Work, Jobcentre Plus; Helen Blake, Regional Work Psychologist, Jobcentre Plus; David Booth, Principal Psychologist, Jobcentre Plus; Takis Christophe, Chartis Medical and Rehabilitation; Colin Ettinger, Irwin Mitchell, solicitors; Andrew Frank, Vocational Rehabilitation Association; Clare Ginders, Ginders Vocational Rehabilitation Solutions; Bob Groves, Sainsbury Centre for Mental Health; Katherine Houston, Healthy Working Lives, and staff of the Dundee pilot NHS VR programme; David Ianetta, Supported Employment, Jobcentre Plus; Robert Little, Employment Judge, Employment Tribunals Service; The Papworth Trust, Cambridgeshire; Joy Reymond, UNUM; Eric Sharpe, Derbyshire NHS Condition Management Programme; Heather Watson, physiotherapist; Brenda Williams, United Kingdom Rehabilitation Council; Matthew Young, Association of British Insurers. I am indebted to the facilities and staff of the British Library Documents Centre Reading Room at Boston Spa, North Yorkshire.

Any errors within the book are mine. It is inevitable, within a changing market, that policies, services and professional skills develop. Of significance during the writing of this book has been the formation of the Conservative/Liberal Democrat coalition in May 2010, following 13 years of New Labour government and a period of substantial reform in the Welfare State.

Clive Langman, Sheffield, 2010

Introduction

There is widespread agreement that the process of vocational rehabilitation (VR) should be '*top-down*' and '*bottom-up*' (Frank and Sawney, 2003). Top-down relates to government policy. To enable people with disabilities/health conditions to engage in work and, at the same time, ensure that those unable to work have income security, New Labour reform (1997–2010) was very much a top-down process, whereby health and employment services were brought closer together, and the benefits system was aligned with employment strategies. This is a process that will become even more evident with the policies being pursued by the Conservative/Liberal Democrat coalition formed in May 2010. Practitioners are more likely to view VR as a bottom-up process, whereby clients are helped to return-to-work (RTW) after illness or injury. This book addresses both '*top-down*' and '*bottom-up*' approaches to VR and their interrelationship, in both the public and private sectors.

From the 1990s until the recession that began in 2007, the United Kingdom enjoyed significant economic growth, contributing to record low levels of unemployment. Yet, in 2002, the Department for Work and Pensions (DWP) recorded that, in the previous 20 years, the number of incapacity benefit (IB) claimants,[1] representing the United Kingdom's sick and out-of-work population, had tripled to a total of 2.7 million people (DWP, 2002). Unless the health of the UK working-age population was seriously declining, at the same time as record NHS expenditure was recorded, the data suggest that something else was happening in the labour market, not least because the DWP report recorded that RTW fitted the expectations of 90 per cent of early IB claimants. In practice, 40 per cent never made that transition, and, once a person had been on benefit for a year, they only had a one in five chance of returning to work within 5 years. Although there is evidence that the ease of claiming IB offers some explanation for the growth in the number of claimants, this does not provide an answer to the question as to why so many claimants should find it so difficult to leave IB once on it. A related issue is the lack of any explanation as to why UK employers should have such high rates of sickness absence compared with their European competitors. In addition to the economic and financial consequences of ill health and worklessness to the nation and to employers, the problems accompanying social exclusion (social justice in Scotland) have also been heard, particularly in the mental health (MH) sector. The United Kingdom has a financially and socially unaffordable problem with the health of its working age population.

The Conservative/Liberal Democrat coalition and the emergence of the Work Programme are likely to fill many VR practitioners with foreboding. Fundamental questions have already been asked as to the outcome of examining 1.5 million IB claimants (using a 'snap-shot' assessment methodology based on medical and not functional criteria), when there is unlikely to be any work available for very many of these people, as an architect of benefits reform recognises (Gregg, 6 July 2010; see www.guardian.co.uk). An independent review of the Work Capability Assessment (WCA) identified many flaws (Harrington, 2010).

Although there is a consensus view that the United Kingdom needs to reduce its levels of public expenditure, making the unemployed and disabled pay for RTW services with money saved on the payment of IB (now changing to the Employment and Support Allowance (ESA)) raises not only moral issues but also issues relating to programme efficacy. Despite the complexity of the services developed by New Labour, evidence suggests that the measures taken to reduce the IB count were beginning to work, and, until the recession took hold, the rise in the number of claimants had been checked (Anyadike-Danes and McVicar, 2008).

Hence, having faced up to the problems arising from years of neglect of the welfare state, the United Kingdom is now again in uncharted waters. David Freud, Minister for Welfare Reform, acknowledged at the 2010 Vocational Rehabilitation Association/ College of Occupational Therapists (Work Section) annual conference that there is no evidence that the proposed service provider funding mechanism (based on an outcome-related performance, with additional payments for hard-to-place service users) will protect the interests of those furthest from the labour market.

Although it might be maintained that the specialist disability services within Jobcentre Plus will continue to serve the interests of jobseekers with significant health conditions, and the VR obligations of the NHS, contained within National Service Frameworks (NSFs), remain in place, already contracts for a successful joint Jobcentre Plus/NHS venture, Condition Management Programmes, have not been renewed.

People with disabilities and health conditions cannot be 'incentivised' into employment by reducing their benefits income when they face structural barriers to employment, such as difficulty in matching themselves against suitable vacancies or the preference of employers for fit employees with recent work histories, and when jobseekers have an inability to fit into flexible working expectations. Hence, having made considerable progress over the last decade, VR services in the public sector currently face major challenges to promoting the interests of the population they serve. Likewise, growth in private sector VR services is not guaranteed to continue at the same rate, as insurers face challenges to keep down premiums and employers need to reduce costs. Both public and private sector services can best rise to the challenges by proving the cost-effectiveness of the services they provide. In this fashion, '*bottom-up*' can begin to influence '*top-down*'.

In the circumstances, having examined the major policy influences and factors influencing the substantial growth in the United Kingdom's VR sectors over the last 15 years, this book addresses how VR can improve service efficacy and provide an answer to the United Kingdom's problems of high levels of sickness, disability and worklessness.

Part 1: Health, disability and worklessness in the UK

Chapter 1 defines VR in relation to the post-war development of employment and disability services within the United Kingdom. It identifies why a 'two-strand development' of VR in employment and health services has contributed to varying definitions and understanding of what VR means. It establishes the relationship of VR to treatment, clinical rehabilitation and workplace disability management, including sickness and absence policies. It identifies core and non-core VR practitioners and considers issues relating to the establishment and monitoring of individual and organisational standards in VR practice.

Chapter 2 identifies the scale of worklessness and costs to the UK economy contributing to post-1997 public sector policy development and the private sector growth in VR services.

Chapter 3 considers the policy response of the incoming New Labour government in 1997 to a post-war lack of reform in the welfare state and the high cost of ill health/disability and unemployment. It identifies the VR strategies adopted by the DWP through its operational arm, Jobcentre Plus, the NHS and the Scottish government and considers the implications of the 2010 Conservative/Liberal Democrat coalition and the Work Programme.

Chapter 4 addresses the private sector VR response to the growing cost of litigation resulting from claims arising from accidents, Employers' Liability Compulsory Insurance (ELCI) and Group Income Protection (GIP) policies. It identifies the business case for employers providing VR services.

Chapter 5 identifies the legal obligations of employers with regard to health and safety and their obligations under the Disability Discrimination Act 1995 and 2005 and the 2010 Equality Act.

Part 2: Employment and disability services in the United Kingdom: models of vocational rehabilitation practice

Chapter 6 considers VR service users and the factors influencing the choices they make. This includes reference to benefits changes.

Chapter 7 identifies the services delivered or supported by Jobcentre Plus. It considers the roles of New Deal for Disabled People (NDDP) and Pathways to Work and their subjugation into the Work Programme. It further addresses the role of disability employment advisors (DEAs), work psychology, Access to Work, residential training colleges (RTCs) and the changing face of supported employment.

Chapter 8 presents private sector VR services, with reference to the modus operandi of a number of large and small service providers. In addition, the long-standing importance of the voluntary sector is illustrated with reference to both generic and condition-specific services.

Chapter 9 reviews VR-related services within the NHS. In particular, it addresses the role of primary care and the implementation of the VR components of NHS NSFs. It reviews the comprehensive VR strategy of the Scottish government for delivering community-based VR within the NHS, and it examines two condition-specific models of VR practice within the NHS for service users with MH problems and for those with an acquired brain injury.

Part 3: The vocational rehabilitation process: the application of skills and knowledge

Chapter 10 addresses the multidisciplinary nature of VR. It considers the role of the VR counsellor (whatever discipline), case management and case recording.

Chapter 11 begins to address the VR process by considering theoretical models of disability underpinning VR practice. Following the presentation of a four-stage, twelve-step VR model, stage 1 of the process is examined, with a view to initial information gathering and the formulation of an assessment and rehabilitation plan.

Chapter 12 considers stage 2 of the VR process: assessment practices, identifying a range of available instruments for assessing physical, cognitive, social and behavioural skills contributing towards a graduated-return-to-work (GRTW) plan.

Chapter 13 develops stage 3 of the VR process: pre-placement support and job development, with reference to rehabilitation services, job search and interview skills, in addition to considering the role of job coaches.

Chapter 14 considers stage 4 of the VR process: improving job placement and retention rates. It addresses placement options, the use of work-site evaluations, the role of workplace adjustments, the development of compensatory strategies, self-management strategies and the use of natural supports at work.

Chapter 15 looks to the future with regard to incentivising VR, supporting small and medium-sized employers (SMEs); public sector expenditure and learning from the mistakes of the past; research; and the needs for organisational and individual accreditation and regulation.

Part 1

Health, disability and worklessness in the United Kingdom

1 Recognising vocational rehabilitation

Key issues

- Post-war separation of employment from health services.
- Definitions and understanding of VR reflecting two strands of development.
- The relationship of VR to clinical rehabilitation and disability management (DM) practice.
- Major stakeholders in VR and their target populations.
- Identification of 'core' and 'non-core' VR practitioners and services.
- The development of service provider and practitioner standards.

Learning objectives

- Understanding the background to the public sector employment and disability services from when New Labour took office in 1997.
- Awareness of the reasons for the development of private sector VR.
- Understanding the differing perspectives and activities describing VR practice.
- Awareness of the Vocational Rehabilitation Association's Standards of Practice (2007), the UKRC's Rehabilitation Standards (2009a, b, c; 2010), and the Publicly Available Specification 150 (UKRC, Dept. BIS, BSI, 2010).

Introduction

Although it has received a great deal of government and private sector attention over the last decade, VR remains poorly understood within the UK. Hence, an obvious starting point for this book is to clarify what is understood by '*vocational rehabilitation*'. As VR has come to mean different things to different people, some historical explanation is required as to how this has arisen. In contrast to the United States, where the passing of the 1920 Smith-Fess Act is perceived to have marked the development of VR (Rubin and Roessler, 2001), the United Kingdom has no comparable legislation establishing VR services and marking operational boundaries. Neither are there are any mandatory organisational or individual accreditation requirements specifying VR practitioner standards and establishing a means of compliance. Although VR in the United Kingdom was given an initial thrust by the 1944 Disabled Persons (Employment) Act, public sector VR essentially describes RTW practices developed by employment and health services for their service users with health-related barriers to work. To understand VR in the United Kingdom, including differences of opinion as to what constitutes VR, is to understand this development, a matter expanded over the last 15 years in the private sector, through the interests of insurance companies. In the circumstances, Chapter 1 starts with a brief post-war history, until 1997, of RTW services for people with health conditions, providing the background for examining the various definitions of VR and its component parts. (Developments from 1997, and from when New Labour took office, are continued in Chapter 3, as these form the basis for the nature of current services.) Chapter 1 concludes with a review of recently developed service provider and individual standards.

Two strands of development: 1941–97 employment and health services

Employment services

Floyd (1997) reports that 'vocational rehabilitation services in the UK were virtually non-existent prior to the Second World War'. Concern for people injured in the war resulted in the Tomlinson Committee being set up in 1941, and its recommendations led to the 1944 Disabled Persons (Employment) Act (Bolderson, 1991). Underlying Tomlinson's recommendations was the proposal that, following medical treatment, rehabilitation back to work should be provided by the Ministry of Labour. Hence, industrial rehabilitation services began to be developed apart from the National Health Service, which was not formed until 1948. The Act, shaping employment and disability practice for the next 50 years, offered four distinct means of promoting employment:

1   A quota scheme, whereby employers of more than twenty people were required to employ 3 per cent of the workforce registered as disabled at their local Labour Exchange – 'the Green card scheme'. Initially, the scheme is reported to have been 'quite successful' (Smith *et al.*, 1991), 'with gradually declining effectiveness' attributed by the government to a failure of disabled people to register enabling employers to fulfil their quota. Organisations representing disabled people maintained that it was the failure to enforce the scheme that resulted in the lack of incentive to register. Prior to the retrenchment of the scheme, preceding the 1995 Disability Discrimination Act (DDA), only eleven prosecutions were made, with fines rarely exceeding a few hundred pounds.

2   The Ministry of Labour was charged with establishing a national network of Industrial Rehabilitation Units (IRUs), renamed Employment Rehabilitation Centres (ERCs) in 1974. By the 1970s, thirty-six ERCs were located in large conurbations, with two residential ERCs, Egham and Preston, serving those unable to attend an ERC on a daily travelling basis. In the 1950s, one ERC, Garston Manor (Watford), was located alongside an NHS Hospital's clinical rehabilitation services, but this development was not replicated elsewhere. The weekly ERC case conference was led by a centre manager and attended by a peripatetic employment medical advisor, who provided an initial screening of referrals and was supported by an on-site nurse, a disablement resettlement officer (DRO), an occupational psychologist (OP), a social worker and the leader of the industrial and commercial staff responsible for the various workshops and offices. Six ERCs also had a physiotherapist attached to them. All referrals were received from DROs (retitled Disability Employment Advisors in 1994) based in Labour Exchanges (subsequently Jobcentres).

For nearly 50 years, ERCs were the most readily recognisable VR service in the UK – the modus operandi contributing to a non-clinical view of VR that continues to prevail in some circles. The rehabilitation process was based on interviews, counselling, psychological assessment and workshop observation. By the mid 1970s, the proportion of ERC clients going into open employment had dropped to less than half. An evaluation was undertaken by the Employment Rehabilitation Research Centre (ERRC), established in the mid 1970s and disbanded a decade later.[1] The report addressed the lack of changes over the previous 30 years, including outdated assessment approaches and even a failure to recognise changed labour markets and types of disability (Cornes, 1982). These criticisms and a National Audit Office (NAO) report (1987), which noted the lack of ERCs in large areas of the country and discrepancies in respect of measuring their occupancy, performance and costs per resettlement, led to changes in the way ERCs operated. The approach to assessment was changed, with the introduction of the VALPAR range of component work samples (VCWS). Effectively, assessment relied on initial interviews and examinations, followed by two days of psychometric testing, work sampling and workshop performance during the remainder of the intake week. Only if it was considered necessary was a programme of rehabilitation offered. This was viewed as a gentle introduction to work and an extended practical assessment, achieved by placement in the ERC's own workshops, commercial, clerical and/or outdoor facilities.

3   An employment placement service, effectively DROs placed in Labour Exchanges, and training at newly formed Government Training Centres (GTCs), renamed Skillcentres in 1974 and closed in the early 1990s. The 1940s also saw the emergence of specialist Residential Training Colleges (RTCs).

4   The setting up of sheltered workshops. Remploy was formed to run a large number of such workshops, although a few local authorities also responded with their own schemes. The other significant strand of the 1944 Act, the Sheltered Placement Scheme (SPS), sometimes in the past referred to as Sheltered Industrial Groups (SIGs), has continued to be based on the concept of disabled people working alongside able-bodied ones in open employment and subsidised through government.

There was little change to the nature of the disability employment services during the next 30 years, although the Piercy Committee, reporting in 1956 and reviewing the 1944 Act, had some success in promoting psychologically trained staff within IRUs.

In 1973, the Employment Rehabilitation Service (ERS) was put under the wings of the Manpower Services Commission (MSC), aligning the service with training and separating it from its referral sources, DROs and Jobcentre services, which remained within the Department of Employment. Within the latter service, the 1970s saw some other developments, and particularly a focus on addressing environmental barriers to employment. The work of DROs was supported with a number of special schemes providing clients with:

- help with fares to work;
- advice and financial assistance with regard to technical aids and with adaptations to premises (the beginning of the Access to Work scheme);
- a personal reader service for blind and partially sighted people;
- a small subsidy to employers for the first few weeks of employing a disabled person (the Job Introduction Scheme (JIS)).

Following 1987 NAO criticisms of ERCs, the Employment Service went on to publish a consultative document, *Employment and training for people with disabilities* (1990). ASSET (Assistance to Employment and Training) teams were initially established, providing a short assessment service prior to three key changes that followed:

1   Beginning in 1992, DROs and the assessment activities of ERCs were combined into Placement, Assessment and Counselling Teams (PACTs), each one with an occupational psychologist. Assessments were based on interviews, psychometric tests and work samples.
2   The network of ERCs was closed down and replaced by nine regional Ability Development Centres (ADCs), with responsibility for monitoring the provision of services to people with disabilities, co-ordinating staff training and research. ADCs were closed during the mid–late 1990s.
3   Tenders were sought from private, public and voluntary agencies to provide around 8,000 Work Preparation (rehabilitation) courses per annum.

The PACTs, renamed Disability Service Teams in 1999, controlled the budgets for agency rehabilitation contracts in their local areas. Work Preparation courses, typically of six weeks' duration, have continued to be run, mainly by voluntary organisations (Lakey and Simpkins, 1994; Banks *et al.*, 2002), although they are now due to be incorporated into a new, Supported Employment programme (see Chapter 8).

Key dates to 1997 in the evolution of policy and practice are indicated in Table 1.1. The policy approach gradually moved from assistance with assessment, rehabilitation and placing, to include the encouragement of labour market participation through tax credits, and anti-discrimination legislation.

Health services

In giving responsibility for employment rehabilitation to the Ministry of Labour, the 1944 Act separated employment services for disabled people from the emergent NHS.

Table 1.1 Post-war evolution of disability employment policy in the UK to the mid 1990s

1944	**Disabled Persons (Employment) Act**: Responsibility for services given to Ministry of Labour, established IRUs, quota scheme (set at 3%), sheltered employment, designated jobs and DROs.
1956	**Piercy Committee**: Introduced psychologists into IRUs.
1971	**National Insurance Act**: Invalidity benefit introduced.
1973	**Employment and Training Act**: Establishes MSC (with responsibility for national skills training), IRUs renamed ERCs and placed under MSC. DROs become disability employment advisors and stay in the Employment Department.
1991	**Disability Working Allowance Act**: Wage top-up for low-paid workers introduced (replaced with tax credits in 1999).
1992	**Closure of ERCs**: (process began in 1991) PACTs established. Work Preparation courses introduced as 'agency rehabilitation'. Ability Development Centres (ADCs) introduced.
1994	**Social Security (Incapacity for Work) Act**: Introduces All Works Test and Incapacity Benefit.
1995	**Disability Discrimination Act**

Smith *et al*, (1991) make no reference to VR within the NHS, although Holmes (2007) and Ross (2007) outline some post-war provision. Chamberlain (2007) records that, post-war, those who ran medical rehabilitation services within the armed forces transferred their skills to the new NHS. However, only one 'of at least 25 rehabilitation centres' had an IRU placed alongside it (Garston Manor at Watford). She observes that, 'this experiment was successful: it allowed graduated entry into the industrial environment or, where this had been too early, allowed the person to receive the required medical or therapy input.' Although the Piercy Committee (1956) recommended extensions, this experiment was never repeated. Chamberlain adds that, although many reports (Tomlinson, Piercy, Tunbridge, Mair) said that rehabilitation needed to be incorporated into clinical practice, they were 'almost entirely ignored'. Despite these periodic attempts within the NHS to promote a commitment towards employment rehabilitation, the lack of any statutory obligation contributed to a situation in which the issue of returning patients to work largely disappeared from both practice and training agendas. A change in the nature of the labour market in the 1960s, away from manufacturing and production, contributed to making it more difficult for patients to find work, and workshops became largely redundant. In the mental health (MH) sector, Industrial Therapy Units (ITUs) were not replaced with adequate community-based alternatives (Wansbrough and Cooper, 1980). The NHS and Community Care Act (1990) led to large numbers of health-care professionals moving out of acute hospitals into community-based services, and the focus of rehabilitation became one of independent living. Throughout most of the 1990s, RTW services substantially remained the responsibility of the Employment Service and its agencies, although both private and NHS development was taking place (Thurgood, 1997). Even so, the British Society for Rehabilitation Medicine (BSRM) reported that 'the NHS has largely lost the culture and skills of facilitating employment as a key element of effective health care' (BSRM, 2000).

An overview of public sector development is indicated in Figure 1.1.

Private sector

Until the mid 1990s, private sector VR rarely existed, outside a tiny number of cases arising from personal injury (PI) litigation and employee assistance programmes (EAPs).[2] However, during the previous decade, the Association of British Insurers (ABI) developed an interest in VR that included funding research, resulting in the publication of the *Vocational Rehabilitation Index* (Cornes, 1990), a tool to enable insurers to make an early identification of personal injury claimants only likely to return-to-work following VR. Both a general lack of enthusiasm for funding VR and a lack of agencies for delivering VR services contributed to such activity being neglected and forgotten.

By the mid 1990s, there had developed a crisis in the public sector relating to the number and costs of IB claimants and associated issues (see Box 1.1).

Although the Conservative government introduced the 1995 Disability Discrimination Act, the provisions were initially restricted to employers of more than twenty people. By the time New Labour took office in 1997, the consequences of years of neglect and lack of reform of the welfare state were reflected, not only in the high cost of paying IB, but also in the high level of sickness, disability and worklessness contributing to the rising cost of Employer Liability Compulsory Insurance (ELCI) and social exclusion.

The 'two strands' of VR development (Employment Service and NHS) have been covered because of the way this contributes to the current understanding of VR within

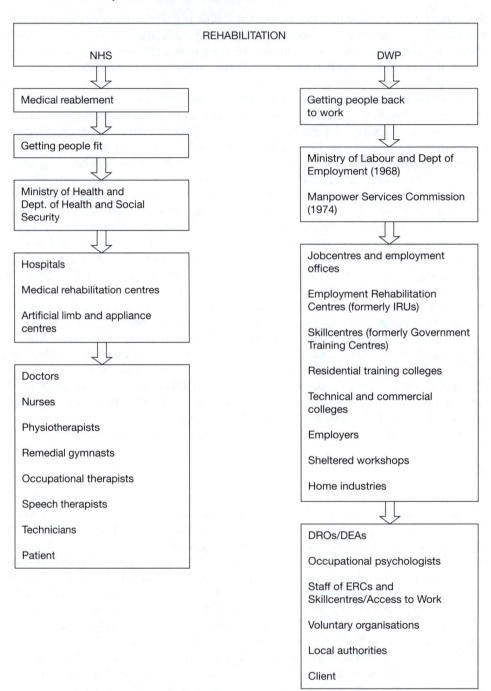

Figure 1.1 Post-war development of VR services

Box 1.1 1990s' crisis in the employment and disability sector

- The number of people claiming incapacity benefits continued to rise
- A policy approach to the employment of disabled people was based on a medical model of disability perceiving people with health conditions as so sick or disabled as to be unemployable (and unable to benefit from employment rehabilitation services). For many years, claimants in receipt of IB were expressly excluded from ERC attendance, on the basis that they were not 'work ready'.
- There was a separation of medical from employment services.
- Geographically and numerically limited VR services failed to keep abreast of both changes in the UK labour market and international practice.
- The private sector became concerned at the rising costs of compensation and premiums.

---

the United Kingdom. The development of VR services in the United Kingdom is continued in Chapter 3.

Defining vocational rehabilitation

A significant characteristic of VR in the United Kingdom is that it is a *voluntary* activity. It remains to be seen to what extent sanctions provided in the payment of the ESA, introduced from 2008, will lead to claimants having to participate in any RTW programme or risk having their benefits reduced. In the private sector, there is no obligation on any organisation or employer to provide VR, although, in PI claims, the courts will sometimes order a defendant to pay for VR if a voluntary agreement between the parties cannot be reached.

When organisations, such as the Vocational Rehabilitation Association (VRA, 2007), and individuals, such as Waddell *et al.* (2008), have defined VR in the United Kingdom, they have relied on perceived main activity, not bounded by reference to organisational or individual accreditation, qualifications, skills or any legislative framework.

Box 1.2 Defining VR: the VRA Standards of Practice (VRA, 2007)

'A process of facilitation, designed to assist people with impairments or health conditions to secure employment and to integrate into the community.'

Box 1.3 Defining VR (Waddell *et al.*, 2008)

'Whatever helps someone with a health problem to stay at, return to and remain in work.'

The first definition implicitly incorporates a case management concept through reference to 'a process of facilitation', whereas the second description, provided by clinicians, could refer to almost any activity, however singular or tangential, contributing to a patient's employment.

This dichotomy, between, on one hand, a case-managed process taking a service user through a series of return-to-work (RTW) steps, and, on the other hand, any work-related intervention, continues to reflect much current understanding and use of the term 'vocational rehabilitation'.

A useful way of understanding how this situation has transpired is to examine the role of 'core' and 'non-core' VR practitioners. VR is widely recognised as a multi-disciplinary process, and, almost invariably, it is non-core practitioners who implicitly reflect the much broader understanding of VR defined by Waddell *et al.* (ibid.).

Core and non-core practitioners

In July 2000, representation was made by the National Vocational Rehabilitation Association (NVRA, now VRA) to Margaret Hodge, Minister with Responsibility for Disabled People, to consider the need to develop qualifications for people with responsibility for providing employment support, information, advice and guidance for disabled people.

HOST Policy Research was commissioned to undertake the research (HOST Policy Research, 2002). The objectives of the project included mapping the diverse occupations covering employment and disability functions in the United Kingdom. Although occupations 'covering employment and disability functions' do not necessarily meet the varying definitions of VR, a feature of the UK market is the piecemeal availability of services, so that even a private sector VR case manager may have to rely on referring a client to a public sector service in order to provide a comprehensive VR package.

HOST distinguished:

- **Core occupations** – where practitioners from a range of disciplinary backgrounds, and in a variety of activities, spend the whole or a substantial part of their time in working with disabled people, or with service delivery staff, with the aim of individuals securing or retaining employment or self-employment.
- **Non-core occupations** – where practitioners may have involvement with assisting the employment or retention of disabled people, but this forms only a small part of the practitioners' work, illustrated by reference to general practitioners (GPs) in primary health care.

HOST proposed five main clusters of core occupations, based on the analysis in Figure 1.2. Across all five areas, HOST found specialists and generalists shared common functions and a training/qualifications gap. HOST used this framework to present an understanding of the constituent occupations in the employment and disability sector, noting:

> the great diversity in skill and skill mixes in the area . . . Actual jobs will involve different combinations of some of the constituent activities, although, for few occupations, employment activities with disabled people will commonly cross several of these clusters (e.g. occupational therapists, case managers, and employment consultants/job coaches).

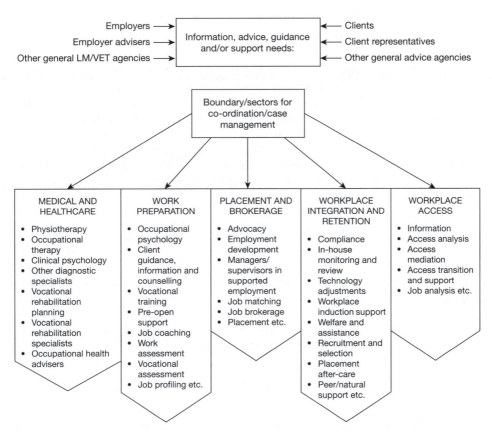

Figure 1.2 Disability and the labour market: defining and identifying occupational boundaries (after HOST 2002)

Overall, the HOST review showed that practitioners involved in employment and disability in the UK operate in a fragmented and complex occupational labour market. At the time, there were around 10,000 'core' practitioners in the UK involved in vocationally related medical and health care, work preparation, placement and brokerage within employment and disability, or in specialist support services in workplace access, integration and retention – all activities that are integral to VR. Since this review, this number is likely to have substantially increased, as a consequence of insurance-funded private sector growth and public sector policies, such as NSFs within the NHS. Many practitioners operate across two or more of the occupational groupings, suggesting a high degree of breadth and job enlargement in practitioners' roles, and a high demand for multi-skilling across many constituent functions. The number of non-core practitioners is now likely to considerably exceed the 70,000 identified by HOST. The difficulty in identifying the VR market is reflected in the way the DWP defined VR when drafting *Building capacity for work: a framework document for vocational rehabilitation* (DWP, 2004). It was thought easier to produce a working description of VR rather than try to define the term (Box 1.4):

Box 1.4 Describing VR (DWP, 2004)

A process to overcome the barriers an individual faces when accessing, remaining, or returning to work following injury, illness or impairment. This process includes the procedures in place to support the individual and/or employer or others (for example, family and carers) including help to access VR and to practically manage the delivery of VR; and in addition VR includes the wide range of interventions to help individuals with a health condition and/or impairment overcome barriers to work and so remain in, return to, or access employment. For example an assessment of needs, re-training and capacity building, return to work management by employers, reasonable adjustments and control measures, disability awareness, condition management and medical treatment.

There was also a difficulty in reflecting polarised views on the role of treatment within VR:

> Some stakeholders see VR as the process of getting people who have a health condition or injury or impairment back to work. Other stakeholders suggest that VR is a process for helping people into a job when they have not worked for a long time and others see it has a distinct secondary process over and above medical rehabilitation.

In producing its working description of VR, DWP discussions with stakeholders highlighted the following common characteristics:

- **Employment goal**: At the heart of VR must be an employment goal, for example to remain in or RTW, or access employment for the first time. An individual's goals could relate to full-time or part-time employment, self-employment or even voluntary work. All stakeholders should start with the basic premise that the individual is 'employable'.
- **Balanced mix of appropriate help**: Any form of rehabilitation needs to consider the personal and social needs of the individual, as well as any functional needs. The necessary medical, social and psychological interventions, to help the individual overcome barriers to work, need to be identified.

Many VR practitioners, particularly those in DWP-funded services and the private sector, are now likely to consider that VR has a number of identifiable service characteristics, such as case management, rehabilitation planning and client-support services. A number of issues are perceived to be key to defining and understanding VR (Box 1.5).

It will be recognised how VR has come to mean different things to different people. This book is primarily concerned with the activity of core practitioners, although it would not contribute to any understanding of how VR operates to ignore non-core practitioners and services.

Box 1.5 Key issues in defining and understanding VR

- The stage post-injury or disability onset when VR is delivered (for instance, definitions arising out of NHS experience are more likely to reflect early intervention, including a treatment component).
- Distinguishing service characteristics, for example client identification, initial planning, assessment, the delivery of rehabilitation services, job resettlement and retention strategies.
- The activity of 'core' and non-core' VR practitioners and services.

Vocational rehabilitation and clinical treatment

Arising from post-war development, some VR agencies and practitioners continue to perceive VR as applying only to RTW intervention taking place following treatment. The United Kingdom Rehabilitation Council (UKRC) reported such feedback to its draft paper on organisational standards in rehabilitation (UKRC, 2010). Various models of the rehabilitation process now start with the onset of a condition, as illustrated in Figure 1.3, although there are authorities that maintain that, instead of being a process arrived at sequentially, VR should occur concurrently with other forms of rehabilitation (BSRM, 2003; Waddell and Burton, 2004). Evidence of good clinical practice to facilitate the RTW process has been established for some time, although it remains the case that clinical intervention is often delivered without a vocational focus, and communication problems remain a barrier to effective rehabilitation for work, not least between occupational-health (OH) professionals and GPs (Beaumont, 2003; Sawney and Challoner, 2003). However, it has been established for some time that clinical interventions work best when they have a relationship to the workplace (Loisel *et al.*, 1997; Van der Weide *et al.*, 1997; Frank *et al.*, 1998; Krause *et al.*, 1998); have access to ergonomic solutions (Heller, 1997); include modified work, for example light duties, graded work exposure, work trial (Krause *et al.*, 1998); and they are managed in a non-adversarial, supportive work environment, characterised by pro-active management, employer–employee co-operation, good communications and a managed RTW process (Habeck *et al.*, 1998).

- Post-1997, New Labour policy influenced a cultural recognition that a sick or disabled person's employment capability is not fixed and can be positively influenced. In practice, it can be an unproductive exercise in attempting to draw a line between clinical and vocational rehabilitation, especially when clinical activity is directed towards facilitating employment. Waddell *et al.* (2008) comment on the difference between VR and '*treatment*', at the same time recognising that VR is connected to treatment, not least because untreated conditions can lead to a separation from work. Many VR services now incorporate a clinically based input, especially shortly post-injury/illness and when RTW is first being considered. However, this is not always the case. For example, staff within Remploy's Third Sector VR service report[3] that, although they have access to clinicians, including OTs and psychologists, they 'hardly ever' have recourse to this expertise. Their employment advisors find

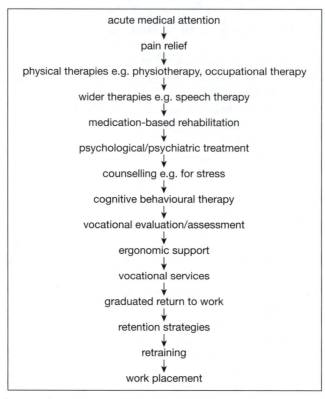

Figure 1.3 The journey from injury or illness to employment

client resettlement invariably requires individual and organisational adjustments to be made, and they have confidence in their own ability to counsel, undertake job and task analyses and identify appropriate supports.

What activity represents vocational rehabilitation?

Given the history, it is understandable that VR practitioners have developed different views on what constitutes VR, ranging from any intervention that supports the RTW process, to a detailed and structured case-managed programme. This situation may only reflect the respective positions of non-core and core practitioners and the nature of the services in which they work. Even if they cannot deliver a complete VR service, all practitioners are likely to recognise the elements in Figure 1.4.

Vocational rehabilitation stakeholders and the target populations for VR services

The UK Framework for Vocational Rehabilitation (DWP, 2004) identified the principal stakeholders as (1) employers, (2) the insurance industry, (3) the individual, (4) government and (5) VR providers (although there are others, such as the legal profession and the Health and Safety Commission/Executive).

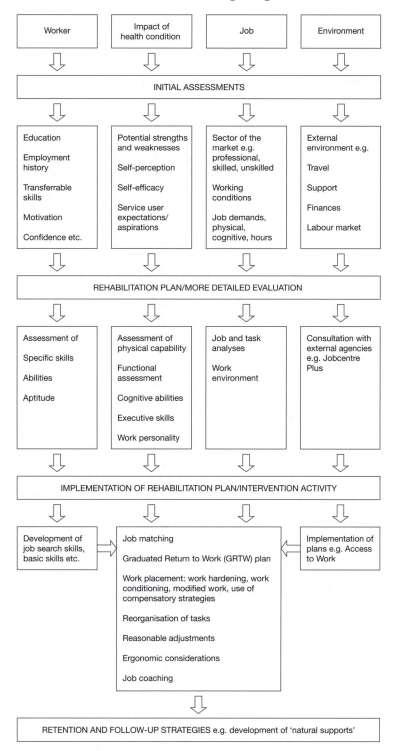

Figure 1.4 Elements of a comprehensive VR service

Box 1.6 Main VR drivers for employers

Perceived benefits:

- managing the costs of employment;
- retention of trained and experienced personnel;
- maintaining employee productivity;
- maintaining a competitive economic position alongside occupational health, sickness-absence management, job retention, and healthy workplaces as a means of achieving such benefits.

---

1   **Employers**: Stakeholders suggested a number of benefits that VR could deliver for employers, for example, in developing a more efficient business through retaining trained and experienced personnel. Employers commented that their main drivers in this area were managing the costs of employment, maintaining employee productivity and a competitive economic position. They suggested that occupational health, sickness-absence management and job retention, and ensuring healthy workplaces are part of the means to achieve this.

In the framework document, there is little reference from employers to VR enabling them to meet their statutory obligations towards disabled employees.

2   **The insurance industry**: The position of the insurance industry is addressed in Chapter 4.

3   **The individual**: Employee representatives, for example the Trades Union Congress (TUC), foresaw VR as vital for those people who fall through the health and safety net. They also saw VR as having a contribution of its own to improving health and safety standards in the workplace, especially when an individual returns to work after injury.

The framework document acknowledges that it is important to remember that individuals whose illness or injury is not work-related, and where no negligence is involved, also need support.

There is often a view, which can be inadvertently reinforced by health professionals, that illness necessarily prevents working. However, for people who are able to work, it can be an important step in the road to recovery and rehabilitation, thereby helping people to enjoy better health and well-being.

4   **Government**: Government interest in VR is argued on several different levels, ranging from helping people who have a health condition or impairment back into employment through to the potential benefits of increased productivity for the economy as a whole. The biggest single driver is to take claimants off sickness benefits. There are many potential benefits to the United Kingdom of increasing the effectiveness of VR. These include a reduction in social exclusion, better health and reduced costs for the NHS. In addition, it is recognised that the government is an employer, and it suffers financially, as well as seeing reduced employee effectiveness, when individuals are absent

from work owing to ill health. The government itself can benefit from measures that can help retain individuals in work or help RTW after ill health or impairment.

5   **VR providers**: The framework document recognises that all of the stakeholders are dependent on the availability of high-quality VR services. It notes that, 'providers have an interest in proving the benefit of VR, as VR demand will inevitably increase as a consequence. It is also important for stakeholders to be confident about the effectiveness of the services on offer.'

Target populations

DWP discussions with stakeholders for the framework document highlighted that one area of contention appears to be whether VR includes helping individuals who have never worked. It can be seen as contradictory to use the term rehabilitation to explain support to restore a capacity that was not previously there. However, many stakeholders saw that providing support to help an individual with a health condition and/or impairment overcome barriers to employment, and so enter work for the first time, as VR. A research overview suggests the target population for VR services might include the people indicated in Table 1.2.

Vocational rehabilitation and workplace disability management

In the United Kingdom, some people refer to VR and disability management (DM) synonymously. On the other hand, there are other authorities, such as Holmes (2007), who recognise conceptual and practical distinctions.

On a worldwide basis, DM owes its origins to self-insured employers in the United States responding to the rising costs of claims for disability and injury during the 1980s. It continues to be an expanding area of practice, and the International Labour Organisation (ILO) has developed a Code of Practice for Managing Disability in the Workplace (http://ilo.org/public/libdoc/ilo/2002/102B09_340_engl.pdf).

At an international level, DM refers to *employer-led* prevention and rehabilitation initiatives ensuring that not only sickness absences but also known health conditions of *employees* are regularly monitored, and that appropriate adjustments are made to accommodate their needs and those of disabled job applicants. For example, when describing the Canadian approach, Harder and Scott (2005) consider that, 'disability management has been primarily concerned with return-to-work post-injury or illness' and describe a model of practice linked to claims management and RTW programmes, adding that, 'it is important that DM initiatives are in line with the corporation's

Table 1.2 Target populations for VR services

People:
1   currently in employment, who are experiencing difficulty retaining employment because of a health condition or impairment
2   temporarily absent from work because of a health condition or impairment
3   with a health condition or impairment for whom absence becomes longer term and who may become unemployed as a result
4   who have not worked for some time, or never worked, because of a health condition or impairment

overall objectives and mandate. The components of the programme include all the important elements of prevention, claim initiation, claims/case management, RTW and accommodation'.

The employer-led approach is reflected in definitions of DM; see, for example, Box 1.7.

Box 1.7 Definition of disability management (Williams and Westmoreland, 2002)

A 'pro-active employer-based approach to a) prevent and limit disability, b) provide early intervention for health and disability risk factors, c) foster co-ordinated disability management and rehabilitative strategies to promote cost-effective restoration and return to work.'

In the UK workplace, DM is perceived by many to encompass a much broader approach than managing a potential or actual compensation claim (CIPD, 2009, www.cipd.co.uk/subjects/dvsequl/disability/disandemp.htm). Figure 1.5 presents an overview of organisational DM, based on the parameters set out in one of the earliest UK publications on DM (Smith *et al.*, 1991), considered just as relevant today as when published.

Hence, within the United Kingdom, DM is used to refer to comprehensive organisational policies ranging from recruitment practices through to training, promotion and medical retirement, as well as including matters familiar to VR practitioners, such as ensuring that not only sickness absences but known health conditions of employees are regularly monitored, with appropriate adjustments being made to accommodate their needs and those of disabled job applicants. The typical aims of a DM policy are indicated in Table 1.3.

In relation to point 7 of Table 1.3, Ross (2007) cites studies indicating that the DM model has been successful for those with musculo-skeletal injuries (Isernhagen, 2000)

Table 1.3 Aims and objectives of a DM policy

Enabling employers to:

1   comply with anti-discrimination legislation
2   ensure 'the best' candidates are not rejected because of unfounded assumptions
3   ensure the workforce remains integrated and motivated
4   identify and promote talent
5   provide a safe working environment
6   manage absence and a return to work
7   facilitate the retention of employees who become disabled or develop a condition
8   develop an awareness of internal and external support
9   increase workforce morale and provide a framework for workforce/union discussions
10 facilitate job retention (particularly during the first year of employment and for an ageing workforce)
11 decrease the cost of health-related absence from work; in particular reduce the number of lost working days
12 increase productivity

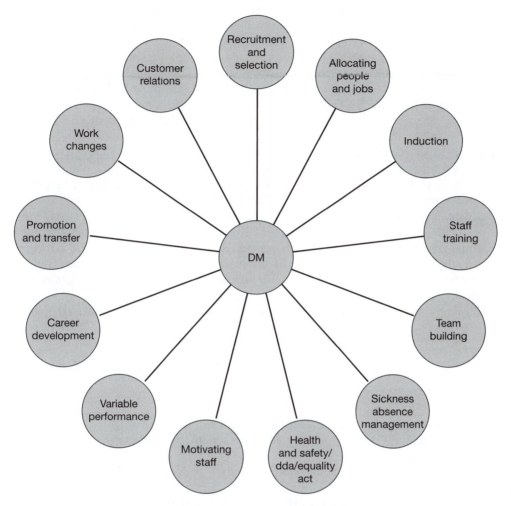

Figure 1.5 Aspects of a comprehensive disability management policy

and preventing work injury (Williams and Westmoreland, 2002), but has been less widely used for people with MH problems (Olsheski *et al.*, 2002).

What is the relationship of VR to DM?

Within the United Kingdom, the Health and Safety Executive (HSE) has identified the link between OH and safety, sickness and absence management, and VR. It perceives VR as a distinct activity within an organisation's overall management of disability in the workplace (James *et al.*, 2003). However, it has been found that only 10 per cent of organisations have a separate rehabilitation policy, although 80 per cent practise some form of rehabilitation process (IRS Employment Review, 2001). The most effective are said to be early intervention, maintaining contact with sick employees and a phased RTW. Other research has found that the three most popular RTW options are an adjustment of working hours, transfer to other work and restricted duties (Nice and Thornton, 2004). Other typical workplace interventions include modified work and specialist referrals, for example to OH, physiotherapy and counselling services.

Within the United Kingdom, evidence suggests that employers are more likely to have stand-alone sickness-absence policies than integrated DM policies incorporating VR. Even when employers have sickness-absence policies, it is rare to find any reference to VR among SMEs. Few SMEs have a provision for occupational health, and, when an employee receives VR, this almost always follows the intervention of an insurance company or, possibly, NHS/Jobcentre Plus. Larger employers are more likely to make reference to VR in sickness-absence policies, but this almost always follows prolonged (at least 6 months) absence. Sickness-absence/attendance management policies often focus on short-term absence rather than the potentially greater problems of long-term absence, normally defined as 4 weeks and above. Although short-term absence is more prevalent, longer periods of absence can account for 75 per cent of costs (Henderson *et al.*, 2005). As a significant proportion of absence is long term, RTW initiatives are essential to any absence strategy, if sickness levels and costs are to be managed effectively (Evans and Walter, 2003). Effective rehabilitation in the workplace is likely to involve the issues identified in Box 1.8 and address common barriers identified in Box 1.9.

A salutary note is that some employees have shown resentment towards an employer accommodating a disabled worker. This has been used as a defence by employers in

---

Box 1.8 Effective rehabilitation processes

- Early intervention and contact with absent employees.
- Provision of rehab support – medical treatment, physiotherapy, counselling, retraining.
- Availability of workplace modifications – reduced hours, alternative or restricted duties.
- Co-ordinated approach to workplace rehabilitation involving all stakeholders.
- Clear policy frameworks relating to rehabilitation procedures.
- Full involvement of all employees in rehabilitation process.

Box 1.9 Common barriers to rehabilitation

- Access to medical treatment due to NHS waiting lists.
- Economic factors – generous occupational sick pay or disability benefits.
- Lack of top-level organisational commitment.
- Cost of workplace modifications and availability of suitable alternative duties, particularly for smaller firms.
- Poor communication and common purpose among key stakeholders.
- Lack of co-ordinated approach among rehabilitation providers.

legal proceedings, a matter particularly recorded in the United States (Paetzold *et al.*, 2008). Although strongly resisted by the courts, this argument illustrates the extent to which co-worker education and training need to be incorporated into effective disability and attendance-management strategies.

VR service provider and practitioner standards

Employers, insurers and groups representing individuals have all identified the need for providers of VR services to adopt agreed standards where they exist and develop standards where they do not. Stakeholders have also expressed the need for the accreditation of providers (DWP, 2004). Although the private sector VR market has grown substantially in recent years, to be worth many millions of pounds a year, and the service users of both public and private sector VR deals have vulnerable clients, standards of VR practice in the United Kingdom are voluntary, implicit and not policed by any regulatory authority. Although agencies contracted to Jobcentre Plus have to provide evidence of their propriety, the focus has invariably been on financial management. Even many individual core practitioners are not subject to mandatory standards set by a professional body. The exceptions are when individual practitioners are members of a professional organisation, such as the College of Occupational Therapy, the Society of Chartered Physiotherapists or the British Psychological Society, and overseen by the Health Professionals Council. However, these bodies are concerned with the professional competence and standards of their members and not VR standards. Rehabilitation providers in countries such as the United States and Canada have long had standards and regulations to follow (the Commission on Accreditation of Rehabilitation Facilities (CARF) Regulations), so that commissioners and service users are aware of the standard of rehabilitation they might expect. In the absence of legislation defining the market, setting the boundaries and establishing a regulatory agency, the United Kingdom is unlikely to develop mandatory standards and accreditation requirements in the immediately foreseeable future. However, there are a number of quality descriptors, although, as yet, little incentive to observe them. Accreditation to a quality mark seems the natural step forward, and then regulation of the rehabilitation field. It seems sensible for the UKRC to take on the role of accreditation and policing, although, at the present time, it does not have the resources to do this.

Standards developed in the VR market relate to: the purchasers of services; the providers of services; and individual practitioners.

United Kingdom Rehabilitation Council (www.rehabcouncil.org.uk)

The UKRC took shape from around 2006 onwards, when like-minded individuals recognised a need for the United Kingdom's rehabilitation sector to speak with one voice.

Although the UKRC remains a small voluntary body, receiving some financial support from the Department of Health (DH) and the Scottish Centre for Healthy Working Lives, it is playing an increasingly influential role in the development of rehabilitation standards. Developed with the aid of a DWP contract, and following extensive consultations, the UKRC's own standards were published in May 2009 (www.rehabcouncil.org.uk). Reflecting initial ABI and DWP support, these standards provide guidance for service providers and cover the issues identified in Box 1.11.

Box 1.10 United Kingdom Rehabilitation Council

Our mission

The UKRC exists to provide an authoritative voice and focal point for anyone with a stake in medical and vocational rehabilitation and to support those who are working to help sick and injured people regain their independence.

The council

The UKRC is a community of rehabilitation associations, rehabilitation providers, clients and other stakeholder groups. Our common goal is to ensure access to high-quality medical and vocational rehabilitation services in the UK.

Acting as an umbrella organisation for this broad community, the council has been established to provide a united voice on issues of importance to us. The council seeks to co-ordinate the efforts of its members, in order that our combined efforts have the greatest possible impact.

Box 1.11 Minimum policies of service providers

- equal opportunity and diversity policy
- user involvement policy
- user care and protection policy
- data protection and confidentiality policy
- health and safety policy
- bullying and harassment policy
- drug and alcohol policy
- customer service policy
- other providers' communications policy, both for internal and external use
- corporate social responsibility policy
- recruitment and selection policy
- continual professional development policy
- quality assurance and feedback policy
- contracting/subcontracting policy
- business continuity policy
- whistle-blowing policy
- environmental policy

Public Availability Specification 150 (PAS 150)

Following on from the UKRC standards, the Department for Business, Innovation and Skills supported the development of a Code of Practice to facilitate the commissioning and purchasing of services. These standards were produced by the British Standards Institute (BSI) and came into effect in April 2010 (www.bsigroup.com). Unless these standards become recognised as the sector norm and kite-marked, purchasers of services will continue to have no ready means of identifying the expertise of practitioners and no means of comparing and contrasting costs and outcomes.

Box 1.12 Scope of PAS 150

- services
- organization
- rehabilitation workforce
- service user involvement
- referral
- induction
- assessment and planning
- intervention
- case co-ordination
- discharge/closure
- follow-up services
- programme evaluation

Individual VR standards

Even though the HOST report (ibid.) found the effectiveness of support services being held back by poor access to, or provision of, practitioner training, skills training and qualification, the United Kingdom still has no requirement for any VR practitioner to hold a specific level of recognised accreditation.

The VRA represents both individual and corporate practitioners. In April 2007, the VRA launched its Standards of Practice (www.vocationalrehabilitation.org). The standards set out service delivery standards (Box 1.13), as well as the required demonstrable standards for VR professionals in respect of service delivery, client protection, professional development, professional knowledge, transferable skills, corporate governance and business development.

At the present time, any organisation running a RTW service can describe itself as a VR agency, and anyone working in such an organisation as a VR professional. Although it may be reasonably maintained that most practitioners have at least graduate-level qualifications and belong, or answer to, professional organisations with their own code of ethics, this does not guarantee that they are able to meet all professional VR standards, such as those outlined in Table 1.4.

Box 1.13 VRA service delivery standards

- Adequate staff training and supervision.
- Clear definition of services.
- Clearly outlined referral procedures.
- A clear understanding of the nature and relevance of any recommended assessments.
- A clear identification of obstacles at individual, organisational and systemic levels.
- Access to understood community-based assessments.
- An action plan aimed at meeting agreed goals.
- Implementation of the action plan 'in a timely fashion'.
- Integrated services.
- Consistent and active monitoring and support.
- Maintenance of counselling skills.
- Avoidance of transferring cases.
- Appropriate closure.
- Involvement of client and employer in the VR process.
- An understanding from 'significant others' that the client is the key decision maker.
- Written service standards, policies and procedures.

Other than the VRA Standards of Practice, the other individual developed standards relate to case management. The Case Management Society of the United Kingdpm (CMSUK) has published Standards of Practice (2005) aimed at practitioner level (www.cmsuk.org).

Summary

The VR sector in the United Kingdom is a broad church. At one end of a theoretical VR continuum, there are organisations and individuals entirely dedicated to providing VR services. At the other end, there are those providing just one aspect of a comprehensive VR service. Moreover, VR in the United Kingdom is at a dynamic and critical stage of its development, emphasising the need for practitioners to be equipped to move with market requirements and the changing needs of service users. In this climate, the identification of VR services and practitioners becomes increasingly important, as the United Kingdom inches towards both service regulation and individual accreditation. This is a difficult process, given the lack of legislation identifying operational boundaries.

The content, focus and context of many services and the work of VR practitioners continue to change, as public policy changes the way in which disabled people are supported in preparing for, remaining in, or seeking work. Indeed, it will be noted in subsequent chapters that the United Kingdom is developing discrete public and private sector approaches to VR, although the skills and knowledge of practitioners have much

Table 1.4 Selected requirements of VRA Standards of Practice

Client protection There should be evidence of:	Professional development/maintenance VR professionals should:	Professional knowledge VR professionals should be able to demonstrate knowledge of:	Transferable skills
Client consent	Have a degree (the VRA will review other education, training and experience to consider 'equivalency')	VR theory and practice	Communication skills
Confidentiality	Have the competencies to complete required tasks	Labour market recruitment and employment practices	Conflict resolution
Support and assistance	Pursue professional credentials in their areas of expertise	Job matching, job retention and return to work	Advocacy
Client protection	Ensure that services are effectively managed, in line with standards, guidelines and legislation	Medical aspects of disability	
Safety and security	Adhere to the Code of Ethics	Psychosocial aspects of disability	
Crisis management	Have regular supervision	Vocational aspects of disability	
Intervention	Participate in an annual performance review	Legislation/benefits system	
Mechanisms for reporting abuse, other concerns	Maintain knowledge and skills	Rehabilitation policy	
A complaints procedure	Be members of an appropriate professional body	Individual counselling	
	Contribute to the field	Family support and advice	
	Conduct research in a professional and responsible fashion	Multicultural issues	
	Have professional indemnity and public liability insurance	Community resources	
		Health and safety legislation	

in common. A particularly significant development is the growth in organisational disability management policies incorporating sickness-absence management strategies with specific reference to VR, a matter encouraged by the insurance market.

Student exercises

1.1 Core and non-core VR practitioners
Starting with yourself in the middle, build an organisation chart (hierarchical or linear) linking core and non-core VR practitioners on whom your service (or the one you would like to work in) relies.

1.2 Standards
With reference to the VRA's Standards of Practice, identify additional areas of knowledge and skills you need to acquire, on top of your own professional training, in order to be able to meet the requirements.

2 The nature of the problem

Sickness, disability, absenteeism, worklessness and a developing compensation culture

---

Key issues

Incidence of sickness absence in the UK

Public sector driven by:

- number of IB claimants;
- costs of worklessness being described as 'unsustainable' and exceeding cost of the NHS (DWP/DH, 2008a);
- social exclusion.

Private sector driven by:

- reducing the consequences of sickness and absenteeism;
- occupational health and safety;
- costs of claims for loss of earnings;
- insurance costs.

Learning objectives

- Awareness of the levels of sickness and absenteeism in the United Kingdom in comparison with neighbouring European countries.
- Understanding the particular *nature of* the United Kingdom's record.
- Recognition of who bears the costs of sickness and absenteeism.

Introduction

In 2006, Dame Carol Black was appointed as the government's National Director for Health and Work, a position bestriding the DH and DWP. Her review of the health of Britain's working-age population reports that, in 2006, an estimated 175 million working days were lost in Britain owing to sickness absence (DWP/DH, 2008a). The estimated annual costs of sickness absence and worklessness associated with working-age ill health were over £100 billion, reported to be greater than the annual budget of the NHS. However, statistics alone cannot convey the full cost to society or the economy of unemployment and disability. Although the burden of paying sickness and disability benefits is a key driver for policy reform, another oft-cited reason is the human cost of disability and long-term absence from the labour market (Burchardt, 2000; DWP, 2001; Office for National Statistics, 2002a and b; DWP, 2002; Prime Minister's Strategy Unit, 2004; Prime Minister's Strategy Unit *et al.*, 2005). The DWP states that, on average, those claiming IB for 12 months will continue to claim for 8 years. After 2 years, they are more likely to die or retire than return-to-work. Someone off work sick for 6 months or longer has an 80 per cent chance of being off work for 5 years (DWP *et al.*, 2005). Although there is good evidence that, in most situations, the benefits of work for an individual's mental and physical well-being outweigh any risks (Waddell and Burton, 2006), by the time New Labour took office in 1997 it is hard to escape the impression that the United Kingdom had slipped into a mentality that sickness and disability are synonymous with an inability to work.

New Labour took office with a programme of welfare reform, coinciding with 'vocational rehabilitation' being heard more often in the academic, voluntary, public and private sectors. By the new millennium, the British Society of Rehabilitation Medicine was calling for more joined-up services and advocated an increased role for the NHS (BSRM 2000, 2003), a momentum supported by the College of Occupational Therapists (COT). Contributing to the public sector change in attitude towards VR was a recognition that employment can help improve a person's health and well-being and help reduce health inequalities (Waddell and Burton, 2006). Conversely, it was recognised that unemployment is linked to higher levels of mortality and psychological morbidity (Mclean *et al.*, 2005). New Labour was particularly concerned with the costs to the public purse arising from disability and unemployment (DWP, 2002, 2003). In the private sector, the small, but significant, insurance-led VR services that began to emerge from the mid 1990s onwards were also driven by financial considerations to control the rising cost of ELCI and reduce compensation payments for the loss of earnings arising from injury or illness.

Although the primary driver for government and insurers remains a perception that an investment in VR will ultimately reduce expenditure, stakeholders began to develop their own positions, reflected in *Building capacity for work: a UK framework for vocational rehabilitation* (DWP, 2004), a document stemming from debate over the rising cost of ELCI. Although the framework document finds no evidence to support any radical intervention in the labour market (such as a compulsory system of rehabilitation analogous to the workmen's compensation systems found in countries such as Australia and Canada), the ABI has continued to promote VR and provide evidence as to the cost-benefits for its membership (ABI, 2006). In the public sector, New Labour took the view that the range of services on offer to unemployed people with health conditions would provide adequate RTW support (see Chapter 8).

Incidence of sickness absence in the United Kingdom

Although there are issues in respect of the accuracy of data on absence from work (Barham and Leonard, 2002; Barham and Begum, 2005), surveys of sickness absence are reported by the Confederation of British Industry (CBI) and the insurance giant Axa, the Chartered Institute of Personnel Development (CIPD) and the Engineering Employers Federation (EEF). Key findings from the CBI/Axa (CBI, 2008) and CIPD (2009) are indicated in Boxes 2.1 and 2.2.

Box 2.1 Key findings on absence and labour turnover (CBI, 2008)

Analysis based on replies from 503 companies who together employ more than 1 million employees, equivalent to 3.6 per cent of the UK workforce.

• In 2007, the direct cost of absence was £13.2 billion, or £517 per employee. Indirect costs add another £263 per employee. The total cost of absence came to £19.9 billion.
• The average employee took 6.7 days off sick.
• Some 172 million days were lost to sickness absence, 12 per cent thought to be non-genuine.
• Five per cent of absence spells became long term (20 days or more), accounting for 40 per cent of all time lost.
• Average absence levels in the public sector were 9 days, compared with 5.8 days in the private sector.
• Organisations that recognised trade unions saw three days' more absence than non-unionised workplaces.
• There were strong regional differences across the UK: the North-West and Yorkshire and Humberside lost most days, southern England the least.
• Minor ailments, such as colds, were the most significant cause of short-term absence; back pain came second.

Box 2.2 Key findings on sickness/absenteeism (CIPD, 2009)

Analysis based on replies from 642 employers, with more than 1.9 million employees:

• The average sickness absence was 7.4 working days per employee.
• The average annual cost of absence of each employee was estimated at £692.
• Absence levels in the public sector remain the highest.
• The main cause of short-term absence for both manual and non-manual workers was minor illness such as colds, flu and stomach upsets.
• Smaller organisations typically record lower levels of absence.
• The main causes of long-term absence (four weeks or more) among manual workers are acute medical conditions, followed by back pain, musculoskeletal conditions, stress and mental health problems.

The 2008 CBI/Axa survey reports absence between 3 per cent and 3.5 per cent of working time over the previous six years, figures broadly in line with CIPD and EEF studies.

In the public sector, absence is generally reported as being higher than in the private sector. The CIPD survey says that 9.7 days per employee were lost in the public sector in 2009, against 6.4 days in the private sector.

Duration of sickness absence

The 2008 CBI absence survey shows that, although 95 per cent of absences last fewer than 20 days, the remaining 5 per cent account for 40 per cent of all lost time. Europe presents a useful comparator to assess the United Kingdom's performance. A report from the International Monetary Fund (IMF) examines absence data from eighteen European countries. It is reported that the United Kingdom has the fourth-worst record, ahead of only the Netherlands, Sweden and Norway. The United Kingdom's performance is well below the main economic competitors, Germany and France (IMF, 2007).

Such data mask a significant absence issue. When comparing short-term and long-term absence, the United Kingdom has the second-lowest proportion of time lost to long-term absence across Europe, behind only Iceland. In most countries, the amount of total absence accounted for by long-term occurrences is much higher than for short-term. However, in the United Kingdom and Iceland, short-term absence is over 50 per cent of the total.

The UK has an unusual pattern of long-term absence (Box 2.3). The 2008 CBI/Axa absence survey suggests that only 6 per cent of all absence occurrences last for over 4 weeks, although they represent 43 per cent of the number of days lost. Given a total of 175 million days lost to all absence in the United Kingdom, this equates to 75.25 million days lost to long-term absence, and 99.75 million to short-term absence. Organisation for European Co-operation and Development (OECD) data make the same point, stating that, in the United Kingdom, only 5 per cent of sickness cases are classified as 'long-term', that is more than 20 days (OECD, 2006, 2007).

Although ill health obviously causes absence from work, overall levels of absence do not necessarily reflect the overall health of the working population. Some people exhibit 'presenteeism', working when not well, and there are people claiming incapacity benefits potentially capable of work but who, for one reason or another, do not work. *The Guardian* newspaper (13 October 2009) reported that 36 per cent of new ESA claimants are being found fit for work under the new assessment criteria (Chapter 6). Although critics suggest that the system is flawed (Harrington, 2010), particularly in assessing performance on a particular day rather than over a period of time, the inference is that large numbers of people in receipt of long-term sickness benefits are capable of some type of work. Indeed, long-term absence is often unaccompanied by major illness: rather, a person has 'drifted away' from work for one of many reasons, an important

---

Box 2.3   Unusual characteristics of United Kingdom's sickness-absence pattern

Compared with other European countries:

1   Sickness absence is high.
2   There is an exceptionally high quantity of short-term absence (less than one week).
3   There is a low number of long-term absences in terms of occurrences.
4   These long-term absences account for a disproportionately large amount of lost time.

factor contributing to the biopsychosocial approach to vocational rehabilitation (Chapter 11). However, it is incorrect to take a view that a large section of the UK IB/ESA population is workshy. It is apparent that, just as the overall level of sickness absence and worklessness reflects certain specific problems in the United Kingdom – high levels of short-term absence, low occurrence of long-term absence having a high impact, and a number of significant public health issues – the individuals falling within these categories are likely to have varying reasons for an absence from work. An understanding of these reasons forms the basis of intervention strategies aimed at addressing such matters.

The costs of sickness/disability absence and worklessness

Although reported data substantially refer to people with an employment history, there are many people with health conditions who have never entered the labour market, although capable of doing so, given the right support. This group of people is included in government data on the overall costs of worklessness. Dame Black's 2008 report (ibid.) into the health of Britain's working-age population presents a stark picture of the cost of poor health. For the government, the losses are estimated at between £62 and £76 billion. These costs are made up of benefits, health-care costs and lost taxes. The costs to the UK economy of poor health and absence among the working age population are calculated differently. A figure between £103 and £129 billion has been estimated, including health-care and informal-care costs, lost production and sickness absence. The high costs of IB/ESA and the impact on people's lives of long-term dependence on state benefits are major policy concerns for government. Around 7.5 per cent of the working-age population now claim these benefits. Claims are still running at around 600,000 per year and cost the taxpayer over £7 billion per year.

Why does the United Kingdom have high levels of sickness absence?

Dame Black's review records a UK working-age population of 36.6m people, with around 25 per cent not in work, 28 per cent in this position because of sickness, injury or disability. On the other hand, the employment rate for disabled people increased from 38 per cent to 48 per cent between 1999 and 2008. Black also reports that as many as 40 per cent of employers have no sickness-absence management policy. Various sources of data suggest some common ground as to the health reasons for sickness absence, although it appears that employees with MH issues are reluctant to self-report this (Table 2.1 and Box 2.4).

Causes of short-term absence

The main causes of short-term absence for both manual and non-manual workers are generally attributed to 'minor illnesses' such as colds and flu, stomach upsets, headaches and migraines. Among manual workers, musculoskeletal disorders (MSDs), such as neck strains and repetitive strain injuries, are the next most significant group. Stress is the second-biggest cause of short-term absence for non-manual workers, followed by MSDs, home and family responsibilities and back pain (CIPD, 2009). Preventing or addressing conditions early, while they are short term, could help to reduce long-term absences.

Table 2.1 Common health problems as causes of disability and sickness absence

	People with self-reported long-term disability (LFS, 2003)	GP sick certification (Shiels et al., 2004)	Self-reported sickness absence due to work-related ill health (HSE unpublished data)	Early retirement on health grounds (Collected literature)*
Mental health conditions	11%	40%	32%	20.5%
Musculoskeletal conditions	34%	23%	49%	15.5%
Cardio-respiratory conditions	24%	10%	—	c10–15%

*Major variation in different occupations and organisations.

Source: Waddell and Burton (2004).

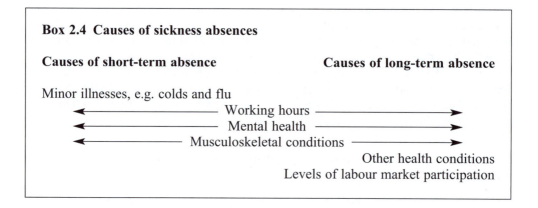

Box 2.4 Causes of sickness absences

Causes of short-term absence   **Causes of long-term absence**

Minor illnesses, e.g. colds and flu

◄——————————— Working hours ———————————►
◄——————————— Mental health ———————————►
◄——————————— Musculoskeletal conditions ———————————►

Other health conditions
Levels of labour market participation

Working hours

The UK has the second-longest working week in Europe, after Iceland, the other European country in the IMF survey with very high levels of short-term absence. The IMF concludes that, 'high sickness absence in the United Kingdom seems to be explained mainly by its comparatively long working hours' (IMF, 2007).

It is not clear what aspects of long working hours cause high absence rates, but a number of factors have been suggested. '*Stress*' of work has been advanced as one reason. The importance of the work–life balance also appears important. The IMF suggests that taking time off to attend to family, household or other personal issues is a 'rational' response to long working hours.

Causes of long-term absence

The major causes of long-term absence are reported in the main absence surveys and produce similar results. Employers rate acute medical conditions, back pain, MSDs and stress as the top four causes of long-term absences among manual employees. Stress is the number-one cause of long-term absence among non-manual employees, followed by acute medical conditions, mental ill health, such as depression and anxiety, and MSDs. Although some acute conditions necessitate a long period away from the workplace, most absences are not predetermined to be lengthy ones. The reason for absence persisting often begins with the way that it is managed in the first place. Leaving an employee isolated from their work is often a contributory factor to lengthy absence.

Labour markets

The IMF report (2007) suggests that rates of labour market participation have a role in levels of sickness absence, maintaining that, in countries where labour market participation grows, absence is likely to be higher. This is owing to the presence of more women and older workers in the labour market. Both of these groups tend to have higher than average levels of absence. Until the start of the recession in 2007, the UK labour market was growing, although hampered by high numbers on long-term benefits. Attempts to increase the levels in the future are likely to lead to a greater upward pressure on absence.

The IMF models indicate that a 1 per cent increase in labour market participation leads to an increase in time lost to absence of 0.05 per cent (IMF, 2007). In the United Kingdom, an increase of 0.05 per cent in time lost to absence is equivalent to losing another 87,500 days, based on a figure of 175 million days lost. If employment levels ever rise to 80 per cent, a government target prior to the recession, from a reported figure of 74.8 per cent (DWP, 2007), another 455,000 days of absence per year can be anticipated, simply as a result of increased labour market participation.

Data on workplace injury also support the view that an expanding labour market results in more injury and, thereby, more lost days. Whysall and Ellwood (2006) note that the dominant influence contributing to an individual's risk of injury is their job. Within the United Kingdom, the five most hazardous occupations are construction labouring; metal, wood and construction trades; vehicle trades; agriculture and animal-care occupations; and store- and warehouse-keeping. Research from the University of Warwick indicates that a 1 per cent growth in gross domestic product (GDP) is associated with a 1.4 per cent increase in major accidents (Davies and Jones, 2005). Such matters are thought to be particularly prominent in construction and manufacturing. The risk of workplace injury declines as job tenure increases. On the other hand, an increase in the number of new workers and overtime is associated with a higher level of reported injuries.

Levels of sickness benefits

The IMF indicates that high levels of public benefits are a possible cause of long-term absence from work. The Netherlands, Norway and Sweden are the only countries with a worse absence record than the United Kingdom in the report's scope and they are exceptionally more generous than the United Kingdom. In the Netherlands, this includes 2 years of sick pay (paid by the employer), 100 per cent of salary paid by the state for 1 year in Norway, and in Sweden, 80 per cent of salary that can be paid by the state indefinitely.

Within the United Kingdom, there is a lack of evidence that the level of benefits has any significant impact on the level of unemployment. On average, UK sickness benefit rates are among the lowest in Europe; hence, this cannot be a convincing explanation for the fact that so many people drop out of work owing to long-term absence from work. However, this situation may provide a part of the answer. As can be seen from surveys of IB claimants, the low paid are very much over-represented, and, hence, benefits represent a much higher proportion of potential earned income (Kemp and Davidson, 2008a, b).

Why the United Kingdom does not deal with its absences

There are a number of possible explanations as to why the United Kingdom has a poor track record in dealing with sickness and absence from work (Box 2.5).

Effects of health status and the 'medicalisation' of absence

A belief that the individual is 'too ill to work' has been highlighted repeatedly when considering the issues surrounding absence from work, participation in labour markets and levels of flow on to sickness and incapacity benefits, although 'no clear relationships have been found between sickness absence and health status' (IMF, 2007).

Most absence begins as a health issue for the person concerned. A problem can arise from a 'sick self-concept' and the way this is reinforced by health professionals and employment practices (Ford *et al.*, 2008). Over a period of time, the absence itself only adds to any perceived inability to return-to-work. Breaking the period of absence through early intervention therefore becomes crucial.

Research carried out at the Unum Centre for Psychosocial and Disability Research at Cardiff University highlights the importance of psychosocial factors – including beliefs, fears and advice from family – in prolonging absence from work (www.Unum.co.uk; press release dated 14 October 2008). The research also demonstrates that employers and health-care professionals need much greater awareness of these psychosocial issues when assessing how to help people return-to-work.

The principle negative influences on RTW are considered to be personal and psychological problems, including the belief that stress is the cause of ill health; social

---

Box 2.5 Explanations for the United Kingdom's poor track record in dealing with sickness and absence from work

1   **Effects of health status and the 'medicalisation' of absence**: a view that a person is either fit for work or they are not fit as a consequence of a health condition.
2   **Sickness certification and the role of general practitioners**: willingness to provide sick notes.
3   **Waiting times for NHS treatment**.
4   **Employers, the NHS and health and safety**: a lack of clearly defined responsibilities.
5   **Historical lack of prevention in UK health systems**.

influences, the most important of which are lone parents, unstable relationships and rented or social housing; and workplace culture and organisation (www.personneltoday.com, 20 November 2007).

Primary care: sickness certification and the role of GPs

In the United Kingdom, the role of GPs is critical in the medicalisation process (Ford *et al.*, 2008). GPs are seen, and often see themselves, as patients' advocates. This is likely to influence the signing of a sick note, particularly if the patient feels that the condition has been caused by work, or is likely to be made worse by it. To make a genuinely informed decision about whether the person can work or not, a GP is likely to need to understand the condition and how it arose; the tasks involved in the person's work; the working conditions, hours, environment and how these might change over time, affecting the employee; relationships with managers and colleagues; and possible alternative tasks that could be done in the person's workplace; and know what OH or well-being services are available at the individual's workplace and communicate with an employer about the individual.

Repeated sick notes often follow the first, depending on the employee's condition and on the GP's judgement. In particular, if the person has been referred to a hospital, a GP is unlikely to recommend RTW before the treatment has been received, regardless of what that treatment is. In the meantime, there is a risk of the individual becoming further isolated from work, and of further conditions adding to the existing one.

The position of the GP resulted in Dame Carol Black's report (ibid.) recommending Fit for Work notes and a Fit for Work service (see Chapter 9).

Waiting for NHS treatment

Waiting times in the NHS are highlighted as a problem by Dame Black in her report. This situation is almost inevitable, as the main causes of absence, MSDs and mental health, are likely to stretch available services, both through their high volume, and because they are unlikely to be an urgent priority, when set against acute and chronic conditions. Data released in February 2008 found that psychotherapy and counselling services had the longest NHS waits, with six trusts recording waits of more than 2 years (BBC News website, 8 February 2008). Waiting times for physiotherapy services can also average at least 60 days. The NHS has an ambitious target of seeing all referred hospital cases within 18 weeks. However, this does not cover community-based or primary-care-trust (PCT) delivered interventions, into which much MH and physiotherapy fall.

Employers, the NHS and health and safety – a lack of clearly defined responsibilities

Occupational Health is non-existent in many parts of the UK labour market. Employers' practices have long reflected a view that the NHS treats everybody, regardless of where or how their illness or injury happened. Employers have never had to make arrangements for employee health care unless they have wanted to do so, even if an employee was injured or made ill as a result of their work. In such a circumstance, the health care is paid for under the NHS Cost Recovery Scheme, through which insurers, who bear costs as a result of ELCI, pay around £200 million per year to the NHS.

In addition, the Health and Safety at Work Act 1974 never made protecting the general (non-workplace) health of workers a specific employer responsibility. Although there is a duty of care, the focus of the legislation is on safety rather than promoting health and well-being. The United Kingdom now has a good safety record, in contrast to many European countries. The impression is that businesses are far more receptive to messages on safety than those on the health of their workers. This is probably owing to the legal implications of failure in this regard.

Promoting the general health of employees has fallen into a gap between the NHS, health and safety legislation, and the workplace. A study of OH services in Sheffield examined what SMEs were doing and their attitudes to OH (Bradshaw *et al.*, 2001). The report concluded that,

> There appeared to be genuine confusion concerning who should be providing occupational health and to what degree employers should be responsible for the health of their employees, particularly when 'non-work-related' ill health was concerned, such as the risks associated with smoking and obesity. Furthermore, certain workplaces used accident rates alone as the marker for the success of occupational health provision and training, and that as a group, SMEs appeared to be orientated towards safety issues in the workplace, rather than health issues.

Decisions to invest in employee health and well-being

In the United Kingdom, the decision to invest, or not to invest, in employee health and well-being is left to employers. The decision is likely to be a financial one. In the absence of legal duties, employers must consider whether the health of their employees is adversely affecting the performance of the organisation enough to warrant investing in programmes supporting health. With regard to individual employees with a particular condition, the employer must decide if they should intervene or wait for the NHS process to run its course.

ABI research (Table 2.2) into why employers do not invest in OH found that employers overwhelmingly failed to see the need for OH services (ABI, 2006). Factors that lie behind this include a belief that this is not an employer responsibility, a lack of appreciation of the costs of poor health and absence, and considering themselves not likely to bear the costs of ill health over the long term.

Table 2.2 Why employers do not invest in occupational health (ABI, 2006)

	Private sector (%)		Public sector (%)		All (%)
	SMEs	Large	SMEs	Large	
Never thought they needed it	54	61	56	25	54
Too small to handle it	28	6	0	0	23
Cannot afford it	21	17	19	50	21
Never thought of it	12	0	6	0	10
NHS good enough	8	22	0	0	8

Base: All employers without OH provision

When making decisions about investing in individual or group health, an employer is likely to consider the return on investment and when this is likely to be realised; whether or not there is a mandatory imperative to invest; how much interventions cost; the costs of not investing; alternative costs such as hiring temporary staff or overtime costs; and whether or not the investment has other results, for example increased loyalty among employees or reduced staff turnover.

It appears that many employers consider there is no case for intervention, although businesses may not have fully assessed the costs of absence to the business. They may feel they have already contributed to the costs of the NHS; that investments in health take too long to feed through into productivity or into greater employee loyalty; or that interventions cost too much, and that the costs of long-term absences do not affect them severely enough to justify action.

With employees staying in jobs for shorter periods, there is less incentive for employers to take action to address public health issues. Obesity, smoking and alcohol consumption can continue for many years or decades before they have an effect on health. Although they may cause some short-term absences, they are more likely to lead to long-term conditions such as cancer, heart and liver disease or strokes. Many employers may decide that the unhealthy lifestyle of the employee will not cause a major problem during their period of employment.

Prevention in UK health systems

The United Kingdom has long lacked investment in preventative approaches. This is reflected in just 1.8 per cent of total spending on health going towards 'preventative' health care, as against an OECD average of 2.3 per cent (Health England, 2007). The United Kingdom spends large amounts trying to repair damage already done.

Who bears the costs of absence from work?

Although it varies as to when costs of absence from work are borne, they fall on the following:

1 employers
2 NHS
3 government
4 individuals
5 insurers (addressed in Chapter 4).

Employers

Employers directly carry the costs of absence through:

- statutory sick pay (SSP) (payable for up to the first 28 weeks of absence);
- occupational sick pay (OSP);[1]
- ELCI;
- cover for an absent employee or the cost of recruiting a new one;
- income-protection policies and, indirectly, lost productivity.

Taking into account direct and indirect costs of absence, the effect of absence on colleagues' performance, the variance of absence levels according to salary levels, and how costs fall on employees, in accordance with rates of OSP, qualifying periods and waiting days, it has been calculated the average daily costs of absence to employers is £120 per day (Sainsbury Centre for Mental Health, 2008). Given a total of 175 million days of absence, this works out at a total cost to employers of £21 billion in a single year. This estimate is similar to two other estimates. The 2007 annual CBI/Axa survey into absenteeism put the figure at £115 per day (CBI, 2007), and the Independent Counselling and Advisory Service Absence Survey 2006 (ICAS, 2006) arrived at a cost to employers of £119 per day.

NHS

The cost of absence to the NHS is difficult to quantify. Each visit to a GP costs over £30, and, although the cost of prescriptions, treatment and medical equipment, and administration could be considered as the provision of normal health care, they may also be considered as the costs of a person not well enough to be working, thereby placing an extra cost on the NHS.

The government/economy

The UK Framework for Vocational Rehabilitation indicates that around 25 per cent of GP consultations are work related; around 7.6 per cent of the working-age population claim IB/ESA; approximately 6.9 million people of working age self-report being long-term disabled; and around 5.4 million declare a work-limiting disability, 50 per cent of whom are in employment. Around 46 per cent of people with disabilities are economically inactive (DWP, 2004).

Throughout the first decade of the new millennium, around 2.7 million people continued to receive IB. Although costs are shared between employers, employees and the government, they arise at different stages in the process of employment or 'employability', turning into long-term sickness and exclusion from the labour market. In the first 28 weeks of absence from work, the government meets the cost of NHS-provided health care and lost taxes, if the person is on reduced OSP or on SSP. However, the individual still pays tax and national insurance (NI) through this period on whatever they receive above the tax and NI thresholds. The employer also continues to pay NI above the secondary earnings threshold. After 28 weeks, the costs of absence shift substantially from the employer to the state. The individual is no longer eligible for SSP and is unlikely to be entitled to any further OSP. The individual then enters the benefits system.

Individuals

The financial costs of absence for the individual obviously vary from person to person, depending on such factors as rates and duration of OSP. Over the long term, eligibility for state benefits is an important issue, as is the loss of any work-related benefits such as employer pension contributions. Shorter periods of absence are unlikely to hit the employee too hard, although, if there are waiting days for OSP, this could be important for low-paid employees.

The loss of skills can be considered a financial cost, but this is difficult to quantify. For those who work where rapidly changing requirements and equipment are common, a period of absence from the workplace can damage their prospects.

Longer-term absence is likely to be accompanied by a fall in income allied to potentially worsening health, including the possibility of other conditions developing, especially those linked to mental health. Absence from work can lead to social exclusion, worsening family and personal relationships, deepening debt problems and to substance misuse issues.

A parent experiencing long-term unemployment increases the likelihood of children being brought up in poverty and the loss of a working role contributing to a cycle of deprivation.

Summary

In both the public and private sectors, sickness absence in the United Kingdom represents enormous state and personal costs. However, the pattern of absence is not typical of Western Europe. The United Kingdom has a comparatively large amount of short-term absence, while a small percentage of long-term absences account for a great number of lost working days. A number of reasons have been put forward to explain this situation, including the 'medicalisation' of absence, compliant GPs and NHS waitng lists. There is little financial incentive for many employers to address long-term absences, as the financial burden quickly passes from the employer to the state.

Although government policy is primarily driven by financial considerations, the social problems for the individual arising from labour market exclusion have been increasingly recognised in recent years. However, given that a major thrust of policy of the Conservative/Liberal Democrat coalition is to reduce the level of benefits paid to sick/disabled people, the major effect this is likely to have is on the standards of living of claimants, not on their level of labour market participation. Evidence suggests that measures are required to address structural barriers to employment, as well as a significant economic growth for this to occur. As low growth is expected in the immediately foreseeable future in both public and private VR sectors, the lessons for service providers are ones of addressing barriers to achieving specific employment objectives, and of preventing job loss through promoting job-retention strategies.

Student exercises

2.1 Sickness absence and the public sector
What explanations are there for the public sector having a higher reported level of sickness absence than the private sector, and what can be done about this?

2.2 Sickness absence and employers
Given that the cost of long-term sickness absence is invariably met by the state and/or insurer, how can employers be encouraged to take a proactive approach towards the benefits of VR?

3   The public sector policy response

Key issues

- Fragmentation of policy responsibility.
- VR merging into the health and well-being agenda.
- NHS National Service Frameworks.
- The search for evidence-based practice.
- A co-ordinated strategy: the response of the Scottish government.
- New Labour and the Third Sector.
- The Work Programme: coalition response.

Learning objectives

- Identification of the government offices with responsibility for developing employment and health policy.
- Understanding of the main policies driving developments in the employment and health sectors.

Introduction

Given the United Kingdom's record on sickness and absenteeism, the scope for a more productive employment of people with health conditions attracted much policy interest as the United Kingdom moved into the new millennium. In addition to the financial and social costs of ill health/disability and unemployment, structural changes in the labour market, such as skill shortages and an ageing population, were seen to add a greater potential for many disabled people to seek work and for employers to recruit them. Increased life expectancy put pressure on pensions and health services, and work came to be viewed as crucial to maintaining living standards. Although economic slowdown has restricted opportunities, job-vacancy levels have remained high, even if there are issues in respect of the 'quality' of many vacancies. Conversely, there are also issues regarding the skills and qualifications required for higher-status positions and the attainments of many of the IB/ESA population.

New Labour (1997–2010) aimed to expand the numbers in employment to 80 per cent by '*incentivising*' people into work, including people with health conditions, and reducing the number of people falling out of work because of ill health (DWP, 2001). From 1997 onwards, the government vigorously promoted changes to the welfare state.

Although some policies and practices have had a direct impact on the development of VR, others have only done so in a tangential fashion. It could be argued that the sheer number of changes contributed to a fragmentation of responsibility and services. On the other hand, it could be maintained that they represent a response to diverse needs. From May 2010, the view of the coalition government is that, while it accepts many changes that have been introduced to promote labour market participation and reduce benefits expenditure, 'simplification' is required.

Organisational responsibility

VR does not operate in a vacuum. While the main public sector strategies for employment and health are driven by the DWP, DH and the Health and Well-Being Strategy introduced by Dame Carol Black (DWP/DH, 2008b, 2008c) the role of other bodies is also important, particularly in the MH field. Prominent among these organisations are the:

- **Office for Disability Issues** (www.officefordisabilityissues.co.uk). The ODI speaks for disabled people within government. It was set up to help government deliver on the commitment made in the report, *Improving the life chances of disabled people* (Prime Minister's Strategy Unit (PMSU) *et al.*, 2005).
- **Social Exclusion Task Force** (and its predecessor, the Social Exclusion Unit (SEU)) (www.cabinetoffice.gov.uk/). The Task Force was set up in 2006 to work with all government departments to ensure that the needs of the most socially excluded are addressed.
- **National Social Inclusion Programme**. The NSIP was a four-year programme established in 2004 to oversee the implementation of the cross-government action plan from the SEU report *Mental health and social exclusion* (SEU, 2004).
- **National Institute for Mental Health (England)**. The NIMHE was established in 2001 to 'coordinate research, disseminate information, facilitate training and develop services' (Bartlett and Sandland, 2007). It was responsible for co-co-ordinating the overall delivery of the Mental Health and Social Exclusion report. The NIMHE has now been disbanded, and a new body, the National Mental Health Development Unit was launched in 2009 (www.nmhdu.org.uk).
- **Equality and Human Rights Commission** (www.equalityhumanrights.com/). In the face of opposition from the disability lobby, fearing the loss of the campaigning Disability Rights Commission (DRC), the EHRC was set up in 2007 as a non-departmental public body (NDPB), replacing the Equal Opportunities Commission, the Commission for Racial Equality and the DRC.
- **Health and Safety Executive** (www.hse.gov.uk/). Workplace disability management and VR are inextricably linked to health and safety. The HSE has long recognised this situation (James *et al.*, 2006). In February 2005, the HSE piloted a service for SMEs called Workplace Health Direct (Lucy *et al.*, 2009). The service has been replaced with various programmes across the UK, such as the Fit for Work service.

Key papers and policies in public sector VR development (Table 3.1)

In the opening paragraph of the Green Paper *A new contract for welfare* (DSS, 1998), the Prime Minister recognised that there had been no comprehensive review of the welfare

Table 3.1 Key dates in policy development, 1997–2010

1998	**New Deal for Disabled People (NDDP)**: pilots innovative schemes, personal advisors and job finders grant.
1999	**Tax Credit Act**: introduces the Disabled Persons Tax Credit, effectively a wage top-up for low-paid workers (merged into the Working Tax Credit in 2002). **National Service Frameworks in Mental Health**: identified need for rehabilitation and work opportunities.
2000	**WORKSTEP**: introduced into the Supported Employment programme with new progression and retention funding.
2002	**Pathways to Work Green Paper (DWP)**: introduces work-focused interviews (leading to incapacity benefit personal advisors), Condition Management Programmes and 'Return to Work' credits.
2003	**Disability Discrimination Act 1995 (Amendments) Regulations 2003**: incorporates EU Directives.
2003	**Employers Liability Compulsory Insurance Review (DWP)**: stated government commitment to produce VR framework for the United Kingdom.
2004	**A UK Framework for Vocational Rehabilitation (DWP)**: aimed substantially at making employers responsible for the rehabilitation of their own employees. **Choosing Health: Making Healthier Choices (DWP, DH, HSE)**: joint strategy document, resulting in first National Director for Health and Work. **A Strategy for Workplace Health in Great Britain to 2010 and Beyond (HSC)**: examines strategies for RTW and sickness absence management.
2005	**Health, Work, Wellbeing: Caring for our Future (DH, DWP, HSE)**: introduces cross government Health, Work and Wellbeing programme.
2006	**A New Deal for Welfare: Empowering People to Work (DWP)**: launches plans for a radical review of the welfare system with an emphasis on work capability.
2007	**Improving Specialist Disability Employment Services** (**DWP** Consultation Paper).
2008	**Working for a healthier tomorrow**: Director for Health and Work Dame Carol Black's review of the health of Britain's working age population. **No one written off: reforming welfare to reward responsibility**: government response.
2009	**Welfare Reform Act**

state since Beveridge (1943). The Green Paper outlined the main policy responses to the costs of people claiming IB as 'work-based welfare', with the mantra '*work for those who can, security for those who cannot*' agenda for developing the environment in which VR operates and services on which many VR providers have come to rely, including private sector ones.

The origins of the New Deal for Disabled People (the first item in Table 3.1) and the development of job-broking services (the contracting out of job-placing services) lie in New Labour policy directions from taking office. A Green Paper, *Pathways to Work: helping people into employment* (DWP, 2002) and *The government's response and action plan* (DWP, 2003) set the major agenda, driving the roll-out of Jobcentre Plus offices, incorporating social security offices within Jobcentres. The Green Paper made a case for change, stating that most people claiming IB did not report severe health conditions. Other obstacles besides health kept people on IB, such as, in particular, a lack of skills and a perceived lack of financial incentives.

The following documents and policies are further considered:

a *Building capacity to work: a UK framework for vocational rehabilitation* (DWP, 2004).
b *A new deal for welfare: empowering people to work* (DWP Green Paper, 2006).
c Health, work and well-being strategy.
d Welfare Reform Act 2009.

Building capacity to work: a UK framework for vocational rehabilitation (DWP, 2004)

This document is a position statement building on widespread consultation. The focus is on employers delivering VR services (rather than the DWP directly or indirectly supporting VR services). Due notice of this intent was given in the Second Stage Report into the Review of ELCI in December 2003. It was considered that the public strategy to help unemployed disabled people was already well developed, 'e.g. Pathways to Work', and that this contained elements of VR.

Absence of evidence

To help produce the framework, DWP analysts undertook a literature review, noting that most research had been undertaken in North America, Australia, New Zealand, Scandinavia and the Netherlands. It was considered that much of the existing work had been undertaken with people who have MH conditions, MSDs and cardiorespiratory conditions, the most common causes of long-term incapacity, and was related to case studies of small-scale VR services. It was difficult to generalise from these. There existed few longitudinal studies tracking the employment and benefit status of people over time and relating this to any VR interventions received. What influenced RTW was poorly understood. However, a number of factors did seem to recur between studies affecting employment outcome (Box 3.1).

The influence that VR services and delivery processes had on gaining or retaining employment, over and above other factors affecting employment outcomes, was unclear. The evidence on what types of intervention facilitate RTW after a period of sickness absence could not provide a definitive guide to effective VR. The conclusion (Box 3.2) is that, although there is some 'good evidence' related to restoring function, especially for some specific health conditions, evidence for what constitutes effective VR is inconclusive.

Many VR practitioners were left disappointed by the framework document, considering that there is a tendentious aspect to it, with the government not wishing to be seen to be imposing any extra duties on employers. In 2002, the HOST policy report (Chapter 1) recognised the lack of UK research and made recommendations to address this situation. The government/DWP did not respond. In the circumstances, the limitations on UK-based research evidence is hardly surprising.

Because of the 'inconclusive evidence' from which to develop VR recommendations, the framework document states that the government was not in a position to produce 'a new approach for VR for the UK', although it considered that it was demonstrating its commitment to VR by proposing structures helping it to work with stakeholders to develop a new approach by:

Box 3.1 Factors that may affect employment outcomes

- Number of dependents, number of children under five, and being younger seem to increase the frequency of sickness absence from work.
- Variables related to work such as long hours, lack of autonomy at work, job insecurity, low level of job commitment and job satisfaction seem to reduce the likelihood of RTW, while being younger, having a higher education and being a non-manual worker and having a higher income seem to increase the likelihood of RTW.
- There is a lag in employment outcomes for those with health conditions or impairment compared with national economic cycles. Local employment rates also affect outcomes.
- People with the same clinical conditions and clinical diagnosis have different RTW rates.
- The extent to which severity of condition and associated measure of pain are factors in RTW is unclear. Some research shows that subjective assessment of pain, illness beliefs and the meaning that work has for the individual are more significant in predicting RTW.
- There is some evidence that being involved in litigation for compensation or in receipt of compensation affects RTW, but the extent to which this is a factor over and above other attitudinal risk factors is unclear.

---

1   improving the VR evidence base
2   addressing standards and accreditation, and
3   examining how the public sector could better use VR.

It was considered that the government had already started improving the evidence base through research initiatives already underway, particularly the Job Retention and Rehabilitation Pilot (JRRP) and the evaluation of the Pathways to Work pilots. In addition, the DWP also commissioned two new qualitative studies to explore:

- the practice of VR in Britain, stakeholders' views of effectiveness and factors encouraging and limiting access (resulting in Andrew Irving Associates' *Developing a framework for vocational rehabilitation* DWP report 224; www.dwp.gov.uk/asd/asd5/index.asp); and
- attitudes of employers to sickness absence and RTW, the policies and services used and barriers affecting service use (contributing towards Nice and Thornton, 2004; www.dwp.gov.uk/asd/asd5/index.asp).

The government also indicated that it was commissioning work to examine the costs and benefits to employers of employing people with health conditions and/or impairments that would support the development of a business case for VR (contributing to Needles and Schmitz, 2006).

Box 3.2 Vocational rehabilitation and employment outcomes (DWP, 2004)

- Research on the impact of VR is contradictory. Some research shows that people receiving VR are no more likely to RTW than those not receiving VR. Other studies found a difference in job placement following VR, but there was no evidence on hours worked, job retention or income.
- Motivation to RTW and a willingness to take steps to achieve this are suggested as explanations for differences in RTW rates between non-participants and participants in some VR programmes.
- Early intervention is considered beneficial.
- Interventions focused on the medical condition and medically oriented treatments can improve functionality and well-being but, on their own, do not significantly affect work outcomes, including job retention.
- Using job and task analysis and functional assessments and ergonomic assessments to match people to jobs does not show conclusive results in facilitating RTW.
- Flexible working hours, adjustment of work demands or lighter work for a short period of time can facilitate RTW and help reduce sickness absence.
- Accelerated job placement and supported employment (SE) and minimal pre-employment services for people with MH conditions have a greater effect than pre-employment psychosocial intervention in time to first job, but make no difference in terms of hours worked or job tenure.
- Whether improvements in psychosocial health increase employment outcomes is not clear. Although cognitive behavioural therapy (CBT) has been shown to affect compliance with treatment for those with psychiatric disorders and improve coping skills for daily living for others, there was no evidence of effect on RTW.
- Case management often forms an important element of VR services. The few studies that have been undertaken show that client satisfaction with services increases with prompt intervention and facilitative caseworkers. However, there is little evidence of the effectiveness of case management in improving employment outcomes.
- Research suggests that better communication between stakeholders, such as the GP, OH professional or VR specialist and employer, focusing on issues relating to the nature of employment and adjustments, as well as capabilities for work and the influence of health and other factors on work, might increase the likelihood of successful RTW.

Next steps

The framework document concludes that stakeholders should be encouraged to develop 'robust evidence' on proven VR interventions in order to inform future progress. Owing to the lack of a conclusive evidence base on the added value of VR, and what works, it was concluded that government was not yet in a position to outline a new approach to VR for the United Kingdom, although the framework document outlined how the government, and devolved administrations, would work with stakeholders to develop a new approach to VR. To enable all stakeholders to contribute to the development of a new VR strategy, the government proposed the following structures to help it take forward the framework:

1   DWP to set up a Vocational Rehabilitation Steering Group to help stakeholders play an active part in the future development of any new approach to VR, and to help manage the delivery of the framework.
2   A Research Working Group to be set up to identify, and agree action to deliver, research priorities.
3   A Vocational Rehabilitation Steering Group to be asked to set up a Standards and Accreditation Working Group to consider how best to increase standards and to consider the case for the accreditation of VR providers.

The government recognised that many stakeholders, such as employers and insurers, were committed to VR but, to maintain this commitment, it was important to meet some immediate needs. New guidance and additional tools were needed and would be delivered in the near future. These included:

*   HSE's best-practice approach to managing sickness absence and return-to-work;
*   the second module of an online DWP distance-learning package for GPs to cover health and work issues; and
*   HSE producing a prototype sickness-absence recording software tool aimed primarily at SMEs to help them record, analyse and manage sickness absence.

Although the framework document has run its course and can be considered to have been subsumed in the health and well-being agenda, there are some important legacies. The HSE has delivered its services. Waddell *et al.* (2008) produced *Vocational rehabilitation: what works with whom and why?*, a comprehensive review of evidence-based practice. Support was given to the development of standards by the VRA and United Kingdom Rehabilitation Council (VRA, 2007; UKRC Rehabilitation Standards, 2010).

A New Deal for Welfare: Empowering People to Work (DWP Green Paper, January 2006)

The Green Paper sought to reform the welfare state, enabling benefit claimants to move from a poverty trap many experience under the benefits system. Various measures were proposed to reform the benefits system (Box 3.3).

Introduction of the ESA

A major thrust of reform was to begin the process of replacing IB with ESA for all new claimants, in return for participating in work-related activity. Claimants would no longer be defined by their condition alone but by the severity of its impact on their ability to function. At least, this is what was claimed; when the final assessment emerged (Chapter 6), arguably it resembled far more of a 'snap-shot' medical assessment than a functional one.

> **Box 3.3 Welfare reforms**
>
> 1 Introduction of the ESA.
> 2 Reform of the entitlement/assessment process.
> 3 Support for OH.
> 4 Increased support for people with MH problems.
> 5 Increased expectations and support for GPs and primary-care providers to encourage patients to RTW.

Reform of the entitlement/assessment process

The government revised the medical assessment (personal capability assessment) of the IB claims procedure to focus on ability and support needs (capability and capacity) rather than incapacity.

Support for OH

The Green Paper proposed that the government, working with employers, employees and health professionals, would aim to create healthy workplaces with good OH support, and also improve absence-management procedures to help support recovery. A helpline (Workplace Health Connect) delivering OH advice targeted at SMEs was to be created. SSP was to be simplified, enabling employers to better manage sickness and the flow of people from SSP to IB.

Increased support for people with MH problems

Pathways to Work and health services were to be geared to meet the needs of people with MH problems.

Increased expectations and support for GPs and primary-care providers to encourage patients to RTW

GPs and primary-care practitioners were to be offered more support to encourage people back to work. Performance targets for specific interventions would be included, with rewards, in primary-care contracts. Training on health and work was also to be offered to GPs, and it was planned to incorporate this into medical training.

Health, work and well-being strategy

This strategy is a partnership between the DH, DWP, HSE, Welsh Assembly government and Scottish Executive. Working alongside employers, trade unions and health-care professionals, the government proposed to create healthier workplaces; ensure the provision of good OH services; enhance rehabilitation support; and provide employment opportunities for those currently not in work owing to ill health or disability, thereby reducing the levels of sickness absence and benefits claims.

As part of the strategy, Dame Carol Black reviewed the health of Britain's working-age population, setting out numerous recommendations for action (DWP/DH, 2008b). Proposals included fit notes instead of sick notes, health, work and well-being regional co-ordinators, helplines for small businesses, funding for local initiatives, review of the health and well-being of the NHS workforce and piloting Fit for Work services, all of which started in 2009.

The government's reply to Dame Carol Black was published together with a Green paper (DWP/DH, 2008b,c*)*. These documents made it clear that the NHS would be asked to do much more to enable people to remain at work.

The Welfare Reform Act 2009

This legislation was preceded by the White Paper *Raising expectations and increasing support: reforming welfare for the future* (December 2008), building on the proposals in the Green Paper *No one written off* and setting out in detail the plan for the future as part of a vision described as 'a personalised welfare state, where more support is matched by higher expectations for all'. The Act paved the way for reform of the benefits system; introduced a regime of benefit sanctions for non-attendance at Jobcentres; required job search by partners of benefit claimants; introduced work-focused interviews for over-60s; and required work-related activity in return for receipt of ESA.

*   *   *

The National Health Service

Following a post-war decline in NHS VR practice, there has been a resurgence of interest reflected in various policy statements, particularly reflected in *Improving working lives standards* (DH, 2000), NSFs (Box 3.4), the *Choosing health* White Paper (DH, 2004a) and the Next Stage Review (and associated policy documents).

Box 3.4 National Service Frameworks

- mental health (DH, 1999), emphasis on severe conditions;
- coronary heart disease (DH, 2000);
- older people (DH, 2001);
- children, young people and maternity services (DH, 2004);
- long-term neurological conditions (DH, 2005), with reference to
  - brain injury
  - epilepsy
  - multiple sclerosis (MS)
  - spinal injury;
- chronic obstructive pulmonary disease (DH, 2008).

(All available at www.dh.gov.uk)

National Service Frameworks

As part of its reform of the welfare state, New Labour began to set out in NSFs specific condition-related targets for the NHS. The two main roles of NSFs are:

1 setting clear quality requirements for care based on the best available evidence;
2 offering strategies and support to help health organisations achieve these standards.

Each NSF sets a target for improving the standard of care and the associated health-care outcomes related to that care. Patients with long-term conditions use a disproportionate amount of NHS resources (DH, 2004a; Hudson, 2005). By targeting support at specifically identified groups, it is planned to reduce such matters as repeat hospitalisations. From a vocational perspective, the most significant NSFs (in terms of the number of people covered by them) are the ones for MH and long-term (neurological) conditions (LTNCs).

Mental health

The NSF for MH includes two standards in which the importance of work is stressed:

Standard 1 requires health and social services to 'combat discrimination against individuals and groups with mental health problems and promote their social inclusion', with work singled out as key to inclusion.
Standard 5 requires that care plans for people with more serious mental health difficulties include 'action needed for employment, education or training or another occupation'.

The implementation of RTW strategies for people with MH conditions needs to be viewed in conjunction with a number of other initiatives. Following extensive consultation, in June 2004, the SEU published the report *Mental health and social exclusion*. Implementation of the recommendations requires:

- the provision of vocational support to be embedded in the Care Programme Approach (CPA; CPA DH 2001);
- access to an employment advisor for everyone with severe MH problems;
- Mental Health Trusts to monitor vocational outcomes for people on CPA and employment rates of people with MH problems in their own agencies; and
- day services to be developed to provide for SE, occupation and mainstream social contact beyond the MH system.

Implementation of the SEU report is monitored by local implementation teams and, at a national level, the joint review inspection framework developed by the Healthcare Commission and the Commission for Social Care Improvement.

National Service Framework for long-term (neurological) conditions

Quality requirement 6 of the NSF for LTNCs highlights the need for services enabling people with a LTNC to enter work, education or vocational training, remain in or return to their existing job or withdraw from work at an appropriate time, all collectively considered to describe VR. The course of a neurological disease differs according to the condition. Some, for example stroke and traumatic brain injury, come on suddenly, whereas others, such as epilepsy, may be intermittent and unpredictable. Some conditions are progressive – for example MS and Parkinson's disease – whereas others, such as cerebral palsy, are stable but with changing needs due to ageing. People with different conditions require different types of VR service at different times. Although services for people with MH conditions are well established, the same cannot be said with regard to LTNCs. The current provision of services for people with LTNCs in the UK is a postcode lottery. Some services are provided by existing NHS rehabilitation services; some are linked to Jobcentre Plus; and others operate within the private or voluntary sector. There are no appropriate VR services in many parts of the UK.

Quality requirement 6 sets out the anticipated standards for patients with LTNCs. These include:

1   a basic vocational assessment, with the aim of helping patients develop work-related skills (assessment is not defined);
2   informed guidance about available options, including advice on welfare rights and benefits entitlements;
3   practical support to manage problems in the workplace;
4   liaison and advice to employers to adjust work duties;
5   advice on retiring on health grounds.

The guidelines recommend how VR should be organised to meet the differing needs of people with a LTNC, building on existing guidelines for people with acquired brain injuries (BSRM *et al.*, 2004) and calling for partnership working between health and social services and statutory (Jobcentre Plus) and voluntary services to bridge service gaps and ensure that people can access services when they need them.

The Department of Health appears to recognise that there is a long way to go before VR is integrated into NHS practice, even for patients with neurological conditions, and that NHS development is likely to need a community dimension in order to be successful. One reason for the lack of vocational activity within trusts may be that a national strategy for VR within the NHS has yet to emerge, and, although practice in trusts varies enormously, VR is not perceived to be a priority other than in a small number of care trusts, sitting between NHS PCTs and local authorities and providing VR MH services. On the other hand, trusts have until 2015 to develop the delivery of the NSF for long-term conditions. In Scotland, the Scottish government, operating through local health boards, has made a robust start. Local health boards also operate in Northern Ireland, where four boards fund eight brain injury programmes (BSRM *et al.*, 2004).

Evidence-based practice

Nothing illustrates the lack of joined-up government thinking on VR more than the approach to the acceptance of research evidence. It will have been noted that, in 2004, the DWP considered that it could not propose a 'new approach' to VR because of a lack of evidence supporting the efficacy of intervention (DWP, 2004). On the insistence of the Treasury, supported by its own influential medical advisors, the DWP sought evidence obtained from the highest standards of research practice.

Despite objections on ethical grounds to the use of randomised controlled trials (RCTs) made by voluntary organisations on the basis of denying 50 per cent of participants a service, and academics such as Floyd *et al.* (2004) noting that comparisons cannot be drawn with medical research and even questioning the insights the data may provide, during New Labour's period of office, the DWP relied on RCTs in its major VR research programmes, such as the Job Rehabilitation and Retention Pilot (JRRP).

Job Retention and Rehabilitation Pilot

JRRP represented a joint initiative between the DWP and the DH, with support from HSE (Nice and Thornton, 2004; Farrell *et al.*, 2006; Purdon *et al.*, 2006). The pilot was open to employed and self-employed volunteers working more than 16 hours per week and absent from work on health grounds for between 6 and 26 weeks. The pilot, beginning in April 2003, was rolled out in six areas of the United Kingdom and was due to run for 2 years (Stratford *et al.*, 2005b). There was a range of contact methods, and those interested in taking part telephoned a 'contact centre'. A series of questions is said to have identified those unlikely to return-to-work without support. The most common health condition found was musculoskeletal (33 per cent) with MH conditions second (30 per cent); 14 per cent of subjects ascribed their sickness absence to an injury. The subjects were randomly allocated to:

1   **a health intervention**: in this group, the most commonly used services were physio-therapy (36 per cent), complementary therapy (30 per cent), psychotherapy (26 per cent) and referral to a medical specialist (23 per cent);
2   **a workplace intervention**: the most commonly used services were ergonomic assessment (42 per cent) and employer liaison/mediation (22 per cent);
3   **a combined (workplace and health) intervention**: health interventions were more common than workplace ones (32 per cent receiving physiotherapy, but just 11 per cent receiving an ergonomic assessment and 22 per cent receiving employer liaison/mediation); almost a third (30 per cent) of the participants in this group underwent CBT;
4   **a control group**.

Because of a low take-up rate, and around 15 per cent of participants withdrawing once allocated, the programme failed to recruit a sufficient number of subjects to support the research methodology. Both the recruitment period and target number of subjects had to be adjusted. In total, 2,845 people entered the trial and were allocated to the four groups. All 2,845 were asked to take part in an interview after the trial. This formed the main source of outcome data.

The case management aspect of the trial was well received by the participants (Strafford *et al.*, 2005b). Staff described it as involving the identification of needs and service responses, facilitating and co-ordinating the use of services, supporting and empowering service users, and providing specific help or treatments (Farrell *et al.*, 2006).

Staff said that important aspects of the service were:

1   being able to intervene early;
2   taking a holistic approach, tailored to the individual;
3   being readily available to clients,

4   flexibility in the use of budgets; and
5   ability to provide flexible and focused interventions.

   Barriers to their work were:

1   getting access to employers: some were unsupportive and inflexible; and
2   getting access to GPs, and 'overcautious' advice.

   Service users' responses varied:

1   Some felt their needs were met very effectively.
2   Others identified types of assistance they would have liked but were not given.

Phased returns and lighter duties were important RTW facilitators.

Outcomes

The primary outcome for the trial was RTW of some 13 weeks or more. The figures
for the four groups were almost identical:

*   health intervention: 44 per cent;
*   workplace intervention: 45 per cent;
*   combined (workplace and health) intervention: 44 per cent;
*   control: 45 per cent.

These figures imply that the JRRP interventions had no impact on RTW. Although small
subgroup sample sizes mean the results have to be cautiously considered, it appears that
the interventions may have actually reduced the prospect of a RTW for people with a
MH problem (59 per cent of the control group returned to work, compared with 47 per
cent in one of the intervention groups). In contrast, the interventions may have been
most helpful to those sustaining an injury (55 per cent in one group returned to work,
compared with 36 per cent in the control).

Explaining the results

Purdon *et al.* (2006) say the '*most likely*' explanations for the results are as follows:

1   the interventions offered were not always seen to be appropriate to the clients or
     fully to meet their needs;
2   some of the primary reasons for returning to work, such as financial, were out of
     the control of the service providers; and
3   service providers faced barriers from employers and GPs, reducing their potential
     success.

They added that, 'other possible explanations such as the high withdrawal rate and the
profile of people who entered the trial seem implausible.' One point not covered is
the fact that the work was contracted out to organisations paid on a per capita basis. In
turn, they recruited extra staff for the programme, and some (not all) had little experience

of such specific RTW activity. When the referral numbers did not come through, a certain amount of disillusion among staff crept in with regards to their own prospects and the research methodology. However, service providers were criticised for not 'always encouraging clients to be proactive and initiate contact'.

Waddell *et al.* (2008) declared that the 'organisation, planning of the JRRP were so bad that they probably foredoomed it to failure'. It is evident from the review undertaken by Stratford *et al.* (2005b) that, not only was the marketing of the programme unsatisfactory, but there were also issues concerning the timing of the intervention (12 weeks' sickness absence); the screening process (one-third of potential recruits were not eligible); the actual interventions offered by six groups of providers (Waddell *et al.* suggest that they did not conform to the best scientific advice); low intensity of contact; and a high drop-out rate.

In contrast to the research reliance on RCTs, in 2005 the DH advanced a number of papers in quality requirement 6 of the NSF for LTNCs relying on other methodologies. These papers include reference to brain injury (Prigatano *et al.*, 1984; Ben-Yishay *et al.*, 1987; Malec *et al.*, 1993; Teasdale *et al.*, 1993; Groswasser *et al.*, 1999; Tyerman, 1999; Klonoff *et al.*, 2001); spinal-cord injury (SCI) (Tomassen *et al.*, 2000); epilepsy (Collings and Chappell, 1994); multiple sclerosis (Rumrill *et al.*, 1996; Roessler *et al.*, 1997; Johnson *et al.*, 2004).

In addition to the legislative and cultural differences between the United Kingdom and countries from where some of this evidence was gathered, a number of these studies contain methodological weaknesses, such as small sample sizes, varying periods of follow-up, the lack of any comparators and varying definitions of employment. Some of the research recommendations for VR practice are even contradictory, or they can only be made by inference. For example, the Tyerman study (see Chapter 9) advocates a great deal of pre-placement preparation, whereas Wehman is a supporter of the SE model of VR, involving little or no a priori evaluation. Johnson *et al.*'s (2004) qualitative research addresses the benefits of work and barriers to employment faced by people with MS, and relies on only sixteen subjects. The report says nothing explicitly about VR, although there are lessons in respect of the benefits of early intervention and adjustments to accommodate MS. It is inexplicable as to why the DH should cite studies not meeting the highest level of research requirements, when the Treasury insisted on large-scale RCTs before supporting DWP investment in VR.

A co-ordinated strategy: the response of the Scottish government

The Scottish government has taken the lead on ensuring that rehabilitation is consistently available within the Scottish NHS (Scottish Executive, 2007). The framework document identifies three target groups: the elderly, people with long-term conditions and those returning to work and/or aiming to stay in employment. The key elements of VR are indicated in Table 3.2.

The model VR team, based in the community, is considered likely to consist of professionals including a case manager (any discipline), counsellor, manual handling trainer, OH advisor, OH physician, physiotherapist, OT, psychologist and support worker.

The Scottish Centre for Healthy Working Lives, based in Hamilton, part of NHS Health Scotland, is overseeing the development of pilot VR projects. The first project, Working Health Services Dundee, opened in April 2008. A significant feature of the way the

Table 3.2 Key elements of VR

1   Assessment of functional, physical, psychological and cognitive work capacity.
2   Vocational assessment and counselling to determine suitable job options.
3   Counselling to support adjustment to disability.
4   Supervised on-the-job training and/or a short vocational course.
5   Fitness and work-conditioning programmes.
6   Confidence building/self-esteem groups or individual sessions.
7   Assessment of workplace suitability.
8   Development of skills for job-seeking.
9   Brokerage and case management.
10   Linkage with community based agencies.

service has been rolled out is the way it is targeted at employees of SMEs with up to 250 employees, and has a focus on job retention.

New Labour and the Third Sector

A significant aspect of the delivery of public sector VR and related services, whether in conjunction with Jobcentre Plus or the NHS, is the development of a reliance on the private sector and, particularly, the Third Sector, for delivering services. Following on from a number of general policy pronouncements (Home Office, 1998; HM Treasury, 2002, 2004; Labour Party, 2005; Third Sector, 2006), the DWP Green Paper *A new deal for welfare: empowering people to work* (DWP, 2006) makes specific reference to including the voluntary sector in employment services.

Changes took place at the same time as the introduction of devolved administrations in Scotland, Wales and Northern Ireland. As Alcock (2009) notes, 'Devolution of policy to promote and support Third Sector activity has been significant and has resulted in the creation of four separate policy regimes for the Third Sector across the four countries of the UK.' He also points out that, despite this divergence in policy regime, the broad direction of Third Sector policy has been 'remarkably similar', in that all of the countries of the United Kingdom have moved towards a partnership approach.

The attraction of the voluntary sector to government

The Conservative governments of the 1980s and 1990s allowed the voluntary sector to fulfil a service role, but it was not seen as a major partner. The focus of the Conservatives was to cut public expenditure and expand the role of the private sector in the delivery of public services. New Labour saw the voluntary sector as the vehicle for resolving what it believed to be the failings of the public sector. Many senior Labour figures shared the Conservatives' analysis of the public sector as suffering from low productivity, offering inefficient, expensive and poor-quality services.

The expansion in contracted and subcontracted DWP services, with private, voluntary and not-for-profit organisations running both specialist and non-specialist employ-ment and disability services, has resulted in a situation in which it is impossible to give any succinct overall picture of who is doing what, or where, in publicly funded services. The nature of the contracting-out process has resulted in diverse regional

---

Box 3.5 The Freud Report (2007)

- Extend private and voluntary sector involvement in the delivery of Welfare to Work.
- Create market incentives to deliver more effective Welfare to Work.
- Expand the market for welfare-to-work provision.
- Transfer to the private and voluntary sectors the question of who is helped.

---

services. Although some large organisations, such as the Shaw Trust, have a network of job brokers in many parts of the United Kingdom, this level of coverage is not typical. To give some idea as to the complexity of the voluntary sector market, albeit not all publicly funded, in 2001 the Social Policy Research Unit at the University of York carried out a survey for the DWP, analysing data for 2,520 disability-focused employment projects: 937 of these served people with a MH problem or another condition; 1,538 MH or learning disability; and the remaining 982 focused on other disabilities (Arksey *et al.*, 2002).

The Association of Chief Executives of Voluntary Organisations (ACEVO) and the Employment-Related Services Association (ERSA) have steadfastly campaigned for a mix of third and private sector services, based on the Australian model of service delivery (Bubb, 2006). They have been receiving around £500 million a year, largely in Jobcentre Plus contracts. A number of the organisations involved in delivering employment services for people with disabilities have substantial operations. In 2006, the largest, the Shaw Trust, reported an income of £65.57million, of which nearly 60 per cent, £38.87 million, came from Jobcentre Plus. Its services included Workstep, Work Preparation, Pathways to Work, New Deal for Disabled People and European Social Fund projects.

Commentators have noted that, although the public is sceptical about private profit-making organisations operating in the sector, it has confidence in the Third Sector (MacErlean, 2005; Mathiason, 2005; Caulkin, 2006). However, around a third of the members of ERSA are private sector organisations.

In 2006, the DWP commissioned David Freud, an investment banker, to review the government's Welfare to Work strategy. Freud recommended that Jobcentre Plus should concentrate on those closer to the labour market, with 'support for the hardest to help being delivered through the private and voluntary sector'.

The contracting out of services raises a number of concerns (Box 3.6).

Better services?

Ministers and service providers claim that contracting services to the private and third sectors results in better value for money for the taxpayer and in a higher-quality service than Jobcentre Plus can provide (Mansour and Johnson, 2006; House of Commons Work and Pensions Committee, 2007). Davies (2007) produces substantial evidence from various Jobcentre Plus programmes (outlined in Chapter 6) to challenge such claims; for example:

Box 3.6 Contracting out services: areas of concern

- Priority of private sector organisations is to maximise profit and not advance public policy.
- Influence of ERSA representing large organisations, and £2,500 annual subscription excluding small service providers (House of Commons Works and Pensions Committee, 2007, Ev. 318).
- Potential conflict for voluntary organisations between their roles as advocates and as service providers.
- Voluntary sector increasingly drawing its executives from the private sector. As Davies (2009) indicates, it is hard not to see this influencing their attitude towards public sector services and to obtaining more work from Jobcentre Plus.

Pathways to Work

A claim by contractors that they are better equipped than Jobcentre Plus to deal with clients further from the labour market, because of the amount of time spent with clients (ERSA/ACEVO, 2006), was rebutted by the NAO, noting third-party perceptions that Jobcentre Plus staff spent only 10–15 minutes with customers did not accord with the 41 minutes average length of a personal advisor (PA) interview (NAO, 2006). A number of reports reflect a positive customer experience of PAs (Moss and Arrowsmith, 2003).

New Deal for Disabled People

Job brokers are cited in the 2006 Green Paper (DWP, 2006) as an example of the advantages of contracting out to the private and voluntary sectors. In their joint submission on the Green Paper, ERSA and ACEVO claimed that the voluntary and private sectors have '*inherent*' advantages over Jobcentre Plus in respect of trust, assisting hardest-to-help groups, time spent with clients and innovative approaches. In evidence to the House of Commons Works and Pensions Committee, they stated that, 'evidence shows that independent providers are producing better results and better value for money than existing statutory providers', and that, 'private and voluntary sectors will out perform the back to work rates achieved within existing Pathways providers' (House of Commons Works and Pensions Committee, 2006). ERSA referred to DWP research (Lewis *et al.*, 2005), which, they claimed, 'demonstrated that NDDP job brokers had advantages over Jobcentre Plus in being able to spend more time with people, providing a more in-depth service, and being independent of government systems'.

Although Lewis *et al.* suggested that job-broking organisations have a useful role to play, the report also says that independent job broking is only 'one element in a concerted multifaceted strategy'; job brokers *felt* that they were able to spend more time with clients and that a number of respondents (service users, job brokers and Jobcentre Plus staff) considered that some job brokers were keen to maximise the number of registrations, with a fee paid per registration, but neglected the more difficult-to-place clients because of funding arrangements, targets and, sometimes, high case-loads. Lewis *et al.* (2005) considered that, 'client choice is not working particularly effectively', a matter echoed by Hasluck and Green (2007), noting that, 'at an individual level the facility of "choice" of job broker has not really worked'.

Far from being innovative, Corden *et al.* (2003) found that, 'there was little evidence from the research so far to suggest that the NDDP extension had generated innovation in services provided by Job Brokers'. The report went on to note that job brokers seemed to work very much like Jobcentre Plus staff, particularly DEAs.

Work Preparation

In respect of the Work Preparation programme, Riddell and Banks (2005) noted that, 'Although relatively small-scale, the rationale for the programme was to help disabled people into employment, but . . . a relatively small number of people progressed into the open employment'.

Workstep

The House of Commons Committee of Public Accounts (2006) reported that there are over 500 contractors delivering disability programmes for Jobcentre Plus, and that the quality and value for money varied considerably. As an example, they pointed to the Workstep programme in which, between 2002 and 2005, 50 per cent of the learning was judged unsatisfactory by the Adult Learning Inspectorate.

Davies (ibid.) concluded that, 'although great claims are made for the Third Sector in terms of superior performance, better results in job placement and value for money compared with in-house provision, the evidence for this is rather thin.' The House of Commons Committee of Public Accounts (ibid.), in a review of various providers of NDDP, concluded that

> There is little robust evidence that the nature of the provider of services, be it Jobcentre Plus, a private sector provider, or some other organisation has a systematic impact on effectiveness. What does appear to be important is the quality, enthusiasm, motivation and commitment of the staff providing the service.

2010 Conservative/Liberal Democrat employment strategy

The Conservative strategy to address unemployment, the 'Work Programme', was announced at the party's 2009 Conference (www.conservatives.com/New/News-stories/2009/10/Radical-welfare_reform_to_Get_Britain_Working.aspx). The Work Programme is to be delivered by a limited number of 'prime providers', that is those large enough to handle volume referrals, with Jobcentre Plus acting as a gateway. Essentially the programme entails:

- a single back-to-work programme for everyone on out-of-work benefits;
- funding to be provided by abolishing a Treasury rule preventing the government paying work providers, using the benefits saved once someone has a job; it is claimed that this will fund support for all IB/ESA claimants;
- paying providers by results, with a focus on sustainable outcomes and rewards for getting the hardest to help into a job.

In the aftermath of the 2010 election, and during coalition negotiations, the Liberal Democrats signalled their support for such measures:

> The parties agree to end all existing welfare to work programmes and to create a single welfare to work programme to help all unemployed people get back into work.
>
> We agree that Jobseeker's Allowance claimants facing the most significant barriers to work should be referred to the aforementioned newly created welfare to work programme immediately, not after 12 months as is currently the case. We agree that Jobseeker's Allowance claimants aged under 25 should be referred to the programme after a maximum of six months.
>
> The parties agree to realign contracts with welfare to work service providers to reflect more closely the results they achieve in getting people back into work.
>
> We agree that the funding mechanism used by government to finance welfare to work programmes should be reformed to reflect the fact that initial investment delivers later savings in lower benefit expenditure.
>
> We agree that receipt of benefits for those able to work should be conditional on the willingness to work.
>
> (www.telegraph.co.uk/news/newstopics/politics/7715166)

At a joint VRA/COT conference held at Nottingham University on 2 July 2010, David Freud, by now Under Secretary of State for Works and Pensions, stated such reforms were necessary because existing programmes were too complex, not reaching enough people and not having a sufficient impact (pointing to a 2 per cent annual attrition rate in the number of IB claimants).

Freud stated that the government's approach to reducing the level of benefits claimants is twofold: through the benefits/tax system and the provision of support services. It is apparent that the government has been much influenced by the work of Brien and the Centre for Social Justice report *Dynamic benefits* (www.centreforsocialjustice.org.uk). However, in tying the receipt of benefits to support, the Conservative/Liberal Democrat regime is making a radical departure from the voluntarism that characterised New Deal and much of Pathways. Despite the introduction of '*price differentiation*' (Freud suggested that such factors as the health condition and time out of work are criteria to be used in assessing the level of payment by results to contractors), there is a fear that the major providers will 'cream off' the easier to place, with more difficult clients being referred to subcontractors.

Summary

From the late 1990s, there has been what many may perceive to be a plethora of government Green Papers, White Papers, policy statements, departmental reforms, research programmes and papers, all covering the employment and disability sector, so much so that any casual observer could not keep track. Emerging from all this is a clear strand of government commitment towards VR, although one bounded by cost considerations and a lack of willingness to impose any statutory obligations on employers.

Tackling the IB (and now ESA) registers has resulted in a situation in which the specialist disability services within Jobcentre Plus (see Chapter 8) have become marginalised alongside mainstream programmes also serving claimants (or customers, to use DWP terminology). The United Kingdom has moved on from public sector VR services focused on clients receiving unemployment-related benefits (that is, assessed as fit for work by their GPs) and almost entirely referred by DEAs to contracted specialist services, and only a small number of people receiving VR support within the NHS, to:

1 mainstream public sector services, funded through Jobcentre Plus, but delivered by contracted organisations, with a focus on incapacity benefit (now ESA) claimants;
2 public sector services funded by the NHS; of particular significance are the 1999 NSF for people with MH conditions and the 2005 NSF for LTNCs, with the accompanying Quality Paper 6;
3 private sector VR services funded by insurance companies and focused on job retention and/or an early RTW.

However, public sector VR services within the United Kingdom remain fragmented. The Conservative/Liberal Democrat coalition has announced plans to simplify mainstream provision by reducing the number of service providers, and the NHS has begun to get to grips with the provision of its VR services (Chapter 4). The Scottish government has begun the process of rolling out services for the employees of SMEs, taking the view that other public sector services exist for unemployed people. Factors that might be considered to be driving public sector VR reforms within the United Kingdom are shown in Box 3.7.

A problem in relation to the provision of public sector services is the limited amount of good quantitative evidence supporting intervention, particularly what works, with whom, and why. It may be considered easier to establish the case for VR in the private sector, rather than the public sector, where savings in the size of a compensation payment or the benefits of an employee returning to work are more obvious. The private sector is the focus of the 2004 DWP UK Framework for Vocational Rehabilitation, with its emphasis on making employers responsible for the VR of their own employees, on the grounds that this ultimately benefits them. The limitations on good quantitative research evidence should not be allowed to detract from the enormous benefit VR provides for many individuals.

Box 3.7 Forces driving public sector VR in the United Kingdom

1 A social commitment to enabling more severely disabled people to participate in the labour market.
2 A recognition that, if the scale of the Incapacity/Employment and Support Allowance registers are to fall, then there is a need for early intervention focused on the most prevalent disabilities/conditions (DWP, 2003; DH, 2005).
3 Certain conditions, such as mental health and brain injury, accounting for a disproportionate amount of NHS expenditure, and small-scale studies indicating the efficacy of VR in returning to work patients with these conditions.
4 The need to provide VR services for employees without private sector cover.

Public sector VR services now face increased pressure on costs from two related sources:

- the impact of the recession and the unprecedented level of public borrowing; and
- the expansion of the competitive model in relationship to service providers when there is a squeeze on public spending and consequent government funding of programmes.

Conservative/Liberal Democrat policy places a great emphasis on tendering for service provision rather than grants, presenting concerns about the appropriateness of the model, the survival of some organisations, the scope for innovation within contracts and the driving down of costs at the expense of quality of service. If New Labour can be accused of making policy pronouncements introducing programmes before evidence-based research became available, then the Conservative/Liberal Democrat coalition stands charged with making radical changes to employment policy and support services in the absence of any evidence at all.

Freud's views on the privatisation of employment services say little about the quality of jobs into which long-term sick and disabled should be placed. As all VR practitioners are aware, achieving 'the best fit' optimises the prospect of job retention. Freud focuses on the numbers placed into work and the length of time they stay there.

Freud's approach is very much a free market one, in which everything is regulated by economic factors. However, Grover (2009) maintains that Freud and the government do not seem to understand that people with impairments are disabled by the structures, institutions and practices of society:

> The issue here is that both Freud and the government are closely wedded to merito-cratic notions of employment advancement that decontextualise social status and class from the socio-economic structure, something that the privatised employment services are likely to exacerbate in their search for profit.
>
> (Grover, 2007)

Although everything will turn on the detail in the Work Programme, there is a fear that a great deal of expertise in working with more disadvantaged and disabled jobseekers that has been built up during New Labour will be lost. For example, there is an argument that, not only are joint Jobcentre Plus/NHS Condition Management Programmes (see Chapter 8) professionally staffed, but also they have been successful in working with 'hard-to-place' clients. Although, generally, placing figures are low (around the 20 per cent mark), given the nature of client problems and the propensity to long-term incapacity/unemployment, a long-term evaluation may well show that they have been more than paying for themselves, that is providing net savings to the Treasury. Are private sector companies, driven by profit and the need to satisfy shareholders, and even Third Sector organisations, driven by the need to trigger payment targets, going to employ the same level of expertise and expend as much time on the more difficult to place clients?

Clearly, much will depend upon the level of price differentiation, but, with a government relying on a one-size-fits-all policy, the complexity and diversity of the market do not appear to have been recognised. Unless the price differentiation reflects the huge disparity in costs between returning to work someone with a common health condition, such as someone with some hearing loss, in contrast to, say, someone with a significant neurological problem, such as an acquired brain injury, then the current expert services that have slowly developed during New Labour's tenure in office are likely to think twice about even wanting to be subcontractors.

Student exercises

3.1 Policy
Whether employed (or planning employment) in the public or private sector, identify the papers and policy issues driving the direction of your (chosen) service.

3.2 Conditions
Choose a neurological condition/disability in which you have a particular interest and identify the strategies for developing services outlined in the relevant NSF.

3.3 Service delivery
Are we developing a two-tier VR service in the United Kingdom: an individual case-managed service for clients funded by the private sector, and, in the public sector, generic programmes that may not meet all client needs? Where does your employment fit into such models?

---

4 The private sector response

The legal profession and insurance industry

Key issues

- Interest of the insurance industry in vocational rehabilitation stemming from:
  – Employer Liability Compulsory Insurance (ELCI)
  – accident insurance
  – income-protection policies.
- Interest of the legal profession in vocational rehabilitation.

Learning objectives

- Awareness of the main papers and developments influencing policy and practice in the insurance sector and legal profession.
- Understanding the cost and benefit issues influencing the support for VR of the insurance sector.
- Awareness of the position of the courts towards funding rehabilitation.

Introduction

Historically, UK employers and employees have looked towards the state to provide out-of-work benefits for long-term injury/sickness and any RTW support. Throughout the latter part of the twentieth century and into the twenty-first century, the process of periodic medical examinations, undertaken by the Department of Social Security and later by Jobcentre Plus, has been primarily driven by the need to police the payment of benefits. This process has failed, both as means of checking the rise in the number of IB claimants (DWP, 2002) and as a means of identifying and referring potential VR candidates.

The same reliance on state benefits without VR intervention does not typify developments elsewhere in the Western world, most notably in North America and Australasia. In Canada, for example, companies are 100 per cent responsible for the cost of workers' compensation coverage and, based on whether or not a disability arose out of work-related activities, pay a premium to the appropriate insurer or Workers' Compensation Board. It may seem that there is some comparability with the United Kingdom's ELCI scheme, but there are major differences. Workers' compensation was established in the early 1990s to provide not only wage replacement but also reimbursement for associated medical treatment and costs. This is provided on a no-faults basis. The United Kingdom operates differently. The United Kingdom has a fault-based system of employer's liability. In Canada, Harder and Scott (2005) report that, although not all companies have to participate, those with manual-labour conditions generally have mandatory coverage. In the United Kingdom, although some injured or sick employees may benefit from private medical insurance, most are reliant on the NHS. Historically, treatment and limited rehabilitation services have rarely had the capacity to focus on a return-to-work (Chamberlain *et al.*, 2009).

The ABI represents over 400 insurance companies. It has long been concerned with the shortcomings in the state provision of VR. It supported the development of a Vocational Rehabilitation Index to enable insurers to identify victims of road traffic accidents (RTAs) unlikely to return-to-work without VR (Cornes, 1990). The index was not widely adopted. This is unsurprising, given limited evidence as to the efficacy of VR, potential costs and the lack of service providers.

The insurance sector's interest in rehabilitation continued throughout the 1990s as a consequence of the rising cost of litigation, associated with the lack of available rehabilitation for claimants and compensation for loss of earnings. By the late 1990s, the ABI was putting on conferences in association with such organisations as the COT in order to develop an agenda for VR development. A growth in the sale of GIP policies showed a way forward with regard to RTW strategies. UNUM, the world's largest income-protection company, opened its UK HQ in Dorking in the mid 1990s. In the absence of a private sector VR infrastructure, UNUM set about establishing its own service, initially recruiting OH nurses and former members of the specialist disability services from the Employment Service, and later establishing its current cadre of occupational therapists (OTs) and OPs.

During 1999, interest in rehabilitation as a means of reducing costs led the International Underwriters Association[1] to produce a voluntary Rehabilitation Code for stakeholders; the code was updated in 2007 (www.expertwitness.co.uk/pdf/RehabilitationCode2007/pdf). Although the code exists to bring together insurers, claimants and their legal representatives, this does not necessarily mean the parties pull together in what remains an adversarial and fault-based litigation system. The common interest of the insurance industry and legal profession stems from a need to compensate, not just accident victims and policy claimants, but also, increasingly, employees covered by ELCI. This particular interest resulted in the government producing the National Framework for Vocational Rehabilitation, focusing on compensation for workplace injury and the benefits of VR (DWP, 2004). As the framework document indicates, insurers want to make potential savings through rehabilitation. Even if this was limited to a 10 per cent saving on compensation within the fault-based ELCI system, this might be as much as £200 million per annum.

The search for ways of managing the cost of ELCI led the ABI to commission Greenstreet Bermann, a company with a primary interest in occupational health and safety, to produce a report addressing the costs and benefits to employers of providing rehabilitation and RTW services (Greenstreet Berman, 2004).The report records the HSE finding that only one in seven workers in the UK has the benefit of comprehensive OH support, although 53 per cent have access to an OH professional (HSE, 2002b). The report:

1   perceives health, safety and VR as inseparably linked; for example, it is suggested that, once it is recognised that there are cases of work-related back injury, while

rehabilitation may support the injured employee, the causes of the injury should be eliminated to prevent re-occurrence;

2   does not attempt to draw any distinction between clinical and vocational rehabilitation, noting that,

> rehabilitation tends to be used in the context of clinically oriented care delivered by health-care professionals, such as physiotherapists and occupational physicians. It is also used in the context of vocational activities such as retraining, job counselling and assistance with job seeking.

3   while concluding that early intervention can prevent minor injuries from becoming serious ones, and acute injuries from becoming chronic, it does not suggest that employers should invest in expensive private health care; on the contrary, it is noted that 'on demand' or insurance-led rehabilitation services may be available through NHS Plus or private health-care services, and that the last issue need not be high cost: 'examples exist of small UK firms making use of low cost fast-track physiotherapy services to successfully manage injuries', although 'a general absence management scheme is more cost-effective';

4   considers that the 'benefits to employers, employees and insurers can be significant with effective RTW and rehabilitation'; early intervention and fewer cases of serious injury (not only through preventing accidents but by preventing conditions becoming chronically disabling) result in fewer ELCI claims, less staff absence, reduced or contained employers' liability costs, fewer injures reportable to the HSE or local authority, less aggrieved employees and fewer compensation claims.

The report notes that a previous review concludes that intervention could lead to a reduction of 10–40 per cent of compensation costs (Greenstreet Berman, 2003). Significantly, it is stated that the majority of employees who are injured or suffer work-related ill health do not seek compensation, and, as employers derive benefits from RTW intervention, such as reduced absence and improved workplace productivity, the ratio of benefit to cost is greater for employers than insurers. A case study of Scottish Power indicated a reduction in absence costs of £8.6 million a year. In addition, there was a fall in insurance claims of thirty a year. With a likely reduction in the value of remaining claims, it is suggested that direct benefits to the employer in the form of reduced absence outweighed the reduction in claims costs by at least 6:1. Scottish Power also reported that its ELCI premium increases were contained. The HSE's *Managing absence* report strengthened the ABI's commitment to VR, assessing the cost–benefit ratio of investing in VR or RTW services at 12:1(HSE, 2004).

The insurance sector now routinely funds VR intervention with regard to:

1   victims of work-based accidents
2   victims of RTAs, and
3   GIP claimants.

Victims of work-based accidents

ELCI has been compulsory since 1972 for virtually all employers in the United Kingdom. (Large public sector services, such as the NHS, are considered to have sufficient resources to fund any claims against them.) ELCI insures employers for the costs of compensation for employees injured or made ill at work through the fault of their employer. It provides protection to firms against costs that could otherwise result in financial difficulty and to employees, ensuring that resources are available for compensation, legal costs and rehabilitation, even when firms have become insolvent. The market for ELCI experiences cycles that can make premiums rapidly more expensive and suffers from the effects of long-tail diseases, which can manifest themselves many years after the causation, for example asbestos-related illnesses.

Most insurers now attempt to offer rehabilitation as early in an absence as possible. However, this remains difficult to implement in practice. Although insurers have made many attempts to incentivise employers to report potential claims at an early stage, it takes, on average, over 400 days for a potential claim to be forwarded. This means that, by the time the insurer realises it has a potential liability, the employee is often in a much worse state of health, on benefits and, psychologically, in a difficult position to assist.

The effective provision of VR relies on early notification, and many insurers have linked this to the RIDDOR system of reporting incidents to the HSE (www.healthand safetyforemployers.co.uk/riddor.asp). This provides an efficient system, fulfilling the duties of the employer and alerting its insurer to an issue that needs to be addressed.

However, systemic failures, such as poor absence recording and lack of OH provision, and attitudinal problems, such as fear of the HSE or higher premiums, have made VR difficult to provide for workplace injuries and illness. (Removing the distinction between a workplace- and a non-workplace-caused absence could assist in reducing the fear of claims against ELCI policies.)

Despite the limitations, the number of claimants being referred to VR services by insurers is estimated to have increased by 50–100 per cent over the 5 years to 2008.[2] From the ABI survey of members, it has been estimated that insurers provided around 11,000 individuals with VR in 2007 in respect of their liabilities under ELCI and GIP, with a cost rising to around £13.5 million.[3] This figure of 11,000 probably represents a fraction of the potential market . . . just how small is impossible to estimate from available data, although the level of long-term-sickness absenteeism in the United Kingdom is well recorded in the various annual surveys (Chapter 2).

Victims of RTAs

Victims of RTAs and other accidents are covered by compulsory motor insurance or other accident policies. Medical rehabilitation has long been a part of insurers' response to claims on motor insurance policies, but the extent to which claims handlers or defendant solicitors refer cases for VR (as opposed to case management in general) is not known. Irwin Mitchell, one of the United Kingdom's largest personal injury (PI) legal practices and rehabilitation case managers, suggests that the incidence is likely to be low.[4] Although an issue is the availability of funding, the identification of claimants requiring VR to return-to-work is also pertinent.

Group income protection

GIP, often known as permanent health insurance (PHI), replaces the income of employees who go on to long-term absence through ill health. Individuals can also purchase income protection insurance directly. GIP is usually provided to companies wishing to provide an added benefit to their staff. The policies usually take effect after six months of absence, when OSP is running out, although it can be provided earlier. GIP is usually paid for a set period, although it can be provided right up to retirement age, depending on the requirements of the employer. Data provided by the ABI[5] suggest that GIP is currently provided to around 20,000 employers with five or more staff, and about 6 per cent of the United Kingdom's working population are currently covered in this way.

GIP insurers will usually provide VR for people who become unable to work through ill health. Unlike ELCI insurers, they provide VR however the condition is initiated. Paying a claim for GIP is not dependent on how or where an absence began. GIP insurers often provide other absence-management tools and OH packages with the insurance to ensure that potential absences are identified and actual absences are dealt with in an effective way. GIP policies are particularly vulnerable to recession. Not only are companies looking for ways to reduce costs when the going is tough, but the prospect of VR services returning a claimant to work are reduced.

Motor insurance and other accident insurance

Victims of RTAs are covered by compulsory motor insurance policies. In cases of uninsured drivers, the Motor Insurance Bureau (MIB) is required by government to 'step in' (and receives a levy based on market share from all other insurers to enable it to do so).

The interest of the legal profession in VR stems from representing claimants and defending such claims on behalf of insurance companies. Solicitors undertaking such work are, respectively, represented by the Association of Personal Injury Lawyers (APIL; www.apil.ork.uk) and the Forum of Injury Lawyers (FOIL; www.foil.org.uk). Together, they have supported the development of an advisory (not mandatory) Rehabilitation Code.

The Rehabilitation Code

The 1999 Rehabilitation Code (Box 4.1) was updated in 2007 (www.rehabcode. org). The Code provides an approved framework for injury claims within which claimant representatives and compensators can work together. A Pre-action Protocol provides that the Code should be considered for all types of PI claims. The objective is to ensure that injured people receive the rehabilitation treatment they need to restore their quality of life and earnings capacity as soon as possible and for as long as the parties believe it is appropriate.

VR effectiveness

The ABI recognises differences in emphasis between professionals, providers and insurers on what exactly the delivery of VR constitutes. There is a pragmatic recognition that what matters is the functional capacity of the individual, and that methods used in any intervention are not restricted to the various definitions of VR and treatment that exist. Hence, as far as the ABI is concerned, VR may *include* certain treatments essential to restoring capacity for work, alongside such approaches as case management, assessment, retraining and adaptations.

Box 4.1 Features of the Rehabilitation Code

1 The claimant is put at the centre of the process
2 The claimant's lawyer and the compensator work on a collaborative basis to address the claimant's needs, from first early notification of the claim and through early exchange of information.
3 The need for rehabilitation is addressed as a priority and sometimes before agreement on liability. Fixed time frames support the code's framework.
4 Rehabilitation needs are assessed by those who have the appropriate qualification, skills and experience.
5 The choice of rehabilitation assessor and provider should, wherever possible, be agreed by the claimant lawyer and the compensator.
6 Initial rehabilitation assessments can be conducted by telephone or personal interview, according to case type, and the resulting report should deal with matters specified in the code.
7 The claimant is not obliged to undergo treatment or intervention that is considered unreasonable.
8 The compensator will pay for any agreed assessment of rehabilitation needs and must justify a refusal to follow any of the rehabilitation recommendations.
9 The initial rehabilitation assessment process is outside the litigation process.
10 Where rehabilitation has been provided under the code, the compensator will not seek to recoup its cost, if the claim later fails in whole or part.

In promoting the case for VR, the ABI conducted a survey of VR activity among its members during 2008 (unpublished). Members demonstrated a belief that VR is successful in delivering benefits to employers and employees: around 80 per cent return-to-work following intervention in ELCI cases, with a range of 70–90 per cent, and, for income protection, a range of 55–67 per cent.[6] Generally, VR service providers have to handle a wider variety of cases in GIP cases, including more serious ones. Around 80 per cent of cases dealt with through ELCI are for MSDs, ranging from 70 to 95 per cent across different insurers. Around 10 per cent of ELCI cases are related to MH, with a range of 5–15 per cent. Non-MSD injuries and accidents are the next major category, averaging around 10 per cent, with a range of between 6 and 20 per cent.

The ABI research shows that 69 per cent of people are returned to work faster with VR, with an average of 28 working days being saved. For absences that were predicted to be very long, 11 weeks were saved on average. The evidence shows that, the earlier an absence is notified and intervention can begin, the earlier a person can be returned to work. However, the ABI maintains that there have to be incentives to employers, employees and insurers to pursue VR, and the financial incentives to pay for VR are small. This is a consequence of the lack of any tax breaks for funding VR, the low average cost of a claim, the low earnings of typical claimants and the cost of rehabilitation as charged by some service providers.

The ABI now perceives access to VR and associated services as key to addressing long-term absence issues, reducing the numbers leaving work and claiming benefits, as well as improving competitiveness and productivity by shortening periods of absence, getting people back to work who would otherwise have failed to return and ensuring that the benefits of work for health and well-being translate to employees over the long term.

Liability insurers are also keen to promote a different perspective on what compensation is for, embracing rehabilitation as a normal part of restitution for an injured party.

To date, the focus of ABI interest has been on promoting VR in ELCI claims. Although the value of premiums in this sector is much smaller than from motor vehicle insurance, it is also an area in which the issues surrounding incentives and disincentives to funding VR can be examined with reference to some consistent variables. Despite the growth in the amount of VR provided in the United Kingdom in recent years, provision is still small in comparison with the potential market, and, for a number of reasons invariably associated with costs, it is often only used after a long delay.

Costs, funding and incentives

The cost of VR varies from case to case, based on the condition, the timing of the intervention and the employment to which the injured party is seeking to return. Some cases can cost many thousands of pounds. Others can require a few sessions of counselling or physiotherapy and total a few hundred pounds. The ABI suggests that the average current cost of a case is about £1,200. This includes all conditions and all types of insurance. The ABI considers that, with better, earlier identification and with greater volumes, this cost could be significantly reduced.

VR can be difficult to provide in cases where liability has yet to be proved. If it is certain that an accident or illness has been caused by work, then VR can be provided without attracting any tax or national insurance as a benefit in kind. If there is doubt, then there is reluctance on the part of the employer and the insurer to provide VR, as it may appear to be admitting liability where there may be none. Without liability, tax and national insurance are applied to VR as a benefit in kind, and employees are reluctant to pay what may be significant costs. Likewise, in PI litigation, any intervention is likely to rest on an admittance of liability, and this can take so long to determine as to lessen the prospects of VR intervention succeeding. Reforms to speed up the compensation system that are currently under consideration by the Ministry of Justice should help to address this problem in part, but they will not address the much larger question of how to ensure intervention as early as possible to get a person back to work.

The Rehabilitation Code concentrates on those cases that are likely to result in a claim. Although this is of significant importance for ELCI insurers, it cannot address the much larger issue of long-term absence, nor does it remove the tax disincentive that exists for employees and employers. Owing to the tax disincentive, VR is currently generally only available to those who have suffered an injury or illness because of work. This applies roughly to 20 per cent of all absences, and 20 per cent of those claiming IB/ESA. The other 80 per cent do not have equal access to VR. The ABI considers this situation to be a major stumbling block to dealing effectively with the United Kingdom's health at work.

In any event, the costs of sickness absenteeism are shared among employers, employees and the government. From analysing where the costs of absence fall, on whom they fall and, importantly, when they occur, the costs of absence fall on the different stakeholders at different times. The cost moves steadily away from employers as SSP is exhausted, to fall on the employee and the government, and this situation influences funding decisions. The longer that an absence persists, the less incentive there is for an employer to intervene to return an employee to the workplace. This may explain why the relatively small number of occurrences of long-term absence in the United Kingdom end up accounting for a wholly disproportionate amount of lost time and a high incidence of claims for incapacity benefit.

Rehabilitating injured employees, saving on compensation and lost working days, and facilitating good employment practice may seem such an obvious course of action that there would appear to be a case for the type of mandatory programmes operating in such countries as Canada and Australia (Harder and Scott, 2005). From an insurance perspective, the situation is not so clear-cut. UK insurers write around one million ELCI policies per year, with a net value of £1.7 billion (this contrasts with the £12 billion value of motor insurance). The average cost of an ELCI policy is £1,700. In what is a competitive market, offering discounts to employers operating disability management programmes, including VR, is not perceived to be financially viable. Anything less than a substantial discount is unlikely to act as an incentive. In addition, the average value of a successful claim is less than £8,000 – not enough to justify substantial VR expenditure. On top of these factors, insurance companies are increasingly selling ELCI as part of a 'rolled-up' package of insurance, including such matters as building and contents insurance, fleet car insurance and so on. Financially, ELCI is a very small part of such packages.

It is also known that the wages earned by those who later go on to claim IB are much lower than the national average. The ABI suggests that only 7 per cent of recent claimants earned more than £25,000 per annum in their last job. Research for the DWP suggests that IB claimants are typically low paid compared with the general population. If one assumes an average 35-hour week and £6.69 per hour (a figure taken from Sainsbury and Davidson, 2006), this gives a weekly wage of £234.15. Given that injury claimants are lower-status workers in general, more likely to be on temporary contracts and working in smaller companies, it can be safely assumed that they are also less likely to receive long periods of any OSP.

In the circumstances, it is not surprising to find that there is no support to change the position found by Greenstreet Berman (2004), when it was noted that there are no rehabilitation duties prescribed in law for employers or employees although, 'this limits the extent to which agencies, such as the HSE or DWP, can influence employers, and also limits the extent to which courts will take account of rehabilitation'. For the foreseeable future, it is likely that voluntary co-operation with rehabilitation will prevail (except in litigation, when defendants are ordered to fund intervention). UK governments of all persuasions have shown themselves loath to intervene in the market, and organisations such as the CBI are opposed to mandatory obligations imposed on employers. Hence, the ABI has to rely on limited UK evidence-based practice and education to promote the cost benefits of VR among its members and, in turn, their insured. To its credit, the ABI has consistently promoted VR, on the basis not only of ultimately reducing the costs of compensation to its members, but also of enhancing the lives of claimants, that is in ensuring that insurance does its job to restore the injured party to a pre-injury position as far as reasonably possible.

Not only does the UK government fail to provide incentives to employers and insurers to intervene and provide VR services, but there is little incentive in the system when, on identifying those absences most likely to result in claims for incapacity benefit (now

ESA) and applying the benefits of VR to them indicates potential savings to the UK economy (65 per cent of the benefit falling on the government, according to the ABI, but less than 9 per cent falling on to the employer; indeed, the benefit to the employer may be lower than the cost of the intervention itself). Apart from large litigation claims involving a substantial future loss of earnings, when resettlement is likely to be difficult because of both the severity of injury and, sometimes, claimant and advisor resistance, there is little incentive for insurers to fund VR on the same scale as found in other Western countries.

Vocational rehabilitation procedure

Reference has already been made to employers notifying insurers in ELCI and GIP claims. Chapter 7 makes reference to a flow chart illustrating the implementation of VR in GIP claims. In PI litigation, there has developed a practice of claimants' representatives seeking (often large) interim payments to fund rehabilitation, to the extent that this process has become routinely accepted following the judgment in *Wright* v *Sullivan* (2005) EWCA Civ. Although rehabilitation in this context almost always refers to clinical rehabilitation and case management services, it may also include VR. The market has not developed as insurers would have liked.

Time scales and mechanisms for the consideration of rehabilitation

PI claims procedure

Claim initiation is the first step in the claims process, when an employee or anyone else covered by income-protection, accident and/or employers' liability insurance experiences an illness or sustains an injury. In the case of a non-work-related injury, the accident has to be the fault, or partly the fault, of the 'other party' to trigger a claim for PI compensation.

Claimant solicitor

From the earliest practicable stage, the duty of every claimant solicitor is to consider, in consultation with the claimant/their family and, if appropriate, treating physicians, the need for rehabilitation and to give the earliest possible notification to the compensator of the claim of a need for rehabilitation. Where the need for rehabilitation is identified by the compensator, the claimant solicitor should consider this immediately with the claimant and/or the claimant's family.

Compensator

The defendant solicitor equally has a duty to consider and communicate at the earliest practicable stage whether the claimant will benefit from rehabilitation. This may seem impracticable, given that the defendant solicitor has never met the claimant or his/her family and reports the defendant commissions are frequently in response to the ones received from the claimant's solicitor (unless experts are jointly instructed). However, insurers have mechanisms for identifying potentially large claims, and Swiss Re, for example, the world's largest reinsurer, has its own in-house rehabilitation team working in conjunction with claims managers. Although members of the team will not themselves deliver a service, they will propose a course of action to their insured.

When the need for rehabilitation is notified to the compensator by the claimant solicitor, the compensator should respond within 21 days. The compensator also has a duty to pay for an assessment report within 28 days of receipt of one and to respond substantively to recommendations to the claimant solicitor.

Parties

Both parties have a duty to consider choice of assessor and object to any suggested assessor within 21 days of nomination.

Assessor duties

Assessment is due to occur within 14 days of the referral letter, and the report is to be provided simultaneously to both parties.

The Rehabilitation Code is clearly a welcome measure, although VR is regarded implicitly within the rehabilitation package. A practice of appointing case managers to co-ordinate and oversee all aspects of the rehabilitation process has developed. However, the courts have only approved the appointment of case managers in catastrophic and other large claims. (Although there can be some rehabilitation input in claims of lesser value, this is more likely to take the form of a telephone triage or the limited and specific involvement of a physiotherapist or counsellor, rather than a longer-term managed rehabilitation strategy.)

It is naive to consider that '*working together*' constitutes collaboration necessarily in the best interest of the injured person. The litigation process remains an adversarial one; rehabilitation support is invariably contingent on full liability being admitted by the defendant; and the legal position regarding the provision of VR remains unclear. Although there are solicitors representing claimants who recognise that helping their client to restore functional capability and return-to-work is in their client's best long-term interest, the profession still has a culture that 'success' is represented by achieving the largest possible settlement, a matter often reinforced by counsel seeking to maximise any claim for loss of earnings. Likewise, although there is some variance in the attitude of individual insurance companies towards funding rehabilitation, the underlying motivation is one of reducing their costs.

Wright v Sullivan (2005) EWCA Civ 656

This case illustrates the control that defendants have sought, and failed to obtain, over the rehabilitation process. A seriously injured claimant asked for a large interim payment to set up a care regime under the supervision of a case manager. The defendant was concerned that the cost would be excessive and agreeing to it would make it impossible for a judge to accept anything else at a trial. The case also raised a question as to what extent the defendant's solicitors could have any input into the case manager's instructions. In a setback for insurers trying to control such situations, the Court of Appeal came down in favour of the claimant. However, in line with guidelines issued by the British Association of Brain Injury Case Managers, the claimant accepted that the defendant could make suggestions to the case manager, as long as the defendant did not seek to impose any indications about what the case manager ought to decide was the most appropriate care regime. The main remaining issue was whether or not communications between the claimant's advisors and the case manager should be privileged. The defendant submitted that appointment of a clinical case manager owing duties to the claimant alone would be inimical to the Rehabilitation Code philosophy of co-operation between the parties. Brooke LJ, giving the leading judgment, found these submissions '*impossible to accept*', saying it was inevitable that the case manager owed duties to the claimant alone and,

> while it will be in the claimant's interest that the case manager should receive a flow of suggestions from any other experts who have been instructed in the case, the case manager must ultimately make decisions in the best interests of the patient and not be beholden to two different masters.

Hence, the courts have accepted that the case manager is an independent professional practitioner and can be unilaterally instructed (or, as the Case Management Society of the United Kingdom (CMSUK) prefers, '*receive instructions*'). Given that the legal obligation of defendants in PI litigation is to restore the claimant as far as possible to their pre-injury position, where does *Wright* v *Sullivan* leave the instruction of VR practitioners? After all, many case managers perceive VR to be a part of their responsibilities.

The situation is unsatisfactory. There can be no doubt that many PI claimants not sustaining catastrophic injuries and not requiring a case manager would benefit from VR. The evidence is there from PHI claims, research undertaken for the ABI (Greenstreet Berman, op. cit.) and the experience of employment experts instructed in PI claims when there is a dispute over the future loss of earnings (although, unless jointly agreed between the parties, there are almost always likely to be difficulties in getting the courts to agree to such instructions). If any instruction to a VR practitioner is undertaken unilaterally by a claimant solicitor, are the defendants subsequently going to concede funding on the basis that the courts will support such activity?

The rationale of *Wright* v *Sullivan* appears to say 'yes'. However, defendants are likely to maintain that such a service is not necessary: public sector services are available (although a counter argument is that *Wright* v *Sullivan* supports claimants choosing their own rehabilitation services and not relying on the NHS and Social Services), and *Wright* v *Sullivan* only applies to *clinical* rehabilitation. Claimant solicitors are not going to run up costs without the prospect of recovering the expenditure.

The reality is that the courts in the United Kingdom have yet to give VR practitioners the same professional recognition as case managers (although they may be one and the same person). Although various changes to civil litigation, beginning with the 1999 Woolf reforms, have contributed to few cases now proceeding to trial, as hard to comprehend as it is (particularly to many overseas VR experts now practicing in the United Kingdom, who have routinely been heard by the courts in their own countries), High Court Judges in the United Kingdom will almost always prefer the opinion of a medical expert for an employment prognosis over that of a VR practitioner, and this attitude permeates the litigation system down to District Judge level, where decisions are made over which experts can be instructed.

To what extent do case managers undertake VR?

Case managers are drawn from a wide range of professions, including nursing, social work, occupational therapy and physiotherapy. Referrals to case managers are made in large PI claims when there is a need to oversee the co-ordinated care of a claimant. In such cases, the severity of the injuries invariably means that there is little prospect of the claimant returning to work. On the occasions that RTW is an issue, there is often an expectation that the case manager will take responsibility for all aspects of therapeutic intervention by instructing independent VR experts, if not undertaking the work themselves. The CMSUK regularly places VR on its conference agendas, although there are no data on the extent to which its members directly undertake VR or are qualified to undertake such work, or the extent to which referrals are made to independent VR practitioners. Thompson (2009) sheds some light on the subject.

In GIP, and some ELCI claims, there is the prospect of a specific VR service being instructed, with a VR case manager delivering and co-ordinating RTW services. In such cases, the initiative is almost always taken by the insurer or reinsurer.

Summary

Insurance-led VR still remains a relatively recent response to claims management in the United Kingdom. Although there is evidence from other countries as to the success of VR, there are dangers in reading across from other jurisdictions, especially on costs and benefits. Given that insurance-led VR has been applied mainly to incidents of work-related injury or illness, legal and compensation systems affect when and how VR is used.

The ABI perceives VR as the main way insurers can reduce costs in ELCI claims and claimants can be returned to a pre-injury position. Owing to the value of insurance premiums and the cost of absence quickly passing from employers to government, there is often little financial incentive in the system for insurers and employers to invest in VR. In the circumstances, it is not surprising to find that the market in the United Kingdom is still small, and there is considerable scope for development. Replacing employees can be costly, and VR programmes that can work in conjunction with employers' sickness-absence management practices have the greatest prospect of success.

The position with regard to the funding of claimants with serious injuries arising from other claims, such as RTAs, is confusing. Whereas the courts and defendants now routinely accept the appointment of case managers, this is invariably in cases in which injuries are so severe as to preclude a RTW. Hence, the evidence in respect of case managers undertaking VR is mixed. Some undertake no VR at all, or, if they do, they subcontract the work to VR specialists. It appears that a large number of claimants with less severe injuries, who would benefit from VR, are receiving no support at all.

The absence of legislation identifying responsibilities and a reliance on voluntary codes of practice have resulted in piecemeal development and a lack of coherence. Whether or not an employee requiring VR to return-to-work receives support may depend upon such a significant but random variable as timely reporting to an insurer. The establishment of liability is critical to the funding of VR arising from other (non-workplace) accidents. Other variables include the appropriate identification of clients requiring VR, the attitude of District and High Court Judges, the commitment of solicitors and barristers to rehabilitation, the response of insurers and their representatives, and the expertise and priorities of case managers.

5 The legal context

Key issues

- Health and safety.
- Employers' duty of care.
- Disability discrimination.
- Requirement to make reasonable adjustments.
- Significance of medical questionnaires in recruitment.
- Seeking legal redress.

Learning objectives

- Understanding of the main legislation covering the employment of people with disabilities/health conditions.
- Ability to identify when someone is covered by disability-discrimination legislation.
- Understanding of what the law requires of employers in making reasonable adjustments.
- Understanding of the Employment Tribunals Service.

Introduction

The United Kingdom has no specific legislation requiring the provision of VR. However, VR operates within the United Nations Convention on the Rights of Persons with Disabilities, which came into force in May 2008. The convention has eight guiding principles, including equality of opportunity, non-discrimination and full participation within society. These incorporate the right to work and full access to employment (United Nations, 2008). The European Union has a non-discrimination directive supporting social inclusion (European Union, 2000).

Within the United Kingdom, the law protects the interests of disabled jobseekers and promotes and safeguards the employment of sick and disabled workers (Box 5.1).

Health and Safety at Work Act 1974

The HSW Act requires employers to ensure the health, safety and welfare of their employees so far as reasonably practical. Employers must also carry out an assessment

---

Box 5.1 Legal framework for VR practice

- Health and Safety at Work Act 1974: ensures that the health and safety of everyone at work is protected as far as reasonably practicable.
- Disability Discrimination Act 1995: prevents discrimination on health grounds and requires employers to make reasonable adjustments to accommodate employees.
- Data Protection Act 1998: if an absence record contains specific medical information relating to the employee, this is deemed sensitive data, and the employer has to satisfy the statutory conditions for processing such data.
- Employment Rights Act 1996: requires employers to adopt fair procedures before dismissing employees on grounds of sickness absence.
- Employment Act 2002 (Dispute Regulations) 2004: adopts statutory minimum dismissal, disciplinary and grievance procedures.
- Disability Discrimination Act 2005: removes the provision allowing justification of failure to make reasonable adjustments.
- Equality Act 2010: harmonises discrimination legislation.

---

of risks to employees' health under the Management of Health and Safety at Work Regulations 1999. The HSE has recommended that this ought to include any threats to employees' psychiatric health, including stress. Employers must take reasonable steps to limit any identified risks and monitor the situation. Since October 2003, employees have been able to bring civil claims against employers in breach of the 1999 regulations.

The obligation to ensure that no employee is unduly exposed to levels of risks can create genuine issues for employers. For example, there are many jobs in which employees are exposed to long periods of static muscular contraction that may have an adverse impact on an impairment such as a MSD. The employer needs to be able to ensure that appropriate screening safeguards the employee and does not expose him or her to hazards when reasonable adjustments are not possible. As a consequence of the need to safeguard the health and safety of employees, tensions have arisen around the boundaries of the HSW Act and the requirements of the 1995 DDA, particularly the need to make reasonable adjustments.

Employers' liability and the 'duty of care'

Employers have a common-law '*duty of care*' to ensure the well-being of their employees. An employee has a valid negligence claim if he or she suffers a '*reasonably foreseeable*' physical or psychiatric injury. It is the question of an injury being '*reasonably foreseeable*' that has resulted in what is known as the Hatton Guidance, set out by the Court of Appeal in *Sutherland* v *Hatton* and others.[1]

The employer has a responsibility for taking the initiative when an employee reports occupational stress (*Barber* v *Somerset County Council*).

Box 5.2 Defining 'reasonably foreseeable': the Hatton Guidance

1   An employer is entitled to assume that the employee can cope with the normal pressures of the job, unless the employer knows something about the job or individual to make him consider the issue of psychiatric injury.

2   An employer is not obliged to make intrusive enquiries and is generally entitled to take what he is told by the employee at face value.

3   No occupation should be regarded as intrinsically dangerous to mental health.

4   To trigger a duty on the employer to take action, the indications of impending harm arising from stress at work must be plain enough for any reasonable employer to recognise the need to do something about it.

5   The employer will only breach the duty of care if failing to take the steps that are reasonable in the circumstances, bearing in mind the magnitude of the risk of harm occurring, the gravity of the harm that may occur, the costs and practicability of preventing it, and the justification for running the risk.

6   The size, resources, and scope of the employer's operation can all be taken into account in determining what is reasonable.

7   An employer may only be reasonably expected to take steps likely to do some good. Expert evidence may be required on this subject.

8   An employer offering a confidential advice service, with referral to an appropriate counselling or treatment service, is unlikely to be found in breach of duty.

9   If the only reasonable and effective step would have been to dismiss or demote the employee, the employer will not be in breach of duty in allowing the employee to continue working.

Intrinsically stressful job

In *Hartman* v *South Essex Mental Health and Community Care NHS Trust*, the Court of Appeal considered six 'stress cases', four of which concerned 'foreseeability'. The Court recorded the views that:

(a) the fact that an employer offers a counselling service should be read as foreseeing the risk of psychiatric injury to employees; and

(b) in line with the Hatton Guidance, the fact that such a service is provided will mean that the employer is unlikely to be found in breach of its duty of care, even if harm is foreseeable (although this is not always the case).

Provision of counselling services

In *Intel Corporation (UK) Ltd* v *Daw*, the Court of Appeal held that an employee's email to a manager that she was '*stressed out*' and '*demoralised*', and including reference to two previous incidents of post-natal depression, was crucial to the issue of foreseeability. Urgent action should have been taken to reduce her workload. The Court

---

Box 5.3 *Barber* v *Somerset County Council*: **case study of the 'reasonably foreseeable' and the consequences of stress**

Barber, a maths teacher, took on extra responsibilities to maintain the same salary following a restructuring. His GP signed him off work with stress and depression. On his return, three weeks later, no one had discussed his illness with him, and so he made an appointment to see the head teacher, to make her aware that he was not coping with his workload. The head was unsympathetic, telling him all the staff were under stress. Likewise, two deputy heads, with whom Barber subsequently arranged meetings, took no action, although one was sympathetic towards him. Barber later broke down and was diagnosed as suffering from depression. He sued in the County Court, and the judge held the employer liable in negligence for B's illness.

When the case reached the House of Lords, their Lordships held that the employer had paid insufficient attention to Barber's absence with stress. In addition, Barber had alerted the employer to his illness and the possibility of a psychiatric injury. Their Lordships stated that budgetary constraints and the fact that other teachers were under pressure were not reasons for finding that the school was under no duty to help Barber: 'even a small reduction in his workload, coupled with the feeling that the senior management team was on his side, might itself have made a real difference'. Barber was awarded compensation of £72,547.02.

---

rejected submissions that, applying the guidance in Hatton, the fact that the employer provided a counselling and medical assistance service was sufficient to discharge its duty of care. Each case turns on its facts, and, in this case, the counselling service could not have alleviated D's problems; only management could do this by reducing her workload.

Bullying and harassment

Employers have a duty to ensure that employees should be protected from bullying, a common cause of workplace stress.

Return-to-work programmes

There is no obligation on an employer to offer a RTW programme, but if there is one and the employer does not adhere to it, then it may be liable for any adverse consequences (*Garrod* v *North Devon NHS Primary Care Trust*).

Damages in negligence cases

Damages in negligence cases are not limited by statute. In *Green* v *DB Group Services (UK) Ltd*, the claimant received £800,000, awarded by the High Court, primarily for the future loss of earnings following two breakdowns and a depressive illness.

Working Time Regulations

Long hours and night working pose an increased risk to health and safety. Employers have a duty to take '*all reasonable steps*' to ensure that the limits contained in the Working Time Regulations 1998, are observed. The regulations impose a 48-hour week and limits on night working, although employees can opt out.

The Disability Discrimination Act (1995)

The DDA (1995) became law in December 1996, when some of the employment provisions took effect. Although the 2005 DDA widened its scope, and the 2010 Equality Act has added to this, the 1995 Act remains fundamentally the main piece of legislation making it unlawful to discriminate against a disabled person in their terms of employment or promotion opportunities, by dismissing them or by subjecting them to any other detriment.

The DDA recognises five different forms of discrimination:

1   **Direct discrimination**: 'it is unlawful to treat a worker less favourably on grounds of his disability'. From October 2004, a new section stated,

> a person directly discriminates against a disabled person if, on the grounds of a disabled person's disability, he treats the disabled person less favourably than he treats or would treat a person not having that particular disability whose relevant circumstances, including his abilities, are the same as, or not materially different from, those of a disabled person.

Direct discrimination does not mean that a disabled person cannot be disciplined or dismissed. In *Greenwood* v *United Tiles Ltd*, a tribunal accepted that a diabetic was dismissed for reasons unconnected to his disability, such as a poor work performance and a bad attitude towards management, not for reasons connected to his disability.

2   **Disability-related discrimination**: 'it is unlawful to treat a worker less favourably for reasons related to his disability'. An employer commits an act of disability-related discrimination if,

> for a reason which relates to the disabled person's disability, he treats him less favourably than he treats or would treat others to whom that reason does not or would not apply, and he cannot show that the treatment in question is justified.

3   **Failure to make adjustments**: an employer is also guilty of disability discrimination if he fails in his duty to make reasonable adjustments, which arises where either a 'provision, criterion or practice' applied by the employer, or any physical feature of the employer's premises, 'places the disabled person concerned at a substantial disadvantage in comparison with persons who are not disabled'.

4   **Harassment**.

5   **Victimisation**.

Box 5. 4 Defining disability (DDA)

There must be a mental or physical condition which has a substantial and long-term adverse affect on the employee's ability to carry out normal day-to-day activities.

Long-term means the condition must last, or be likely to last, more than 12 months.

The ability to carry out normal day-to-day activities was made with reference to mobility, manual dexterity, physical co-ordination, ability to lift or otherwise move everyday objects, speech, hearing or eyesight, memory or ability to concentrate, learn or understand, and understanding the risk of physical danger. This reference was removed in the 2010 Equality Act.

Meaning of disability

The DDA defines disability for the purposes of the Act (Box 5.4).

Examples of impairments set out in the Guidance include developmental, such as dyslexia, learning difficulties, MH, respiratory conditions such as asthma, cardiovascular diseases and conditions with fluctuating or recurring effects, such as rheumatoid arthritis, myalgic encephalomyelitis (ME), fibromyalgia and epilepsy.

When impairment ceases to have a substantial adverse effect, it is treated as continuing to have that effect if the effect is '*likely*' to recur. In *SCA Packaging Ltd* v *Boyle*, a Northern Ireland case, the House of Lords rejected case law developed in England and Wales to the effect that '*likely*' in these provisions means '*more probable than not*'. Their Lordships held that '*likely*' refers to an outcome that '*could well happen*'.

Substantial and long-term effect

Examples of 'substantial' given in the Guidance include an inability to walk, or difficulty in walking other than at a slow pace, and difficulties reading or asking questions. However, these examples are illustrative only, and the determination of 'substantial' and 'long-term' has been subject to much argument. Impairment is deemed long term if it has lasted at least 12 months, is likely to last 12 months or is likely to last for the rest of the person's life.

Recurring conditions

People with such conditions as epilepsy and rheumatoid arthritis experience remissions during which they would not be able to satisfy the definition of disability. To ensure such people are covered, a person is treated as continuing to have an impairment if that condition is '*likely to recur*' and have a substantial adverse impact. In *European Wellcare Lifestyles* v *Crossingham*, the Employment Appeal Tribunal (EAT) held that, in assessing if the substantial adverse impact would recur, taking the situation at the time of the alleged discrimination, a tribunal could refer to what subsequently actually happened. However, this appears contrary to a further ruling in *Spence* v *Intype*.

Progressive conditions

As soon as a person with a progressive condition, such as muscular dystrophy, has *any* symptoms affecting their normal day-to-day activity, they are deemed to have a disability, providing (a) they can show some adverse effect on their activity, and (b) in future this is likely to be substantial. In such cases, a medical prognosis is required.

Coping strategies

The Guidance recognises that the effects of a disability can be mitigated by the use of coping strategies. Tribunals should take account of the extent to which an applicant can be reasonably expected to reduce the effects of impairment.

Mental impairment/learning disability

In *Dunham* v *Ashford Windows*, the EAT gave guidance on how a tribunal should deal with a learning disability. The EAT said that medical evidence is not required in every case, but what is important is evidence from a '*suitably qualified expert*'. In this instance, it was not open to the tribunal to reject the evidence from a senior psychologist with substantial experience of learning difficulties because he was not a doctor.

Mental illness

The DDA 1995 originally stated that a mental illness would only amount to a mental impairment if it was '*clinically well-recognised*'. Although the 2005 DDA removed this requirement, tribunals still need to be satisfied as to the existence of an alleged condition.

In *Goodwin* v *The Patent Office*, the EAT issued guidance on deciding whether or not a person has a disability within the meaning of the Act:

1   Does the applicant have a physical or mental impairment? (If in doubt over a mental impairment, tribunals are to make reference to the International Classification of Functioning, Disability and Health (WHO, 2001).)
2   Does that impairment affect the applicant's ability to carry out normal day-to-day activities?
3   Is the adverse effect of the impairment substantial? The EAT reminded tribunals that substantial means more than minor or trivial, rather than very large.

Dispute over existence of a condition

In a tribunal claim, when an employer disputes the existence of an employee's disability, parties may instruct a joint expert. In *Hospice of St Mary of Furness* v *Howard*, the EAT considered the circumstances in which the respondent (employer) might subsequently instruct its own expert witness. Even though *College of Ripon and York St John* v *Hobbs* established that a claimant does not have to identify the conditions giving rise to his or her physical symptoms in order to establish the existence of a physical impairment, such a claim is more open to attack in the absence of an identifiable cause. In *J* v *DLA Piper UK*, the EAT gave guidance on the correct approach to determining whether or not a disability is established, stating it will not always be necessary to identify a specific 'impairment' if the existence of one can be established from evidence of an adverse effect on a claimant's abilities.

Need for employer to be informed

In *O'Neill* v *Symm and Co. Ltd*, a tribunal concluded that ME is a disability but, because the applicant had not informed the employer of her condition, the decision to dismiss her could not be related to the disability, a decision upheld by the EAT. An employer cannot be expected to make reasonable adjustments if it is unaware, or could not be reasonably expected to be aware, of a particular condition.

Job requirements

In *Chief Constable of Lothian and Borders Police* v *Cumming*, the EAT established that a person's inability to meet the physical requirements for entry into a profession does not amount to a relevant adverse effect on that person's ability to carry out normal day-to-day activities.

Development of the DDA

Enforcement of the DDA has been through a process of evolution. The DDA 1995 (Amendment) Regulations 2003 came into force on 1 October 2004 and introduced certain key amendments (Box 5.5).

The Disability Discrimination Act 2005

Prior to the 2005 Act, various amendments introduced in October 2004 removed the prospect of employers justifying a failure to make reasonable adjustments and also set

---

Box 5.5 DDA: key 2004 amendments

- Removes small-business exemption for employers with fewer than 15 employees.
- Makes it clear that the employee is required to establish facts from which it may be presumed that discrimination has taken place, after which the burden of proof is placed on the employer to establish that there has been no discrimination.
- Specific prohibition of harassment based on disability.
- Removes justification defence in direct discrimination cases where the reason for that treatment is based merely on the fact that the person has a disability, rather than on a consideration of the individual's abilities.
- Extends protection in certain circumstances beyond the end of the employment relationship from acts of discrimination (including harassment).
- Removes justification defence in respect of a failure to make reasonable adjustments.

new time limits for lodging complaints. Among the 2005 Act's main provisions are extending the DDA 1995 to cover, from the point of diagnosis, people with HIV infection, cancer and MS; ending the requirement that a mental illness must be '*clinically well-recognised*'; and placing a duty on public authorities to promote equality of opportunity for disabled people.

Equality Act 2010 and disability-related discrimination

One of the last acts of New Labour was to oversee the passing of the Equality Act in April 2010. The plan of the government was that most of the Act would come into effect in October 2010 (the time span can be found on www.equaliteshumanrights.com), although some disagreement between the coalition partners on certain aspects, such as 'positive action', was likely to affect the final outcome.

Protected characteristics

One of the key aims of the Act is to harmonise discrimination law across age, disability and gender. The grounds on which discrimination is deemed unlawful are all brought together as '*protected characteristics*', largely replicating the criteria found in the existing legislation.

Definition of disability

A new definition of disability contains few changes from that found in the DDA (1995). Existing guidance on determining whether a claimant has a disability is largely retained, although the requirement for an impairment to affect a person's ability to carry out normal day-to-day activities was dropped.

Direct discrimination

Two major disability discrimination issues from 2008 contributed to the most significant considerations within the Equality Act. The first is the difficulty in proving disability-related discrimination as a result of the House of Lords' decision in *London Borough of Lewisham* v *Malcolm*. The second is whether the Disability Discrimination Act 1995 can cover those discriminated against because of their association with a disabled person.

Proving disability-related discrimination

The Court of Appeal in *Clark* v *TDG Ltd t/a Novacold* approved a broad approach to the DDA (1995), holding that there was no need for the non-disabled comparator to be in the same relevant circumstances as the claimant. The correct approach to addressing sickness absence was established in *Cox* v *The Post Office*. The tribunal said that the reason for dismissal in this case was absence, absence was caused by disability, and someone who did not have the absences would not have been dismissed. The disabled person had therefore suffered '*less favourable treatment*'. The tribunal had then to consider whether it was justified for a '*substantial and material reason*'. Mr Cox had been absent on average for 8.5 days per annum. This was not substantial. The implication of this case is that an employer may well have to accept a higher level of absence than would be acceptable for a non-disabled person. Hence, an employee dismissed for lengthy sickness absence related to his disability could be compared with a non-disabled employee who had not been absent at all, rather than to an employee absent for a reason unrelated to disability. As the comparator would not have been dismissed, it was possible to show less favourable treatment.

However, the House of Lords disapproved of this approach in *Mayor and Burgesses of the London Borough of Lewisham* v *Malcolm*, a case brought under the housing provisions of the DDA. Their Lordships held that the appropriate comparator in cases of disability-related discrimination was a non-disabled person otherwise in the same circumstances as the disabled claimant. In the case of sickness absence, this translated to comparing the treatment of the disabled person with a person without a disability who had taken a similar amount of sick leave. The impact of '*Malcolm*' was dramatic. In short, the comparator for direct discrimination became a non-disabled person in the same circumstances; for disability-related discrimination, it became a disabled person compared with a non-disabled person. By way of illustration as to the significance, the success or failure of many claims of unfair selection for redundancy has hung on the comparator. In *Kirker* v *British Sugar*, an employee with very poor vision was awarded £103,000 (largely to compensate him for the limited prospect of future employment) because of subjective scoring in a redundancy exercise. Points were deducted for absence due to disability. If compared with an employee absent for other reasons, the claim may well have failed.

The Equality Act establishes that disability-related discrimination occurs when a disabled person can show that, for a reason related to his or her disability, the employer has treated him or her less favourably than he treats or would treat others to whom that reason does or would apply (Box 5.6).

The employer (A) has a defence if he or she did not know, and could not reasonably have been expected to know, that the employee (B) had the disability.

A disabled person is no longer required to establish that his or her treatment is less favourable than that experienced by a comparator. This provision avoids the main issue in *Malcolm*, namely, who the comparator should be. The explanatory notes state that this change is

> aimed at re-establishing an appropriate balance between enabling a disabled person to make out a case of experiencing a detriment which arises because of his or her disability, and providing an opportunity for an employer or other person to defend the treatment.

Box 5.6 Discrimination arising from disability (dealing with the post-*Malcolm* fall-out)

- No need for a comparator.
- A discriminates against B if
  - A treats B 'unfavourably because of something arising as a consequence of B's disability', and
  - A cannot show that the treatment is a proportionate means of achieving a legitimate aim.
- A knows, or could reasonably be expected to know, that B is disabled.

Indirect discrimination

In the Equality Act, the government also opted to include disability among the protected characteristics covered by the indirect-discrimination provisions. A number of responses to the consultation exercise opined that the complex nature of indirect discrimination is not suited to disability. In short, indirect discrimination is established when an employer's policy puts those who share a protected characteristic at a '*particular disadvantage*' when compared with those who do not share it. Since the way the same disability manifests itself varies from person to person, it is hard to imagine how a disabled person can demonstrate a group disadvantage. In any event, it is difficult to foresee a situation when the application of an employer's policy is considered indirectly discriminatory, but is not covered by either discrimination arising from disability or the duty to make reasonable adjustments.

Discrimination by association

On a literal reading, the DDA 1995 is designed to protect from discrimination only those who are actually disabled. However, in *Coleman* v *Attridge Law*, the European Court of Justice held that the EU Equal Treatment Framework Directive requires national law also to protect those who suffer discrimination or harassment because of the disability of a person with whom they associate. When the case returned to the employment tribunal, the tribunal found that this effect could be achieved by reading the DDA as if it included reference to discrimination and harassment on the grounds of a person's '*association*' with a disabled person.

On appeal, the EAT agreed with the effect the tribunal had sought to achieve. However, the EAT was concerned that use of the term '*association*' risked tribunals becoming enmeshed in an analysis of what '*association*' means. The Equality Act makes it clear that associative discrimination is covered, without the need for tribunals to adopt non-literal interpretations of the legislation. This means, for example, that carers of disabled people enjoy protection from less-favourable treatment that they may receive because of that disability.

The Act protects employers from accusations of less-favourable treatment arising from able-bodied employees over the making of reasonable adjustments to a disabled employee's working conditions. It is not discrimination to treat a disabled person more favourably than a person who is not disabled. The Act states: 'If the protected characteristic is disability, and B is not a disabled person, A does not discriminate against B only because A treats or would treat disabled persons more favourably than A treats B'.

Pre-employment health enquiries

Pre-employment enquiries about health issues are thought to be one of the main reasons why disabled job applicants often fail to reach the interview stage. The Equality Act states that an employer must not ask about a job applicant's health (including any disability) before offering him or her work or, when not in a position immediately to offer work, before including the applicant in a pool of persons to whom he intends to offer work in the future. An employer does not commit an act of disability discrimination simply by asking about a job applicant's health (Box 5.7). There is no blanket

---

Box 5.7 Pre-employment questions on health

- Where an employer questions a candidate on health before making a recruit-ment decision, the burden shifts to the employer to disprove discrimination.
- But, questions are not unlawful if necessary to:
    - establish if the duty to make adjustments arises;
    - monitor diversity;
    - enable the employer to take positive action;
    - establish whether the candidate has a particular disability, if that disability is an occupational requirement for the post.

---

ban on pre-employment health enquiries. However, an employer's conduct in reliance on provided information might lead a tribunal to conclude that the employer has committed a discriminatory act. In such a circumstance, the burden of proof is on the employer to show that no discrimination took place.

It remains lawful to ask necessary questions to establish whether the applicant is able to comply with a requirement to undergo an assessment (such as an interview or selection test), whether a duty to make reasonable adjustments arises or whether the applicant will be able to carry out a function intrinsic to the job. The employer is also entitled to ask questions necessary to monitor diversity among job applications in order to promote positive action; or to establish whether the applicant has a particular disability, when having that disability is an occupational requirement. In the latter respect, by way of illustration, the explanatory notes state that, 'an organisation for deaf people might legitimately employ a deaf person who uses British Sign Language to work as a counsellor to other deaf people whose first or preferred language is BSL'.

When it comes to litigation arising out of information provided during the application process, it is almost always the (former) employee suing the employer to recover compensation for loss or damage suffered in the course of their employment. However, any job applicant who is less than truthful when applying for a job may find that, where misrepresentations have induced the employer to enter into a contract of employment, the contract is likely to be terminated. Another remedy, albeit rarely used, is for the employer to claim damages for any losses incurred as a result of the misrepresentations.

Reasonable adjustments

When examining reasonable adjustments, there are essentially two aspects to take into consideration:

- The law and employers' statutory obligations. There are potentially substantial damages for the failure of employers to make reasonable adjustments to accom-modate disabled job applicants and employees.
- Identifying the need for, and, making reasonable adjustments.

This chapter concentrates on the first bullet point (the second is addressed in Chapter 15, when we examine placement and retention strategies).

Disclosure

In order for an adjustment to be made, the condition needs to be disclosed to the employer. It is not only in the case of MH that there is evidence of a reluctance to do this. It has been reported on a major VR pilot programme for employees with a wide range of health conditions that around 30 per cent of employees off work for health reasons did not want their condition reported to their employer.[2]

Employers are exempt from the duty to make reasonable adjustments if they can show that they did not know, and could not reasonably have been expected to know, that the disabled person had a disability and that he or she was likely to be placed at a substantial disadvantage as a consequence of it. In *Secretary of State for the Department for Work and Pensions* v *Alam*, the EAT held that two questions must be answered in the negative, if an employer is to be excused the duty to make reasonable adjustments:

- Did the employer know both that the employee was disabled and that his or her disability was liable to affect him or her in the manner set out in Section 4A(1) of the 1995 Act?
- Ought the employer to have known both that the employee was disabled and that his or her disability was liable to affect him or her in the manner set out in Section 4A(1) of the 1995 Act?

The Act expressly states that the duty to make adjustments does not apply when the employer could not reasonably be expected to know that a disabled person has a disability and is likely to be placed at a disadvantage, or, in the case of job applicants, that an interested disabled person is or may be an applicant for the job in question. The government rejected suggestions that the duty to make adjustments should be anticipatory in nature, requiring employers to make changes before they know, or ought to know, of a specific employee's disability.

The Equality Act consolidates the various provisions arising from the 1995 and 2005 DDAs relating to reasonable adjustments. The duty to make adjustments substantially replicates the DDA (1995), namely where a provision, criterion or practice (PCP) or a physical feature of premises puts a disabled person at a substantial disadvantage in comparison with persons who are not disabled, the person to whom the duty applies must take such steps as it is reasonable to have to take to avoid the disadvantage. The DDA (2005) clarifies the circumstances in which it is considered reasonable to make adjustments.

The following list of examples illustrates the steps that may need to be taken in order to comply with the duty to make reasonable adjustments:

- making adjustments to premises;
- allocating some of the disabled person's duties to another person;
- transferring to fill an existing vacancy;
- altering hours of working or training;
- assigning to a different place of work or training;
- allowing absence during working or training hours for rehabilitation, assessment or treatment;

Box 5.8 DDA 2005 reasonable adjustments

In determining whether it is reasonable for a person to take a particular step in order to comply with a duty to make reasonable adjustment, regard shall be paid, in particular, to:

(a) the extent to which taking the step would prevent the effect in relation to which the duty is imposed;
(b) the extent to which it is practicable for him to take the step;
(c) the financial and other costs which would be incurred by him on taking the step and the extent to which taking it would disrupt any of his activities;
(d) the extent of his financial and other resources;
(e) the availability to him of financial and other assistance with respect to taking the step;
(f) the nature of his activities and the size of his undertaking;
(g) where the step would be undertaken in relation to a private household, the extent to which taking it would:
    (i) disrupt that household, or
    (ii) disturb any person residing there.

- giving, or arranging for, training or mentoring (whether for the disabled person or any other person);
- acquiring or modifying equipment;
- modifying instructions or reference manuals;
- modifying procedures for testing or assessment;
- providing a reader or interpreter;
- providing supervision or other support.

Training

The legislation also covers the training of disabled employees. All disabled employees should have equal access to a company's training programmes. This might include providing individual training for disabled employees to use any adaptations or special equipment used in the workplace; providing training over a longer period for employees who can only attend a training course for a limited number of hours per day; retraining employees who become disabled to allow them to remain in their present job or take a different job; providing training material in different formats; making sign language interpreters available; and allowing trainees to bring a personal care attendant on a course, as well as changing training locations.

Employers should also ensure that they train other staff to understand their policy towards disabled people, provide disability equality training for all staff having contact with the public, set standards within the organisation and ensure the services they are providing are accessible to disabled people.

An added requirement of the Equality Act is that, when a disabled person is placed at a substantial disadvantage, save for the provision of an auxiliary aid, there is a duty to take reasonable steps to provide that aid. Where the PCP or auxiliary aid relates to the provision of information, the steps include measures for ensuring that the information is provided in an accessible format. An employer under the duty to make reasonable adjustments is not entitled to pass on the costs of compliance to the disabled person (subject to an express provision to the contrary).

Interpreting the wording of the legislation has been subject to much debate. Common questions relate to the following.

What is a PCP?

Provisions, criteria and practices include arrangements for determining to whom employment should be offered, and the terms, conditions or arrangements on which employment, promotion, a transfer, training or any other benefit is offered. The duty to make reasonable adjustments applies, for example, to selection and interview procedures and the premises used for such procedures, as well as to job offers, contractual arrangements and working conditions.

What is an adjustment?

An adjustment, in the context of the DDA, is a change. This can be a physical change or a change in the way something is done.

What is meant by 'substantial disadvantage?'

Substantial means simply 'more than minor or trivial' (DDA 1995 Code of Practice).

What does 'reasonable' mean?

The DDA does not define 'reasonable'. Ultimately, it is up to the courts to decide. This is because an adjustment is related to a particular individual, their experience of their impairment and the situation they are in. However, it does set out four tests of reasonableness:

1   **The effectiveness in preventing disadvantage**: The more effective an adjustment is in reducing disadvantage, the more reasonable it is likely to be.
2   **The practicality of the step**: It is more likely that an employer will be expected to take a step that is easy than to take a step that is hard.
3   **The financial and other costs and the extent of any disruption caused**: The duty to make adjustments is bounded by cost, cost–benefits, the scale of disruption and other matters likely to arise from the exercise. Cost is not just about the price of making adjustments, but also relates to the experience and skill of the employee, the cost of replacing that employee, how long the employee has been with the company (it is more likely to be reasonable to make an expensive adjustment for a permanent member of staff than a temp) and whether the adjustment may be of benefit to other employees (disabled and non-disabled).
4   **The extent of an organisation's financial and other resources**: Although tribunals will take into consideration the resources of an employer, they are also familiar with

---

Box 5.9 Examples of reasonable adjustments for some people with MH conditions

- altering the work content
- providing support
- shortening or altering work hours
- increased tolerance of absenteeism
- allowing extra holiday or unpaid leave
- permitting absence for treatment
- allowing rehabilitation following absence

---

the Access to Work scheme (Chapter 8). They will take into account whether or not an employer has approached Jobcentre Plus for assistance in both the identification of any adjustment and for financial assistance if this is required.

The full financial resources of an organisation are also taken into consideration, not simply those of a particular site where an employee or service is based. It is no good a large retail chain maintaining that a particular site is losing money, if the company is otherwise financially healthy. However, if the company indicated plans to close the branch in question, and the adjustment would entail considerable expenditure, a tribunal would have to consider the practicality of the measure.

The reality is that most adjustments for disabled people cost little or nothing, and changes made for disabled people often make working life better for other employees or service users.

Other matters to consider when deciding what is reasonable

Although the DDA does not specifically mention any further factors, other issues may be relevant, depending on the circumstances, for example:

- **The effects on other employees**: If a reasonable adjustment may affect other employees, their needs may need to be considered. For example, if an employee uses speaking software, it may be necessary to wear headphones to avoid disrupting other members of staff.
- **Adjustments made for other disabled people**: If there are a number of disabled staff who find some aspect of the working environment difficult, then there is a greater need for an employer to make a significant change.
- **The extent to which an employee is willing to co-operate**: If an employer offers a fair, reasonable adjustment to reduce any possible adverse effect, but the employee does not like the adjustment, the employer need do no more (if the adjustment is not fair, then this does not apply).

Key cases on adjustments

In *Environment Agency* v *Rowan*, the EAT stated that, before finding an employer in breach of its duty to make reasonable adjustments, a tribunal must identify:

(a) the PCP and/or physical features of premises that have placed the claimant at a substantial disadvantage;
(b) the identity of any non-disabled comparators (where appropriate); and
(c) the nature and extent of the substantial disadvantage suffered by the claimant.

The causal link triggering the duty

In *Tarling* v *Wisdom Toothbrushes*, the applicant (to the tribunal) had worked for the respondent for 18 years. She was in increasing pain from a club foot, and her productivity dropped. The employer sought advice about special chairs but did not install one. Instead, Mrs Tarling was dismissed. Her complaint to the tribunal was upheld, and her reinstatement was ordered. The employer subsequently bought a chair costing £1,000, of which £800 was paid for through the Access to Work scheme.

In *Morse* v *Wiltshire County Council*, the applicant was a road worker who could not drive. He had limited movement and grip in his right hand, stiffness in his right leg and a susceptibility to blackouts. These limitations led to his being selected for redundancy. The employing council preferred qualified drivers. The Industrial Tribunal dismissed his application.

On appeal, the EAT said that the provisions for making reasonable adjustments apply to arrangements for considering whether an employment continues or is terminated, and the tribunal had not considered this possibility properly. The EAT also set out a series of sequential steps for tribunals to follow in deciding adjustment cases:

1   Decide whether there is a duty on the employer in a particular case, that is, whether or not the employee is at a substantial disadvantage in comparison with able-bodied employees.
2   If so, whether the employer has taken such steps as it is reasonable in all the circumstances to prevent the substantial disadvantage occurring.
3   If not, enquire as to whether the employer could reasonably have taken any of the steps set out in the Act (as examples).

Lower level of productivity

An important decision came from *Mulligan* v *Inland Revenue*, when it was determined that the duty of reasonable adjustment does not require the employer to accept a lower level of productivity. Mr Mulligan, with the use of one arm, had contended that targets should not apply to him because these represented a detriment. The employer had made a number of adjustments but successfully maintained that these should not extend to lowering the minimum performance standards.

Significance of medical reports

In *Jones* v *The Post Office*, the Court of Appeal established that it is not for a tribunal to assess the '*correctness*' of medical evidence, only to assess its reasonableness, that is, even if disagreeing with it, it has to be respected, provided it is plausible. The implication appears to be that, if an employer refers an employee to a medical advisor, such as an OH physician, who provides inaccurate or unhelpful advice, such as stating no adjustments can be made, the employer is entitled to rely on this information, and a tribunal should not accept contradictory evidence provided at a later date. Medical assessments that are not accepted need to be challenged at the time with alternative evidence.

Retraining

Mrs Archibald was a road sweeper who could no longer sweep roads. She was retrained as a clerk. However, every time she applied for a post in the council, she was not selected as the most suitable applicant, and she was dismissed after unsuccessfully applying for 100 posts. The House of Lords, in *Archibald* v *Fife Council*, said that an example in the Act of reasonable adjustments is transfer to other work, but it does not say at what grade, and held that there was nothing to prevent the council from promoting Mrs A, and this would have occurred had it not been for the policy of competitive interviews. A disabled employee *can be treated more favourably*, for example, by exempting them from competition.

In allowing Mrs Archibald's appeal, the House of Lords stressed that the DDA may require a difference in treatment to attain equality of outcome. The reasonable-adjustments provisions are the mechanism for achieving this. The judgment made it clear that the reasonable-adjustments provisions are very broad in scope. They cover the situation where a person becomes incapable, through disability, of carrying out his or her job. Employers may have to make adjustments to their usual policies (such as a redeployment policy requiring competitive interviews).

Recruitment

The case of *Williams* v *Channel 5*, emphasises the need for the employer to act swiftly. Mr Williams did not complete the third day of a retuning training programme, because it involved a video without subtitles. He later completed the course with one-to-one training, but, by then, all the jobs had gone. The tribunal held that failure to make adjustment to the training course was an act of discrimination. The employer's argument that no duty arose until the training was completed was rejected. Employers should plan ahead. Likewise, a deaf applicant succeeded in *Murphy* v *Sheffield Hallam University* because no interpreter was available at the interview.

Dismissal

In *Smith* v *Carpets International UK plc*, the employee was a warehouse operator who developed epilepsy. The company doctor concluded that it was dangerous for him to work because of the amount of heavy machinery and forklift activity. A risk assessment concluded that no adjustments could be made to the work. The following year, his consultant reported he was fit to return, but the company doctor disagreed, arguing that the consultant did not know the specific dangers of the workplace. The employee was offered alternative work, but refused and was eventually dismissed. The employer accepted that this was less favourable treatment because of his disability but this was justified. The tribunal held that the reasons were material and substantial, and that reasonable investigations had been carried out regarding adjustment. It was not reasonable totally to adjust the way the work was carried out.

The carrying out of assessments and consultation

A key case is *Spence* v *Intype Ltd*, in which the EAT ruled that an employer's failure to obtain an up-to-date medical report before dismissing a disabled employee was not, in itself, capable of amounting to a breach of the duty to make a reasonable adjustment. The issue was whether or not the necessary adjustments had been made.

In *Mid Staffordshire General Hospitals NHS Trust* v *Cambridge*, the EAT held that a proper assessment of what is required to eliminate the disabled person's disadvantage is a necessary part of the duty to make reasonable adjustments. In a later case, *Tarbuck* v *Sainsbury's Supermarkets Ltd*, the EAT rejected this analysis, noting that, if there was separate stand-alone duty to make an assessment of a disabled person's situation, then one would have expected it to be expressly mentioned in the DDA list of various reasonable adjustments.

The EAT in *Tarbuck* also endorsed *British Gas Services Ltd* v *McCaull*, in which it was held that there is no automatic breach of the duty to make reasonable adjustments simply because the employer is unaware of the duty; the key question is what steps that employer did or did not take. In this case, the EAT held there was no basis for making a distinction between an employer's failure to consult a disabled person and its failure to obtain an up-to-date medical report. Both are part of the procedures that an employer will sensibly adopt when determining what adjustments are reasonable. However, if a failure to consult cannot, in itself, constitute a breach of the duty, then neither can a failure to obtain a medical report. The issue is whether reasonable adjustments have been made; whether by luck or judgement is immaterial.

The carrying out of an assessment itself does not comply with the duty to make reasonable adjustments. However, it will make an employer better informed of the steps to be taken. The DDA is not concerned with how these steps are determined. This means that an employer who has not carried out an assessment may nevertheless make all the necessary reasonable adjustments. However, the EAT in *Spence* went on to state that the carrying out of an assessment is always a good practice, and in many cases a failure to consult will result in a finding of unfair dismissal. Accordingly, employers are well advised to conduct an assessment, regardless of whether they are strictly required to do so under the DDA.

Following adverse OH assessment

In *Paul* v *National Probation Service*, the EAT established that the duty to make reasonable adjustments can extend to making adjustments to a job to overcome difficulties identified by an adverse OH assessment. In *Secretary of State for Works and Pensions* v *Wakefield*, the EAT stated that a finding of failure to make reasonable adjustments could not stand, because the Employment Tribunal, in concluding that the employer had delayed unreasonably in implementing the recommendations of two OH reports, had failed to properly identify how the proposed measures would have prevented the claimant from being placed at a substantial disadvantage. Tribunals should not uncritically accept health reports, nor find an unreasonable delay, without setting out what a reasonable time frame would have been (IDS, 2010b).

Sick pay

In *Nottinghamshire County Council* v *Meikle*, the Court of Appeal further developed the principles established in *Archibald*. On the facts of the case, Mrs Meikle would not have been off sick if reasonable adjustments had been made by her employer. The Court of Appeal held that her reduction in sick pay, in line with the employer's sick pay policy, was both a failure to make a reasonable adjustment and unjustifiable less-favourable treatment. Mrs Meikle received £196,000 compensation. The judgment makes clear the importance of reasonable adjustments in relation to the question of justifying less-favourable treatment. This case establishes that constructive dismissal is covered by the DDA's discrimination provisions, and that the payment of sick pay is subject to the reasonable adjustment provisions.

Time limit for a complaint

In *BUPA Care Homes (BNH) Ltd* v *Cann* and *Spillett* v *Tesco Stores Ltd*, the EAT established that section 32(4) Employment Act 2002 is no absolute bar to a tribunal considering a discrimination complaint where a grievance was submitted more than 4 months after the alleged act of discrimination. The tribunal is entitled to exercise its general discretion under the DDA to consider a discrimination complaint outside this time, where it is just and equitable to do so.

Lack of employer willingness to make adjustments

In *Fareham College Corporation* v *Walters*, the EAT held that a dismissal that occurs because the employer is unwilling to make reasonable adjustments is itself a failure to make the required adjustments. Accordingly, an employer who dismissed an employee rather than allow a phased return-to-work from sickness absence subjected her to disability discrimination.

The 'proper approach' to take to a DDA reasonable adjustments claim

In *Smith* v *Churchills Stairlifts Plc*, the Court of Appeal clarified the approach to take in a DDA reasonable adjustments claim and provided guidance concerning identifying the steps to consider when assessing whether the duty arises: (1) first, it is necessary to identify the arrangements (or, since October 2004, the PCP) that place the disabled person at substantial disadvantage, and this should be given a very wide meaning; (2) the next step is the identification of a comparator with reference to the disadvantage caused by the PCP. The DDA does not require comparison with the population generally; instead, there must be a focus on the disadvantage. This is followed by (3) a decision on whether or not it is reasonable for the employer to have to take any particular step by way of adjustment. Ultimately, it is the tribunal's view of what is reasonable that matters.

How far the employer has to go

It is apparent that the issue of how far they have to go troubles employers. In *Holmes* v *Whittingham and Porter*, the tribunal held that the employer failed to justify the dismissal of a disabled person because it relied on medical opinion from a GP who acted as the company doctor, rather than seeking specialist advice from an OH practitioner or specialist in epilepsy. The tribunal considered that advice on adjustments ought to have been sought, and the question rose as to whether the employee required more time to bring the epilepsy under control. However, the claim for unfair dismissal failed, on the basis that reliance on the GP's opinion was within the band of reasonable responses.

Handling dismissal

Illness is a potentially fair reason for terminating employment, as it relates to the employee's capability to do the job. The first step for the employer is to establish the true medical position. Second, case law has established that, before dismissing for long-term absence, an employer must consider whether or not an alternative position is available, or whether steps can be taken that would allow the employee to return to his/her existing job. An employer is under no obligation to 'create' a job for a disabled employee, and 'bumping' another employee (terminating someone else's employment) is expressly forbidden. However, in *Jelic* v *South Yorkshire Police*, the EAT supported a tribunal's decision that the employer should have transferred an able-bodied policeman from a sedentary position inputting crime data in order to accommodate a policeman retired on health grounds (IDS, 2010a). The EAT noted that the circumstance in which such a prospect occurs is likely to be exceptional. In this instance, the terms of employment required all uniformed officers to be transferable at the employer's discretion.

Employers are guilty of disability-related discrimination if they dismiss an employee for a reason related to their condition, when they would not have dismissed others to whom the reason does not apply, unless they can show the dismissal was justified. Factors that might be taken into account when considering if dismissal was justified include lengthy absences, health and safety risks, and whether all reasonable adjustments have been carried out.

Adjustments or employment termination on the grounds of capability?

An issue facing many employers when an employee develops a chronic condition is the extent to which they have a duty to make adjustments in order to continue the employment relationship, or, alternatively, to determine at what point dismissal or early retirement commences on the grounds of capability. Many employers will want to '*go the extra mile*' with a valued employee, but there are questions in respect of identifying and implementing adjustments in such circumstances and the potential consequences. Employees need to be aware that it cannot be assumed adjustments are automatically incorporated into a contract of employment. Indeed, if working a shorter week as part of a RTW plan, they may not want this to occur. An employer is entitled to take into account changing business circumstances. Claims for constructive dismissal, on the grounds that reasonable adjustments have not been made, may not succeed if the processes of assessing and addressing such needs have not been exhausted. (The prospect of an anticipatory breach of contract succeeding is likely to be remote without strong supportive evidence.) All parties are well advised to document all proceedings regarding the consideration and making of adjustments, including their contractual status, stating exactly why these proposals/adjustments are being made, for how long they are intended, and when they are to be reviewed.

Employment tribunals

Claims are made to regional Employment Tribunals (www.employmenttribunals.gov.uk). It must be remembered that taking a case to a tribunal represents a failure to resolve matters at a local level.

New procedures for dealing with grievance and discipline issues came into force from October 2004, and the majority of disability-discrimination cases are subject to these rules. It is important that the rules are followed, because there are penalties for failing to do so, and, in some cases, the tribunal complaint will be rejected, or compensatory awards can be reduced. Time limits can be extended by following the rules.

If an employee alleges disability discrimination has occurred, they must lodge a letter of grievance with their employer. This must be done within 3 months of the alleged act of discrimination. This has the effect of extending the time limit for lodging a complaint with a tribunal by a further 3 months (6 months from the date of the act being complained of). Any tribunal application cannot be submitted until at least 28 days after the letter of grievance has been lodged. If an employee fails to send the grievance letter and submits a tribunal complaint, the tribunal application will be automatically rejected. They must then submit the grievance letter within 1 month of the normal 3-month limit, and they have 3 months to resubmit a tribunal complaint (but not within 28 days of sending in the grievance).

Although there is no need for an applicant to an Employment Tribunal to instruct a solicitor or barrister, appropriate expertise helps parties to focus on the legal issues a tribunal must consider. However, legal aid is not available, and, even if successful, the remedy (compensation) in some cases may not meet the legal costs. If ESA or IB has been received, pending a hearing, these have to be repaid if the applicant is successful. Some solicitors will work on a 'no win, no fee' basis, and, unlike PI litigation, the law allows solicitors to work for a fixed percentage of any compensation.

Trade unions provide free expert support for their members. Others can consult the Citizens Advice Bureau, and expert support is often freely provided. ACAS provides impartial advice to applicants and employers. A number of human-resource companies and freelance HR consultants act for applicants and respondents. They have a range of fee-paying arrangements.

Tribunal membership consists of an Employment Judge, a solicitor or barrister employed by the Employment Tribunals Service, or a part-time chairperson drawn from private practice but with extensive experience of employment law. They are accompanied by two lay members selected from a competitive procedure run on behalf of the Department for Constitutional Affairs. Historically, the members have been nominated by the TUC and CBI, so that every tribunal has a 'trade union' and 'employer' member. These days, there is open competition, and applications are invited. The members do not 'take sides', but consider the merits of the arguments. Their role is to advise the chair on non-legal issues and contribute towards the judgment. Members receive specific training for hearing DDA cases.

Tribunals follow procedural guidelines in determining the validity of a claim. The arrangements prior to any hearing are subject to a case management discussion (CMD) and, sometimes, a pre-hearing chaired by the employment judge. Typically, such hearings occur when an employer denies a disability. This process requires the parties to make explicit their case and meet deadlines for providing information. Failure to comply may result in a case being struck out. Cases are run in the normal court procedure of evidence in chief and cross-examination.

Remedy

In claims that succeed, a tribunal will:

- make a declaration, that is, a statement of the decision;
- award compensation; some employers may need advising, that unlike unfair dismissal, compensation in discrimination cases is awarded on a tort principle (that is, not arising out of a contract), and there is no upper limit to the amount that may be awarded;
- consider an award for injury to feelings;
- consider aggravated damages when an employer has behaved in a particularly unseemly fashion; on the other hand, a tribunal will take into account prompt remedial measures, including an apology and steps to prevent a recurrence;
- make an award for losses, that is, to put the claimant in a position he or she would have been in but for the discriminatory act.

It should be noted that, under the DDA, employees of the discriminating company who have knowingly aided the employer, or carried out discriminatory acts, may be treated themselves as joint tortfeasors.

When considering remedy (compensation), the first question a tribunal must ask a successful claimant is if they wish to be reinstated. The employer is also given the option of taking back the person. It is rare for both sides to respond positively.

Summary

The main legislation covering the employment of disabled people and those with health conditions is the Health and Safety at Work Act 1974, Disability Discrimination Act 1995, Employment Rights Act 1996, Employment Act 2002 (Dispute Regulations) 2004, Disability Discrimination Act 2005 and the Equality Act 2010.

The requirement on employers to make reasonable adjustments to accommodate disabled employees frequently concerns VR practitioners. This aspect covers recruitment and job termination, as well as everyday employment practices. There are potentially unlimited penalties for employers who fail to get this right. Although case law provides guidance, every case turns on its own characteristics. Evidence suggests that employers have some difficulty in determining what they should do, and how far they should go, in accommodating employees. In this respect, employers are likely to benefit from expert guidance. Particularly troubling matters are the relationship of adjustments to health and safety requirements, the level of acceptable productivity and dealing with sickness absence.

Student exercises

5.1 Productivity
What is the case for and against arguments that providing reasonable adjustments is unfair on other staff, because provision shows favouritism and lets an employee 'get away' with a lower level of productivity?

5.2 Case study: IW
IW had worked in a staff restaurant for a contract catering company for a period of 15 years as a cook, when she injured her back after being asked by an employee of the host company to move a sack of potatoes left by a fire exit. Following 3 months' continuous absence from work, a medical report indicated that, although the damage arising from the incident itself was unlikely to be more than muscular, there had been (more difficult to determine) exacerbation of a pre-existing back condition (of which the contractual employer was unaware). The OH advisor, to whom IW was referred by her employer, considered that she would have difficulty in undertaking the bending and lifting required in a commercial kitchen and recommended '*lighter work*'. In such a circumstance, her condition might be expected to '*settle*' within a '*reasonable period of time*'. When IW returned to work after a total of 4 months' absence, she was given lighter duties. For a period of 2 months, she put food out at the counter and undertook some work on the till as a cashier, alternating between standing and sitting. However, this caused some problems, with other food-preparation staff complaining that IW was not '*pulling her weight*', and a cashier complaining that she was being asked to prepare/serve food. IW returned to her former cooking activities. She was then 'on and off work' for 6 months. The regional manager took the view that the company could not afford to 'carry' IW, and there was no suitable post for her. The company employed seven staff on this site: four cooks, including the supervisor (one cook doubled as a counter assistant at lunchtime), another counter assistant, one cashier and a washer-upper. IW was dismissed while off sick on the grounds of capability and without consultation. She was very upset by this. She liked her job, it was 5 minutes' walk from home, and the hours suited her. IW brought a claim for disability discrimination on the grounds of a failure to make a reasonable adjustment and direct discrimination, citing the counter assistant and cashier as comparators.

(a) Does IW have a disability as defined by the DDA and Equality Act?
(b) The employer was unaware of IW's condition at the time of the accident. In this case, does it still have a responsibility under the DDA?
(c) Given the medical prognosis that IW's condition would 'settle', was it reasonable to expect her to return to her usual work after a period of 2 months?
(d) If you had been consulted by the company while IW was 'on and off work', what advice would you have offered on 'reasonable adjustments'?
(e) Did the employer have a responsibility to consult IW and/or obtain a further medical report before dismissing her?

Part 2

Employment and disability services in the United Kingdom

Models of vocational rehabilitation practice

6 The vocational rehabilitation service user

Key issues

- Factors influencing choices and outcomes.
- Characteristics of IB/ESA claimants.
- Identification and management of barriers to employment.
- The difficult client.
- The role of family and culture in the VR process.
- Personal injury litigation and benefits.

Learning objectives

- Knowledge of research relating to predicting VR outcomes.
- Understanding issues influencing VR service user participation.
- Identification of common barriers to resettlement.
- Understanding the role of families and culture in the rehabilitation process.
- Knowledge of compensation and benefits influencing client choices.

Introduction

Little is known about the characteristics of VR service users in the United Kingdom. There are no published data from the private sector on the health condition, demographic or occupational status of service users. Some public sector programmes have occasionally collected data, but, by and large, information on service users has to be extrapolated from the characteristics of IB claimants. There is a serious research omission. Anyone out of work and experiencing health and employment problems is likely to fall within one of three groups:

1 likely to spontaneously return-to-work, that is, without any assistance;
2 unlikely to return-to-work in any circumstance; and
3 only likely to return work if given VR support.

VR service providers need to have some understanding of the main factors influencing outcomes for their clients: whereas some factors may be positively influenced by intervention, others may not. At the very least, an understanding of such factors contributes to an understanding of the barriers to resettlement. This chapter explores various factors known to influence service user participation and outcomes in VR programmes, as well as considering how barriers and difficult clients can be addressed.

Predicting VR outcomes

For decades, researchers have sought to identify group 3 above and deploy the most efficient use of VR resources. When identifying predictor variables, researchers have tended to adopt one of two strategies for synthesising the results of a large number of independent investigations, meta-analysis and judgemental procedure. Meta-analysis requires the statistical results of all investigations on a particular topic to be converted to a common denominator known as the effect size, ultimately giving an overall picture of the effectiveness of a particular intervention strategy or procedure (Parker and Bolton, 2005). An early example of the use of meta-analysis from the brain injury field is Crepeau and Scherzer (1993). The second strategy, judgemental procedure, relies heavily on the ability to appraise the relative merits of a set of studies and judgementally integrate and synthesise into a series of conclusions or observations.

Given the number of variables influencing outcomes, and the fact that many correlate with each other, even multifactorial analyses cannot provide definitive guidance in individual cases. The work of Saunders *et al.* (2006) illustrates the complexity of the problem. From hundreds of studies, Saunders *et al.* identified 118 studies conforming to the research criteria. These studies investigated nearly 200 independent variables in relation to employment outcomes for disabled people. Studies were classified into eight non-exclusive categories of: (1) client/consumer; (2) counsellor; (3) medical/functional; (4) work environment; (5) measures; (6) programme interventions; (7) services; and (8) financial. Some notable client variables included age, education, gender, marital status, race, education history, employment history, number of months in longest job, technical knowledge, motivation to work, employment expectancy, family support, perception of severity of disability, perception of occupational health services, personality and interpersonal skills, litigation, transportation and wage expectancy.

Given the multiplicity of interacting variables potentially influencing outcomes, it is not surprising to find that much research has moved on from identifying predictive models towards establishing what works with whom.

The VR service user and factors contributing to work problems and influencing the RTW process

There are many common factors contributing to the work problems of disabled people, and they can be analysed with reference to Figure 6.1.

With most conditions, there is a relationship between the severity of impairment and related barriers to employment. For example, the nature and frequency of epileptic seizures will have a bearing on employment prospects. However, it is wrong to consider any condition in isolation from associated impairments; in the example, medication can influence intellectual and neuropsychological functioning. Another example is SCI, when (potential) VR service users experience secondary medical problems, such as urinary-tract infections and pressure sores.

In addition to utilising clinical services to address medical issues, activity limitations need to be analysed with regard to personal, environmental and social factors. A positive

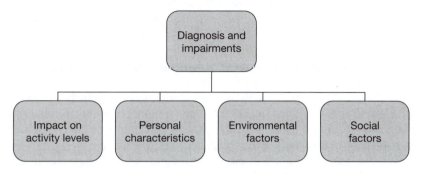

Figure 6.1 Common factors contributing to the work problems of disabled people

work attitude, optimism and sense of personal achievement are all associated with improved RTW rates. For people with physical disabilities, environmental barriers to employment can be found, such as access to public transport and buildings. People with progressive conditions may face increasing problems in undertaking the physical aspects of their work. Social factors do not only affect people with MH problems. Although legislation exists to protect the rights of those falling within the ambit of the DDA, discrimination can still result in disabled people choosing not to reveal their condition.

Whatever the circumstances of the individual, one factor is clear: taking sick leave for problems originating at work is rarely the solution. Indeed, the problems associated with work re-entry may only exacerbate the situation.

For those without a job, analysing the issues affecting their prospects produces different issues. Instead of an examination of a specific work location, there is a need to take a broader view of the capability of the person concerned with regards to knowledge of the local labour market and the identification of suitable employment. Only then can environmental and social factors be taken into consideration. In particular, there is a need to understand the service user's perspective on returning to work (column 2 in Table 6.1).

The literature on factors influencing the RTW rates of disabled people in general highlights the variables identified in Table 6.1 (Frank and Sawney, 2003).

Table 6.1 Factors influencing the RTW decisions of people with a disability/health condition

1 Factors outside individual	2 Individual factors	3 Employer-related factors
Societal beliefs and attitudes	Self-confidence	Sector
Labour market	Self-esteem	Size
Housing	Motivation	Absence-management policies
Transport	Illness beliefs and attitudes	Culture
Family and level of support	Education	Physical environment
Legal processes	Literacy	
Government policies	Social skills	
Benefits	Gender	
	Comorbidity	

A common response to the question of 'who uses VR services?' is an answer that describes clients in terms of commonly found disabilities. When considering the nature of services, there is a need to consider who is paying for the service and the extent to which this influences the characteristics of the clients with regard to the nature of the disability, the period of unemployment or incapacity and whether or not the client has a job or employer to return to (a retention case).

There are two distinct strands of VR clients: the employed (whether in employment or 'off sick') and those without work. This distinction invariably reflects the major difference between service users from the private and public sectors, although this is not always the case, particularly with regard to NHS VR clients.

This situation affects the nature of employment and disability services in the United Kingdom and the question of who takes responsibility for any VR intervention. In theory, the NHS is there to support everyone whose VR needs start with clinical diagnosis and treatment, and Jobcentre Plus and its contracted agencies take responsibility for jobseekers with a work-related health condition (although it also supports some employees in 'retention cases' through Access to Work). In practice, employers operating GIP schemes and sickness and absence policies incorporating VR will invariably turn towards private sector service providers operating a case-managed service, as will lawyers and insurers in PI litigation cases.

The lack of a statutory basis for ensuring the delivery of VR services in the United Kingdom has contributed to a situation in which service provision is not necessarily based on the needs of the individual but on such random matters as the employment status of the person; type of benefit received; the priorities and resources of NHS trusts; circumstances of an injury; employer insurance cover; employer resources; and the position of the insurer towards funding VR. Other factors also intervene, such as geographical location and the expertise of a solicitor. For example, the Scottish government has recognised that many SMEs have limited resources, and the pilot Scottish NHS VR service has been designed for the employees of such companies. Although members of the APIL should be aware of VR protocols, it remains the case that many non-PI specialists continue to run claims. Even if a person with a health condition is within a system that can establish their need for support, such as receiving benefits, the nature of contracted-out services and the lack of any national accreditation mean that there are no means of ensuring that an appropriate, recognised quality service is available or received. Although Jobcentre Plus sets standards for contractors, historically the priority has been one of financial probity.

Characteristics of IB/ESA claimants

Because of the length of time it takes for many VR referrals to be made, both in the public and private sectors, VR service users are invariably in receipt of IB/ESA. The DWP has published two reports (Sainsbury and Davidson, 2006; Kemp and Davidson, 2008) examining how people make the journey into incapacity benefits and their characteristics. Some key findings are indicated in Boxes 6.1 and 6.2.

Health conditions

In respect of benefit claimants, it is known that 35 per cent on the IB (now ESA) registers are said to have depression, anxiety or other neuroses, with only a small number having severe MH conditions such as schizophrenia or severe learning difficulties. A further

---

Box 6.1 Personal characteristics of new IB (now ESA) claimants

- Ethnicity of recent claimants in line with the UK population.
- Claimants disproportionately male and single. Lone parents also over-represented.
- Recent claimants poorly qualified academically and vocationally.
- Those renting from social landlords more than double the proportion usually found in the UK population.
- 37 per cent of recent claimants with children under the age of 19.
- 37 per cent of those usually living with a partner reported partner also not working, with a further 6 per cent reporting that partner off work sick.

Box 6.2 Employment situation of new IB (now ESA) claimants

- 70 per cent of recent claimants had spent most of their working lives in steady employment.
- 56 per cent had been either in work or off sick from their job immediately before claiming IB.
- There was a high level (about 14 per cent) of self-employment among recent claimants.
- 63 per cent of recent claimants who were not in work or off sick from work, had actually worked at some point in the last 2 years, and only 7 per cent had never worked.
- 40 per cent of claimants had been working in firms with less than 50 employees (this contrasts to a figure of 26 per cent of all employees working in firms of this size in the United Kingdom).
- The job tenure of claimants tends to be much shorter than in the general population, with 26 per cent reporting they were in their last job for less than 6 months.
- 59 per cent of claimants worked in an SME (fewer than 250 employees), compared with 38 per cent of the UK population; 73 per cent of recent claimants worked in the private sector, with 23 per cent in the public sector.
- Recent claimants to IB were generally low paid.

---

22 per cent are affected by MSDs, with the large majority having back/neck pain, rather than conditions such as severe arthritis; and 11 per cent have a disorder of the heart or a circulatory or respiratory disorder, such as high blood pressure, angina or chronic bronchitis, with only a small number having severe conditions. Among the most severe conditions, 0.7 per cent of recipients have had a stroke, 0.2 per cent have tetraplegia, and 0.9 per cent have MS (DWP, 2002). Langman (2007) considers that DWP data do

not reflect the incidence of brain injury when contrasted to other statistics, particularly from the Department of Health, noting that symptoms and not the causation can be recorded.

Barriers to employment

An issue regularly occurring in policy approaches to RTW is an emphasis on the medical condition of claimants. Evidence invariably points to other factors acting as barriers to work, particularly after a lengthy period out of the labour market (DWP, 2002). For VR service users with an employer, typical barriers to RTW include the:

- nature of injury or health condition and its impact on (usual) work;
- lack of support from managers and colleagues;
- psychological obstacles, e.g. fear of re-injury through work activities, loss of confidence, lack of motivation;
- work pressures (for example, arising from fear of not being able to undertake 'light duties');
- lack of suitable adjustments (both physical and to hours/duties);
- lack of appropriate advice/treatment/rehabilitation programme;
- management belief that worker should be 100 per cent fit before RTW;
- financial and legal concerns;
- fear of returning to the place where an accident occurred; and
- fear of an inability to cope with the pre-injury/accident/illness job.

VR service users without a job may face additional issues such as restricted labour market opportunities, redundant skills, lack of a financial incentive, age and disability discrimination, lack of references/indifferent CVs, domestic responsibilities and a lack of transport.

VR counsellors need to understand the factors motivating a client, while maintaining their responsibilities to their client, employer, the employer's customers and their own professional standards. For example, if the counsellor is working directly or contractually for an insurance company, there is a need to ensure that the relationship between all the parties remains one that reflects the best interest of the client, while meeting the expectations of all concerned. The case study provided by the independent VR practitioner (Chapter 7) illustrates the need for regular consultation and liaison. There is a need ethically to manage what may at first appear to be conflicting aims: for example, when a client gives the impression of seeking to maximise a future loss of earnings, rather than make a genuine attempt to return-to-work, or when he/she appears unable to take any resettlement steps, despite expert medical evidence indicating there are no physical reasons for this.

The skilled counsellor needs to recognise the client's perspective. Fears over their future financial security may be justified, or a fear of failure may be subconsciously influencing their judgement. The counsellor who can reflect the client's perspective, while helping them address such issues and, at the same time, maintaining a professional independence, is the one most likely to be able to identify and implement an agreed RTW strategy. Potential conflicts of interests should not occur, or, if they do, should be subject to measures to produce some mutual understanding. In order to be able to address barriers, in the first instance, it is necessary to be able to identify them and

Table 6.2 Barriers to employment checklist

Clinical	Yes/no	Comments	Response
Still receiving treatment/therapy Operation pending Negative impact of medication Functional capability not defined Possible behavioural/interpersonal issues Does not accept limitations/poor insight Fatigue Pain issues not resolved			
Demographic/social	*Yes/no*	*Comments*	*Response*
Age Lack of family support Marital issues Lack of incentive to work Lack of confidence Lack of child-care arrangements Presentation Transport Court convictions			
Financial	*Yes/no*	*Comments*	*Response*
PI litigation Level of benefits income Wages being offered Risk of returning to work upsetting steady income Potential retirement with financial gain Cost of looking for work			
Skill related	*Yes/no*	*Comments*	*Response*
Over-qualified Under-qualified Lack of IT skills Language barrier Lack of other skills Lack of experience Lack of specific training Limited organisational skills Limited communication skills Patchy work history Capacity to learn and retain new skills			
Job search related	*Yes/no*	*Comments*	*Response*
Limited job search experience Lack of CV Interview skills Lack of references Lack of jobs in the field No/not sure of job goal			
Other	*Yes/no*	*Comments*	*Response*
Does not function well independently Requires aids/adaptations Believes he/she is unemployable Does not wish to retrain Transport problems Possible alcohol/drug dependency Cultural issues			

help the client work through them. It is always good practice to keep a record of intervention, and a barriers checklist is one way of identifying problems and measures taken to resolve them.

The 'difficult client'

As a VR counsellor, it is easy to get into a way of thinking that perceives the health condition as the one requiring a 'solution'. (This does not necessarily mean adopting a medical model of disability, because the 'solution' may be the identification of an adaptive mechanism.) It is easy to forget that the nature and meaning of work and unemployment are different for different people. The experience of work and unemployment, coupled with cultural values, support systems and the role of work in a person's life, shapes how they perceive and respond to work and unemployment. The United Kingdom has experienced substantial immigration in recent years. Little is known about minority perceptions and responses to disability, unemployment and work.

There are also some conflicting messages. On one hand, UK workers are told that, because of a pensions crisis, they are going to have to work until they are approaching 70 years of age; on the other hand, age-discrimination legislation has been introduced not least because many employers associate rapid changes in the labour market, particularly technological ones, with a younger, flexible workforce.

The whole situation triggers a number of difficult questions, realities and dilemmas that can confront counsellors working in this field. Some of the more frequent issues heard from VR service users are:

1   Why should I work at all?
    * If I return-to-work, my compensation will be reduced.
    * I'm getting my money 'made up'. It doesn't make sense to go back when I'm going to struggle.
    * 'They' are not interested in me. All they are interested in is saving money.
    * 'They' are responsible for my injury. Why should I do them any favours?
2   Why should I have to take a low-paid, rubbish job when I have been on 'good money'?
3   Why should I work in a job that is going nowhere and doing nothing except frustrate me and cause stress?
4   Why should I have to take a low-paid job when I can get as much money in benefits?
5   What's the point in retraining, when younger and fitter workers can't get jobs?
6   There are no jobs for which I'm trained.
7   It's your responsibility (counsellor/agency) to get me a job.
8   I can't get a job without experience. I can't get experience without a job.

This list is not exhaustive, and neither are a number of questions or issues readily answered. A primary concern in addressing such questions lies in assessing the precise nature of the client's reality regarding work and unemployment, and then assisting the client in seeking employment. A frustrating reality may well be the job market and job availability, but only by exploring issues can the VR counsellor differentiate between fact and rhetoric and develop an intervention strategy aimed at facilitating job-seeking behaviour. A simple matrix can assist this process, by being shown to the client, with the directional arrows being 'filled in' to represent progress – see Figure 6.2.

	Job searching behaviour	
Factors related to the nature of work	**Not looking for work**	**Looking for work**
1. Doesn't want to work		
2. Can't find work		
3. Needs retraining		
4. Income/benefits issues		
5. Litigation issues		
6. Domestic issues		
7. etc.		

Figure 6.2 Assessing the nature of work/unemployment and job searching behaviour (after Holesko, 1987)

The list on the left of the figure can be changed as appropriate. The inherent bias in this approach is that it implies that all clients, regardless of their situation, should be able to progress to the looking-for-work category. It also implies that, if the client is looking for work, the activity should be meaningful and not one of going through the motions to satisfy an insurer, the counsellor, family or some other body. It also helps to establish concrete goals to facilitate appropriate job-seeking behaviour.

The role of the family and culture in the VR process

Families can aid or hinder the resettlement progress in a number of important ways. Every family is a system of relationships, and anything that upsets the balance, whether internal (for example, a divorce or death) or external (for example, the loss of a job or a move to a new area), throws the family out of balance. There is then an instinctive response to right the balance, often by establishing new roles.

An injury, particularly a serious one, to a family member can dramatically alter the balance within the family, with time, money and energy being spent on the injured person. Relationships are altered, not just with the injured person, but between family members. As time goes on, the family faces the task of reallocating roles to acknowledge the changed capacity of the injured person.

Some families are successful at this; others continue to struggle with changed circumstances. This is understandable when, for example, a married sister takes responsibility for her injured brother, because her parents are too old for this, but, in the meantime, the needs of her own family come second; or the prime wage-earner can no longer keep his/her family in an accustomed fashion; or parental expectations and ambitions in respect of their son/daughter are dashed overnight.

Two common responses from families

1   **A lack of realism**: Some families are so unrealistic that they attempt to push their injured relative into programmes and situations that are simply beyond their capability.

2   **Overprotection**: Conversely, some families become so protective that they foster dependence. In turn, this works against rehabilitation efforts to promote independence.

How such responses develop is understandable, and there are often predictable stages in responding to the injury. In the case of a serious one, such as brain injury, initially all resources are focused on survival and medical recovery; this is followed by worrying over the extent of 'recovery' but being encouraged by observable gains; there is generally relief once the injured person is able to return home, and expectations of extensive 'recovery' tend to be heightened at this time; as the months go on, however, and the joy from having the injured person back home begins to subside, the irritating and difficult changes in the person become more noticeable; and, subsequently, both frustration and anger can begin to set in when there is a realisation of living with a very different person. This period can be trying for both the injured person and the family. It is often marked by trying to find 'the right solution' within the system.

At this stage, three things can happen:

1   Getting 'stuck'.
2   Forgetting the 'old person' and accepting the new one (hence, anger and frustration can subside).
3   Reorganisation, in which the family, having accepted the 'new' person, rearranges its life in the most adaptive way, albeit such adaptation is often painful and difficult.

Cultural issues affecting VR

Given the wide range of ethnic groups and nationalities now found in the United Kingdom, it would take a considerable amount of study to familiarise oneself with all the various cultural aspects affecting work integration. However, there are a large number of common factors to consider, and, if uncertain as to their implications, there is a sensible course of action:

•   ask the client and/or his/her family;
•   seek expert advice, for example from a community relations office.

Above all, there is a need to find out specific factors influencing individuals and not to make assumptions.

Personal injury (PI) litigation

Many clients of private sector VR services are likely to have PI claims with a future loss of earnings large enough to trigger intervention. For some people, pursuing a claim, which involves attending medical examinations, meetings with advisors, putting aside time for court dates and so on, while simultaneously looking for work, is too demanding for them. Many High Court judges recognise this, and they may give a full loss of earnings up to the date of a hearing and for some months afterwards, allowing for a job search period. However, there are problems with this approach. Not only does the claimant leave themselves vulnerable to accusations of failing to mitigate loss (in other words, a judge may take the view that they could have got a job had they tried and deduct from

---

Box 6.3 Aspects of daily life and VR that may be influenced by culture

Daily life	*VR*
Personal history/heritage	Education history and qualifications
Communication/language	Employment history
Investigations	Understanding of disability/condition
Family relationships	Consent and confidentiality
Gender roles	Assessments
Child-care issues	Role of family in support
Naming systems/forms of address	Placement considerations
Religious beliefs and practices	Attitude to Western medicine
Food	
Fasting	
Clothing	
Modesty and privacy	
Body space, politeness	
Jewellery/make-up	
Washing	
Concepts of cleanliness	
Importance to family/individual of education, religion, cultural activities, work role for male/female	

---

damages what he/she considers the claimant could have been earning), but, once a person has been out of the labour market and 'on the sick' for a prolonged period, it can become very difficult to acquire another job (DWP, 2002).

By its nature litigation is adversarial. In the United Kingdom, parties have moved on from a position caricatured by claimant advisors telling their client that a return-to-work will reduce their damages and defendants taking the view that every claimant is contriving to maximise their loss. There is now a rehabilitation protocol (Chapter 5) and good reason for claimants to participate in VR programmes. Many solicitors, acting for both claimants and defendants, now recognise that the quality of an injured person's life includes resuming some form of employment and make recommendations to insurers to instruct a VR service. In turn, claims assessors are likely to be more sympathetic to such requests, although there remain occasions when solicitors acting for claimants have to make a request for VR funding to the courts.

In addition to being seen to mitigate loss, there are other good reasons for PI claimants participating in VR programmes. Future loss is assessed on a multiplier/multiplicand basis. The multiplicand is the net annual earnings a successful claimant is likely to lose, based on their pre-injury earnings or assessed earning potential (an allowance for future inflation is not built into this). The multiplier is the number of years this sum is multiplied by to produce the total sum for the future loss of earnings. Even for a claimant unlikely to work again, the compensation is not calculated on the annual loss times every remaining year of working life. This is because the money is received in advance of when it would have been earned, and it is maintained that the lump sum can be invested to produce an annual income equivalent to what could have been earned. The applied multiplier is gradually reduced, as the person gets older. In addition, there are sound social arguments for returning to work, such as the resumption of 'normality', a productive use of time, perceiving work as rehabilitation and social stimulus.

Expert VR reports

Although the evidence of VR counsellors on the employment prospects of claimants is accepted in most Western countries, in the United Kingdom, judges will almost always prefer the evidence of medical experts. In any event, legal changes have substantially reduced the reliance of the courts on experts (Woolf, 1996). The reforms established single joint experts, appointed by the courts to provide expert impartial advice. In the VR sector, the Law Society maintains a list of companies and individuals specialising in providing employment reports, including detailed earnings assessments. In general, even if VR practitioners are asked to prepare a report, there is only a small likelihood of being called to give evidence.

The outcome of most PI cases is negotiated between the claimant and defendant's legal representatives. When there is a dispute over the future employment and earnings prospects of a claimant, parties can be well served with an objective report. However, VR practitioners should not consider PI work without additional training on the role of the single joint expert. They should also note that evidence addressing earnings and career prospects can be given a higher priority than employment capability.

Referring clients to solicitors

It is impossible these days to attend any VR conference without passing a solicitor's exhibition table. The legitimate business objectives are to make contacts and foster referrals. Referring clients to solicitors requires careful consideration. Should service providers, including voluntary organisations, accept a fee for this (£500 for every referral, to use a figure offered to one voluntary VR service provider)? Making a referral can comply with the VRA's Standards of Practice, providing it is one that is done in the service user's best interest. This includes full consultation with the client and their family. Anyone making a referral to a solicitor needs to ensure that the firm specialises in PI litigation and that it has the requisite expertise with regard to the client's circumstances. Many voluntary organisations maintain lists of 'recommended solicitors'. For instance, Headways (the National Society for Brain Injured People) keeps a list of solicitors known to have developed an expertise in handling brain injury cases. Such firms will make arrangements to provide the kind of case management services their clients require, although liability for the injury will need to be established.

Benefits

Although VR counsellors may not wish to be involved in their client's financial affairs, income is invariably of paramount importance to them (Grewal *et al.*, 2004). While being able to point the client 'in the right direction' to get expert advice is one way of dealing with such matters, the counsellor who does not understand the financial implications of changing activity, and/or sends their client chasing an answer they could have addressed themselves, is unlikely to retain the confidence of their client.

At the present time, the nature of benefits is 'in the air', the Prime Minister having announced at the October 2010 Conservative Party Conference that the government plans to introduce a single benefit payable by one agency, to replace existing unemployment/sickness-related benefits. The ultimate aim, of course, is to reduce benefits payments. The coalition's strategy appears to be based on the questionable assumption that there are plenty of jobs in the labour market that the unemployed can fill, if only they are willing or compelled to do so. This position appears to involve a disconnection between the realities of a depressed labour market, reflected in the nature of many vacancies, and an ideological belief that those without work have chosen this situation. The government's strategy is causing some concern, even among the architects of the bipartisan Welfare to Work strategy. Professor Paul Gregg has voiced his anxiety at the way in which thousands of disabled jobless are being put on the lower rate of ESA (*The Guardian*, 6 July 2010). VR agencies will be put under pressure, as thousands of people with health problems are forced to enter the labour market.

For the time being, the major benefits with which VR counsellors and their clients are likely to be concerned are as follows:

Incapacity benefit (IB)

The payment of IB follows on from SSP and depends on NI contributions (the number of years is complex but explained in the handbook recommended in the section on 'Additonal reading and sources of information' at the end of the book).

The process of phasing out IB in favour of the ESA began in October 2008. However, those receiving IB prior to this date will continue to receive it.

What work can a person do while on IB?

1 **Work trial**: a client receiving IB can:
    - try out a job for up to 15 working days;
    - continue to receive any benefits to which they are entitled (e.g. Jobseeker's Allowance, IB, Income Support);
    - be paid travel expenses and meal expenses, subject to a limit.

    It is advisable first to consult Jobcentre Plus before a work trial. If anyone is made a job offer at the end of the work trial, the decision to accept does not automatically mean an end to all financial assistance. Jobcentre Plus can advise about possible 'in work' benefits.

    Eligibility: Normally, to be eligible for a work trial, the client would need to be aged 25 years or over and have been out of work for 6 months or more (although there are some exceptions to this).

2 **Permitted work**: the rules for IB and ESA are the same. There is no need to obtain permission to do permitted work that meets the requisite earnings ceiling for the permitted work lower limit (although it is best to inform Jobcentre Plus of any changes that might affect benefits). As the potential earnings figures periodically change, readers are advised to consult Jobcentre Plus or see the recommended reading for this chapter at the end of the book for up-to-date figures. The permitted work higher limit has a much higher earnings ceiling, as the name implies, although

the work must be undertaken for less than 16 hours a week. If in the work-related activity group (see below), this work can only be done for a maximum of 52 weeks, as it is designed to test the ability for work before moving into regular employment. If there is a break of more than 12 weeks, the 52-week period can begin again.

Supported permitted work (work that can be carried out as part of a treatment programme, under medical supervision, while an in-patient or regular out-patient, or work done under the supervision of a person employed by a public or local authority or voluntary organisation engaged in the provision of work for disabled people) also has hours and earnings limitations.

Linking provisions

Rules have been designed to encourage people with health conditions to try work or undertake training, without the fear of losing benefits if their efforts fail. Hence, 104 weeks of linking protection apply where:

- the person has been continuously sick for 28 weeks;
- the person has taken up work or training within a month of leaving benefit; and
- the benefit did not end as a result of an assessment.

Employment and Support Allowance (ESA)

Since October 2008, ESA has gradually been replacing IB. Currently, the aim is to transfer all existing IB customers to ESA by 2013. The government considers that the previous assessment system, based on dividing people into those capable and incapable of work, could act as a disincentive to return-to-work. ESA is paid when a claimant is found to have a 'limited capability for work'. Claimants are then divided into two groups: the 'support group' and the 'work related activity group'. ESA has two components:

- a contributory allowance;
- an income-related allowance.

At the outset, there is a detailed questionnaire to complete. During the first 13 weeks of a claim, the 'assessment phase', ESA is paid at a basic rate and at a reduced rate for those under 25 (equivalent to the age-related rates of the Jobseekers Allowance). After this period, and a WCA, there are additional payments for those placed in the work-related activity group and those in the support group. The WCA is more complex than the Personal Capability Assessment (for IB) that it replaces.

Work-focused interviews (WFI)

Most new ESA claimants are expected to attend an initial 'work-focused interview', which usually takes place during the eighth week of a claim. At this interview, a PA talks about work prospects, the steps a claimant is willing to take to find a job and the available support. The interview can be waived if the PA considers that it is inappropriate because of the condition. If in the work-related group of claimants, a further five interviews will follow, the second one usually at 14 weeks and then, usually, one a month.

These interviews are mandatory. It is possible that, after the first interview, the advisor will be from a private or voluntary sector organisation contracted to do this work. The WFI has a number of purposes, including assessing and encouraging with regard to job prospects, identifying activities such as education, training or rehabilitation to improve job prospects, and identifying current or future opportunities.

Work Capability Assessment

There are three elements:

1   **The limited-capability-for-work assessment**: This part of the WCA is a points-related assessment awarded on the basis of any physical, cognitive or MH limitations. If the points total reaches 15 points or more, then the claimant is placed within the limited-capability-for-work support group, receives a higher rate of payment and does not have to undertake work-related activity unless they choose to do so. Within each physical, cognitive and MH category, there is a list of descriptors, with scores ranging from 0 to 15 points. Points are awarded when a claimant is not able to perform a described activity. If a claimant is unable to perform a number of descriptors within an activity, then only the highest-scoring one is recorded. The physical and mental descriptors in the limited-capability-for-work assessment are grouped into the activities shown in Table 6.2. Although there are a number of circumstances in which claimants are treated as automatically having limited capability for work, for example having a terminal illness or carrying a notified infectious disease, the assessment process has left critics questioning where the process leaves people with fluctuating conditions, such as MS or cystic fibrosis.

2   **The limited-capability-for-work-related-activity assessment**: The second part of the WCA determines whether or not a claimant is placed in the *support group* (not requiring any work-related activities) or the *work-related-activity group*. It also determines the level of benefit received. If placed in work-related-activity group, the claimant must meet certain conditions, including attending six WFIs. The assessment has a similar list of descriptors to the limited-capability-for-work assessment.

Table 6.3 Physical and mental descriptors in the limited capability for work assessment

Physical descriptors	Mental, cognitive and intellectual function descriptors
Walking	Learning or comprehension in the completion of tasks
Remaining conscious	Awareness of hazard
Bending and kneeling	Memory and concentration
Reaching	Execution of tasks
Picking up and moving things	Initiating and sustaining personal action
Standing and sitting	Coping with change
Manual dexterity	Getting about
Speech	Coping with social situations
Hearing	Propriety of behaviour with other people
Seeing	Dealing with other people
Controlling bladder and bowels	

3   **Work-focused health-related assessment (WFHRA)**: This applies only if placed in the *work-related-activity group* (although claimants in the support group can volunteer to participate). Failure to participate can result in the ESA being sanctioned. The assessment looks at barriers to work and available support. It also collects information about any health-related or other interventions that could improve functional capacity and support a move back into work. This includes the use of aids and adaptations. The information required for the WFHRA is collected in a separate interview, following the medical assessment for the first two elements of the WCA, with a report subsequently being made available to the claimant.

It is possible to do voluntary work and claim ESA as long as no payment is received.

In an independent review of the WCA for the government, Harrington (2010) concluded that, 'the WCA is not working as well as it should'. In particular, he considered that,

> the pathway for the claimant through Jobcentre Plus is impersonal, mechanistic and lacking in clarity. The assessment of work capability undertaken for the DWP by ATOS Healthcare suffers from similar procedural problems. In addition some conditions are more subjective and evidently more difficult to assess. As a result some of the descriptors may not adequately reflect the full impact of such conditions on the individual's capability for work.

Harrington made a number of recommendations, including correcting what he perceived to be an imbalance between the authority given to the ATOS report when allocating claimants to the respective groups and the opinion of Jobcentre Plus staff.

Summary

Little is known about the characteristics of VR service users in the United Kingdom, other than from occasional data collected from some public sector programmes. This is in contrast to a wealth of information on disabled people in general and IB (now ESA) claimants. However, it is well established that health conditions on their own rarely present barriers to employment, even for the long-term sick/unemployed. Other factors, such as environmental and personal issues, come into play. Such matters as the level of support, position taken by the employer, motivation of the service user, the identification and the availability of adjustments all have a part to play in the RTW process. If more was known about the characteristics of VR service users, then training of VR service providers could be organised to address the needs more commonly found among service users, and databases could be established identifying 'the best' RTW strategies.

As it is, service providers respond to the individual circumstances of service users and their barriers to work in a variety of ways, reflecting the source of referral, client circumstances and their own organisational or practitioner expertise. The position regarding the payments of benefits and financial incentives to VR service users is complex. Although current announcements to simplify the benefits system will be welcomed by many, a large influx of people with health conditions into the labour market in coming years is likely to produce considerable challenges, while resources for service providers are restricted, particularly in the public sector.

Student exercises

6.1 Involvement in domestic circumstances
Staff at a VR agency have a brain-injured client residing with an older sister. The amount of time the sister spends getting her brother organised, ensuring he attends the agency etc. is resulting in domestic problems. Her husband has approached the agency for assistance. What strategies should the staff employ in providing support?

6.2 Ethical considerations
If instructed by a solicitor acting for a defendant, what ethical considerations do you consider arise when:

(a) in your judgement, based on objective evidence, the claimant is not yet ready to participate in a rehabilitation programme, nor return to work, even though a medical expert instructed by the defendant states otherwise? What would you do?
(b) it appears that the client's potential earning capacity is less than their benefits income?

6.3 Case study: MW
MW is a 39-year-old senior sales supervisor in a large high-street retail company. She has recently separated from her husband and has a 7-year-old daughter. She has been referred to you because, a little over 6 months ago, she received a whiplash injury while travelling as a passenger. MW returned to work the day after the accident but was sent home later in the day after complaining of pain and stiffness. Extensive examination has not revealed any physical reason for her continuing problems, but two part-time attempts to RTW have failed. On both occasions, MW reported that she could not cope on the second day. Under the company insurance scheme, MW continues to receive her full pay.

MW is highly regarded in the company. She has worked there since she left school aged 16 years. She prides herself on her appearance and her organisational capability. On one occasion, when the company was opening a new store, MW worked a 12-hour day, 7 days a week, for a period of 2 months. A colleague has had to stand in for MW in her absence, increasing her own hours to do this, and has made an evident success of it.

At the initial interview, MW presents as tearful and resentful – both of the driver who hit the car in which she was travelling, her employer for 'failing to understand ... I've worked for them for 23 years and now they just want me out', and the VR counsellor, whom she sees as being recruited to either force her back to work or into another job. She refuses to talk about her domestic situation: 'it's nothing to do with work, it's none of their business, did they tell you to ask me?'.

Identify the barriers to employment and how you would address them.

7 The vocational rehabilitation service provider

Key issues

- The public/private sector divide.
- New Labour and the Third Sector.
- Examples of service providers.

Learning objectives

- Understanding of the way the VR market in the United Kingdom has developed.
- Understanding of the common ground to VR practice.

Introduction

In the post-war period, VR services in the United Kingdom were mainly provided by public sector employment services. Limited NHS provision mainly served patients with MH problems. There is a long history of the specialist disability services within Jobcentre Plus contracting with voluntary organisations, typically ones with expertise in a particular area, such as the RNIB. This process was given a thrust by the closure of Employment Rehabilitation Centres in the early 1990s, the need to find providers to deliver Work Preparation programmes and also by the arrangements for the delivery of the Supported Employment programme (Chapter 8).

New Labour's endeavours to address the problems arising from unemployment and the growth in the IB registers created a new ball game. Existing agencies could no longer deal with the volume of potential referrals. New programmes were required (New Deal for Disabled People and Pathways to Work), and new service providers were required to deliver programmes en masse. The creation of Jobcentre Plus from 2002, incorporating social security offices, resulted in the majority of benefits claimants having health-related work problems. There began a remarkable transformation in the nature of service delivery, the process of *favouring* Third Sector and private sector service providers. This is a matter that will continue under the Conservative/Liberal Democrat regime, albeit with a reduced budget and far fewer service providers. Although many of the new service providers cannot be described as delivering VR, because of an emphasis on placing rather than preparation, they are part of the jigsaw of RTW services for many people with health conditions.

Hence, what changed from the late 1990s in the public sector is the contracting out of RTW services and the *extent* to which the Third Sector became preferred service providers for people with health conditions. (There is no precise definition of the Third Sector. It is a loose term referring to a wide range of voluntary and not-for-profit organisations.) In addition, the new millennium saw the development of a closer working relationship between Jobcentre Plus and the NHS, and the continuing development of private sector services catering for the insurance market.

The UK has quickly developed discrete approaches to delivering VR in the public and private sectors (Table 7.1). Despite a divergence in services, the knowledge and skills required of public and private sector service providers have much in common.

Public versus private sector services

Figure 7.1 provides a simple overview of what has been happening in the public sector VR market.

Not included in Figure 7.1 is an additional column, job-placement activity. In this respect, private sector VR services often have an advantage over public and Third Sector services. The clients are more likely to have a job or an employer to return to, and,

Table 7.1 Overview of main reliance for delivering VR services

Circumstance	Lead taker	VR service provider
Employee		
Accident at work	Employee	NHS/Jobcentre Plus[a]
	Employer (human resources/ occupational health)	NHS/Jobcentre Plus or private sector VR service
	Insurer	Private sector VR service
	Solicitor	Private sector VR service
Long-term sickness absence (not covered by specific insurance arrangements)	40% of UK employers with no policy (DWP/DH, 2008a)	May refer to/take advice from occupational health (if available)
	Employer Employee	Reliance on NHS
PHI	Employer Insurer	Private sector VR service provider
Employee or not employed		
Accident other than at work, e.g. RTA		
Third party liability for accident (covered by employer's PHI insurance)	Self Employer Insurer	NHS/Jobcentre Plus or private sector VR service NHS/Jobcentre Plus
Not liable	Solicitor/ insurer	
Not employed		
NHS patient	NHS	NHS
In receipt of ESA or IB	Jobcentre Plus	Jobcentre Plus specialist disability services and contracted agencies
In receipt of Jobseeker's Allowance	Jobcentre Plus	Jobcentre Plus gateway to contracted services

a Whether or not the NHS and/or Jobcentre Plus have appropriate support services are separate issues from the question of reliance.

VR process ⟹

	NHS	Condition management programmes[1]	Jobcentre Plus	Jobcentre Plus contracted agencies
Service user				
	Unemployed, or off work sick following onset of condition/ disability	High proportion of mental health (neuroses) and MSDs	Unemployed/health problem, likely to be long-term sick. Few retention cases[2]	Unemployed/health problem, likely to be long-term sick. Few retention cases
Distance from labour market				
	Variable	Usually not close	Close	Distant
Intervention				
	Heavily clinically influenced emphasis on assessment functional and cognitive skills. Treatment may be involved	Disability management	Assessment based on psychological evaluation Job matching Work preparation Supported employment	Variable ... ranging from providing work experience (work preparation) to emphasis on placing, job brokers
Skills				
	Medical experts/ therapists e.g. clinical psychology, physiotherapy, occupational therapy		Employment counselling Work psychology	Job coaching Job development Human resources

Figure 7.1 Perspectives on the public sector VR process

1 CMPs are included as a contracted service sitting between the NHS and Jobcentre Plus. Although successfully bridging this gap at the time of writing contracts are not being renewed. Unless replaced evidence suggest that a section of the population that has long been excluded from RTW support will again find itself long-term sick/unemployed.

hence, the VR process can be focused on specific placement techniques, such as job and task analysis. Other than in the Supported Employment programme, one aspect of placement activity that has been undertaken in a limited way in the United Kingdom, in all sectors, is that of providing *in situ* support, such as job coaching and developing natural supports (Chapter 15). All VR counsellors can benefit from learning more about such activity, even if the opportunities for on-the-job evaluations are restricted.

Although Table 7.2 cannot be an exact reflection of a diverse market, it does indicate some major differences between the public and private sectors. For instance, clients of

Table 7.2 Similarities and differences: private and public sector VR

Private or insurance sector	Public sector
Philosophy	
Rehabilitate injured workers as near as possible to their level of functioning prior to injury (implies focus on short-term goals)	Maximise each client's potential level (implies long-term goals, for example training or education)
Client population and eligibility	
PI claimants	Benefits claimants
Employer insurance policy determines eligibility	must have disability/health condition presenting as barrier to employment
Size of potential claim must justify degree of intervention	Inability to focus on clients only likely to RTW given support and may be disproportionate expenditure of resources on clients least likely to RTW
Functions, duties and services	
More personalised case management	Larger case-loads or lack of case-load management
Smaller case-loads	Less individual contact with client
Top 5 services	
Case management	Health/condition management
Assessment	Work preparation
Job analysis	Work experience
Job restructuring consultation	Job placement
Labour market surveying	Vocational counselling

public sector services are more likely to have longer-term conditions, and there is likely to be a higher percentage with MH problems and learning disabilities. The skills of VR counsellors and their intervention strategies need to reflect such circumstances. Table 7.2 reflects the need for a wide range of skills and knowledge, with the operational requirements of the employer and the needs of the clients foremost.

Examples of public and Third Sector service providers

Chapter 8 illustrates the Derbyshire Condition Management Programme. The contract for the service was not renewed after December 2010. Chapter 9 contains an example of the implementation of the individual placement and support (IPS) model of SE for people with severe mental illness. Although the Third Sector will be a main provider of the Work Programme, the extent to which services will be subcontracted to specialists remains to be seen. An example of a comprehensive service comes from one of the longest-established VR programmes in the United Kingdom, the Papworth Trust in Cambridgeshire (Figure 7.2). Funding is received from a variety of sources, including Jobcentre Plus and insurers. Although it is unrealistic to expect new VR service providers to match the same level of service provision, even the smallest services need to recognise the value of pre-placement support (Table 7.3).

The private sector VR service provider

Employers' liabilility, PI and the health insurance sectors are now driving a significant amount of the increased demand for VR services and changes to the way services are

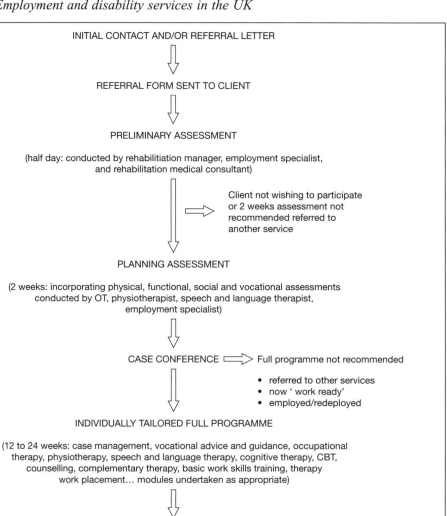

Figure 7.2 Papworth rehabilitation flowchart

Table 7.3 Papworth programme sample

	Morning	*Afternoon*
Monday	9.30–11.30 Computer training 11.30–12.30 Reflexology	1.30–2.30 Speech therapy 2.30–4.30 Communication training (numeracy/literacy)
Tuesday	9.30–12.30 Therapy work placement	1.30–4.30 Therapy work placement
Wednesday	9.30–10.30 CBT 10.30–12.30 Pain management	1.30–2.30 Physiotherapy 3.00–4.30 CBT
Thursday	9.30–12.30 Social therapy	1.30–4.30 Independent living skills training
Friday	9.30–10.30 Counselling 10.30–12.30 Job Club	

delivered. Changes to the civil justice system (Woolf, 1996) and the disappearance of legal aid in PI litigation (except for clinical negligence) have encouraged more co-operation between parties. Additionally, there has been a growth in health insurance covering an employee's need for medical attention and providing income protection if unable to work.

Group Income Protection and VR: the UNUM model

Unum is the United Kingdom's leading provider of GIP insurance. The company can trace its US origins back to the 1840s. A UK head office was established in Dorking in the mid 1990s. By 2006, it had established more than 18,600 schemes in the United Kingdom and paid total benefit claims of £285 million, of which more than £191 million related to income-protection claims. The company is influential in promoting VR in the United Kingdom in a number of ways, not only by providing income-protection schemes, incorporating VR intervention for sick and absent employees (Table 7.4), but also by promoting VR education, training and professionalism. In the early days in the United Kingdom, Unum experienced the lack of a private VR infrastructure and a public sector that did not respond to 'retention' cases. The first VR consultants (VRCs) Unum recruited were OH nurses and staff from the disability services of the Employment Service. It now has an established cadre of OTs, occupational psychologists, nursing and OH specialists operating on a peripatetic basis throughout the United Kingdom, although it has 'Open Door' Vocational Assessment and Guidance Centres in Dorking, Leeds and Bristol. The training arm of UNUM, Work Matters, has enabled VR staff to pursue the NIDMAR Certified Disability Management Professional (CDMP) qualification by supporting this course at Brunel, Huddersfield and Glasgow Caledonia Universities working in conjunction with KPMG Health Partners.

Role of Vocational Rehabilitation Counsellors

Unum considers that the role of the VRCs is to support the employer and employee and to interact with their GP and any other medical specialists. Working collaboratively, they work to identify what the employee can do, barriers to work and means of closing

Table 7.4 Unum's 'Premier' system

Week 1	Employee begins a period of sickness absence.
Week 4	Premier referral (if considered appropriate). Guidance is available when, for example, an employee is absent with no planned RTW date and/or showing signs of stress-related or musculoskeletal problems.
Week 6	Once referral documentation completed, including employee consent form, a VRC is allocated to the employee to facilitate the RTW process. This can entail a home or worksite visit.
Week 10	If RTW not imminent, claim process triggered.
Week 10–26	VRC continues to work with employee.
Week 23–26	Decision on claim notified.
Week 26+	Benefit continues to be paid, as long as employee continues to qualify under the terms of the policy. If unable to provide a rehabilitation service because of the employee's condition, the rehabilitation services team may subsequently get involved to assess motivation and suitability if there is any noted improvement.

Box 7.1 Unum GRTW plan

- Identification of the gaps between what the employee can do and what the job requires them to do.
- Identification of the barriers (medical, personal or work-related) that may prevent the employee from returning to work.
- Construction of a flexible GRTW plan that may include reference to such matters as:
  - number of hours worked in the past and any need to reduce these;
  - travel arrangements;
  - the nature of the condition and whether or not there are any additional physical or psychological needs to be met;
  - any mentoring or support required;
  - what the work involves and the impact of any long-term condition;
  - the work environment and the need for any adjustments;
  - the support and flexibility of the employer.

---

the gaps and overcoming the identified barriers through the construction of a flexible graduated return-to-work (GRTW) plan (Box 7.1). In the event of an employee being unable to return to a former position, the VRC will offer advice and guidance on alternative options, including retraining.

Responding to ELCI insurers: Chartis Medical and Rehabilitation (formerly AIG Medical and Rehabilitation)

Chartis is a case management and OH company established in 1998. It is typical of a number of companies now offering VR services. It provides a nationwide service delivering case management, vocational consultancy and assessment services, over the telephone or face to face in an injured persons' home, hospital or preferred environment. There is a professional employee base of registered nurses, physiotherapists, OTs, OH advisors, OH technicians, vocational consultants and psychologists. In addition to an OH service providing a proactive absence-management and health-surveillance service, Chartis provides the following:

Immediate needs assessment service

This is an assessment of an individual's immediate needs, relating to multiple pathology and catastrophic injuries and illnesses. The assessment identifies the severity and consequences of the injury and the physical, psychological and vocational impact. It includes an outline of the injured person's medical and vocational needs and a costed rehabilitation plan, provided to all parties, in accordance with the Rehabilitation Code.

Medical and vocational case management assessment services

This service is embedded within Chartis Insurance UK employers' liability products. When a workplace injury or illness occurs, a completed RIDDOR form is forwarded to the HSE, and a copy is sent to the Chartis case manager who handles workplace injuries for that company. The case manager contacts the employer for information and then the injured person, requesting consent to approach the person's treating practitioners to ascertain the nature of the injury, treatment and prognosis, in order to develop an overall case management plan. Recovery is speeded up by arranging private treatment if it is recommended because of NHS waiting lists. The case manager works with key parties to ensure that there is a co-ordination of treatment, to enable the injured person to return, as far as possible, to their pre-injury lifestyle or to an optimum level of health. The case manager ensures that treatment and GRTW plans are appropriate and in the best interest of all parties. For employees who do not return-to-work following treatment, or are unable to continue in their pre-injury role, the injured person is referred by the case manager to a vocational consultant (VC) to assist the person and employer in developing a RTW plan, explore alternative roles, give advice on reasonable adjustments and adaptations, which can include retraining, and help the parties utilise government-funded programmes such as Access to Work. VCs produce vocational-assessment reports, making training and RTW recommendations based on the medical history, transferrable skills and work available in the injured person's locality. The case study provided by Chartis illustrates a simple and cost-effective intervention.

Case study: Example of redeployment using 'job carving'

Service user
A 49-year-old male, employed as an injection-moulding technician injured his leg at work. As a result of this injury, he was diagnosed with peripheral vascular disease. Because the injury would not heal and it affected his legs, he underwent an above-knee amputation of the right leg and below-knee amputation of the left leg.

Rehabilitation
The employer contacted the medical case manager by phone, requesting the provision of vocational and medical rehabilitation services to assist the employee to return to work in some capacity, as the employer was not sure how to accommodate the employee. The employee was undergoing a medical rehabilitation programme that included gait training, balance re-education and strengthening. The employee was mobile; he could walk independently using two walking sticks. The medical case manager referred the employee to the VC, as no further medical treatment had been recommended. A home visit was arranged, to carry out a vocational assessment and to ascertain the employment outlook. The assessment indicated that the employee was highly motivated to return to work and had come to terms with the loss of his legs, but had yet to recognise what he could do physically. He was very willing to consider all available roles.

A Job Demands Analysis carried out at the workplace indicated that the role could not be adapted, and that many of the physical requirements were no longer possible. The VC advised the employer that they were not expected to create a job; however, retraining the employee to fill an existing vacancy would be a reasonable adjustment. The employer advised that they had a temporary position as an assembler available; however, it would be a race against time as to whether the employee could reach his goal of walking unaided before the role came to an end.

The VC asked the employer whether it was possible to amalgamate a number of existing small roles to create a full-time post. The employer said this was not possible. However, within a few weeks, the employer advised that a sister plant located nearby was to be closed, and that some of the functions were to be moved to the employee's workplace. The employer advised that they would arrange a meeting with a number of process managers to see whether some of the functions could be combined to create a post for the employee. At a later stage, the employer confirmed that a new role as a technician trainer/telephonist had been created, whereby the employee could use his existing skills to advise, support and train other technicians within the group.

The benefit
The VC supported the employee throughout his rehabilitation process and provided advices and assistance to the employer, enabling them to retain the services of an experienced technician. The VC supported the employee to secure his employment future with his employer, using many of his existing skills in an alternative role.

Physiotherapist in private practice

Case study: Use of GRTW plan

Service user
A 53-year-old man, an LGV driver for a mining explosives company, was referred by his company for assessment of fitness for work because he had been off work for 6 weeks owing to back pain, with radiating pain and occasional pins and needles into the right leg aggravated by sitting.

Initial assessment
A clinical examination concluded there was probably a lumbar disc prolapse causing nerve root pain. Factors that may have contributed to the condition included an employment history of manual work and long-distance driving, previous smoking and a height above the ninety-fifth percentile for the United Kingdom. The Roland Morris and Oswestry Disability Index questionnaires were used, giving results of 20/24 and 52 per cent (moderate–severe) disability scores, respectively. The Acute Low Back Pain Screening Questionnaire was used to screen for psychosocial yellow flags, and the score was 118/210, confirming that this employee was at risk of long-term absence of over 30-day duration.

Rehabilitation
The following advice was given to the employer:

•   At the date of the assessment, the employee was unfit for normal or alternative duties owing to the severity of the problem.

- Physiotherapy treatment was recommended to start as soon as possible to treat the back condition, provide advice, reassurance that physical activities would not make the condition worse, and strengthening and work-conditioning activities. The severity of the condition also warranted a caveat that, if the patient failed to respond to treatment as expected, an MRI scan and/or a referral to a spinal surgeon might be required.
- An initial action plan was provided, and reviewing fitness for work in 4 weeks, after physiotherapy had begun, was suggested, and the company was asked to begin to consider whether any alternative duties would be available to facilitate a return to work in 4 weeks' time.

The company decided to fund private physiotherapy treatment, which commenced almost immediately. This enabled prompt advice and action on managing the pain, and a rehabilitation programme was started that included active home exercises and an emphasis on building sitting tolerance for driving.

The employee was reviewed 1 month later, having received four sessions of physiotherapy.

Repeated disability tests gave much reduced levels of discomfort and disability: Roland Morris Questionnaire–1/24; Oswestry Disability Index–14%–low disability.

Repeated psychosocial screening questionnaire: 65/210 – no longer at risk of long-term absence.

Subjectively, the employee was reporting much less pain, and the previous nerve-root symptoms had resolved, leaving some spinal stiffness and lack of muscle control, which was continuing to improve with treatment and rehabilitation.

GRTW plan
A GRTW plan was agreed. The company had decided to provide some on-site driving and maintenance work for up to 4–6 weeks, and so this was integrated into the programme. The programme began with reduced hours and alternative duties, and built up to normal hours and a return to long-distance driving over 8 weeks. The company and employee were advised that, if there were any problems with the RTW plan, he should remain at the previous week's level of duties for another week, and then try to progress again.

The company was offered an on-site, ergonomic assessment of the work environment; however, this was not taken up.

The company was advised to review its policies and training on manual handling and risk assessment for drivers, and to ensure risk assessments were completed regarding back pain and driving, especially when new lorries were being purchased. The employee returned to work as planned and had a further four sessions of physiotherapy over the following 5-week period. He followed the return-to-work plan and had returned to normal duties by the 8-week target date. A follow-up with his manager some months later indicated he had had no further problems with his back, had remained at work and had taken up kayaking.

Costs
- Cost of absence for 11 weeks in total (6 weeks prior to assessment and 5 weeks while treatment commenced and worked towards fitness for work) was approximately £9,000.

- Cost of intervention (assessments, reports, treatment, basic home-exercise equipment) was approximately £1,000. (Had the employee been referred earlier, it might have been possible to save 1 month of absence, saving approximately £3,000.)

Because the referral was made relatively early on, it was not necessary to involve any other health professionals in the RTW planning process and treatment provision, and the situation was managed by the employee, employer and physiotherapist.

Certified disability manager in private practice

Case study: Co-ordinating services and client support

Service user
J, a 45-year-old married man, was crushed in a printing press and fractured his left clavicle. His shoulder was pinned and plated. He received physiotherapy but, after approximately 9 months of pain and restrictions, a review by the treating surgeon identified that the pinned fracture had not united. Further surgery necessitated a bone graft. J also suffered with depression. He was reported to be desperate to return to work. With the approval of the solicitor handling his claim, J was referred to the independent VR practice by the ELCI insurer. The initial step was a VR assessment.

Initial assessment
J had been employed by this company for 9 years as a machine operator. The work involved heavy lifting, pulling and pushing at various heights. J enjoyed his work in isolation on night shifts, a preferred working pattern. He liked to work in a clearly defined and repetitive role. J did not like change and stated early on in the VR process that he could not stand the thought of having to return to work in a new job with a different employer. J had no formal training or qualifications. The firm continued to pay J's salary during his absence. Prior to referral to the VR service, J had attempted to return to work on full duties on night shifts, which he managed for just a few days. He struggled for a while before reporting the pain and difficulties he was having to his line manager.

Summary of intervention sequence and RTW events
- J was seen in his own home for an initial assessment relating to his injury, work situation and motivation. J presented as keen to get back to work, although still suffering with pain and restrictions in his left (dominant) shoulder.
- The VR case manager visited the employer. Line and HR managers were keen to do what they could, although unsure that J could work safely and productively.

- Job analysis was undertaken. One of the heaviest aspects of the role involved pulling by hand a half-ton of card on a manually operated pump truck across the workshop floor. Operators were also required to lift and manoeuvre large metal or wooden frames, which had to be inserted into the machines at chest height when setting up the machine. Other physical demands required reaching, pushing, twisting and crouching. It was identified that the employer had a new member of staff joining the team, and it would be useful to have J train this person, providing a useful, lighter initial role for J.
- Following a meeting with the employer and J, the VR case manager compiled her recommendations and estimated costs. The report was sent to the insurer and solicitor, J and his employer for their approval. Key recommendations were:
  - VR case manager to compile a GRTW plan in consultation with the treating specialist, to build hours and duties. Lighter duties to include training and, once on his own, machine operating with co-worker support.
  - To avoid heavy pulling of pump truck, case manager suggested an electric pump truck. The employer investigated trucks, and VR case manager supported application to Access to Work. Access to Work agreed to part-fund, and VR case manager obtained funding from insurer for the outstanding balance.
  - VR case manager suggested a full health and safety risk assessment be completed when J returned to work, to assess and identify all risks and to provide J with advice on safe working practices. In addition CBT was arranged by the VR counsellor.
- All relevant parties reviewed and approved the VR plan. The VR case manager proceeded to implement, involving negotiation and liaison with the treating orthopaedic consultant, line manager, HR manager and general manager, J and his wife (J was struggling with his low moods; both J and his wife could not understand the purpose behind the GRTW plan, and time was spent 'selling' this concept to them), GP and CBT provider, Access to Work, insurer and claimant solicitor (both parties were regularly informed of progress via emails and more formal 5–6 week progress reports).
- Once GRTW plan completed and approved, VR case manager arranged for a RTW meeting with J, the line manager and HR. J subsequently returned to work in line with the reduced hours and lighter duties.
- VR case manager monitored good initial progress. Following a period of 5 weeks on lighter duties, J was ready to return to full hours and adapted duties using his new electric pump truck and with no heavy lifting/handling over shoulder height.
- Unfortunately, less than 2 months later, J was involved in an unrelated accident at work. J's treating consultant was hopeful that a period of 6 weeks' rest would help to heal the injury, which had exacerbated his previous one. J was angry and frustrated, as he was enjoying being back at work, and this was having a positive effect at home.
- During the second absence, the employer was less sympathetic than previously, informing the case manager that it was not at fault with this accident, and, hence, it was not happy about being as accommodating. J's pay was stopped,

and he received SSP. The employer was reminded that, regardless of liability, there is still a duty in line with the DDA to support J with his return to work, and that it would help improve relations if full pay continued. This was refused. J began to feel further frustration and, now, anger towards his employer.

- During J's absence, it was also suggested to the employer that it keep in touch with him to ensure he was not isolated from the workforce and to help keep relations positive. This did not occur.

- Following 6 weeks of rest, J's reported pain was said to be unmanageable. Relations with his wife became severely strained. J was angry with his employer, and his motivation to return to work declined.

- The VR case manager advised the insurer that J return to CBT to help him cope with the current situation, and also suggested that J may require further medical case management, but the insurer said that it was happy with VR case management at this stage and would see how things progressed. VR case manager liaised with the treating consultant and asked him to review J, to advise.

- Treating consultant suggested that the fracture was healing well, although the plate was causing him the most pain; however, the plate could not be removed for some time. The consultant made some suggestions for pain relief.

- Treating consultant agreed a RTW date on light duties and graduated hours. VR case manager then brought in an OT to conduct a work-site assessment in order to identify any further potential work-site considerations and adjustments. Her assessment and recommendations were included in the revised GRTW plan, again developed in consultation with J and his line manager and passed to the treating consultant for approval.

- All parties approved the revised GRTW plan. On returning to work, the line manager questioned J's account of the second incident. VR case manager spoke to the line manager and advised to stay focused on supporting J with his return to work. J was provided with CBT arranged by the VR counsellor.

- After RTW, J was assessed by a medico-legal expert (upper limb specialist) for the insurer. The views of this expert conflicted with the treating consultant. He suggested to J that there was a missed fracture, and he should be X-rayed immediately. J reacted badly, broke down and said he could no longer cope with the ongoing pain and, now, confusion as to what was wrong. VR case manager reassured J that this expert may not have had all the history, and he should be led by his treating consultant at this stage.

- J also reported the comment from the defendant expert to his line manager, who then reported to the general manager. The general manager called the VR case manager to say that he was going to send J home on sick leave because of concern about any health and safety risks. VR case manager maintained that they should be guided by the treating consultant and that they should seek advice over sending home an employee on sick leave without GP, employee or treating-practitioner approval. The employer was convinced enough to let J stay in work, but on the basis that the VR case manager would liaise with the treating consultant for his opinion in relation to the points raised by the defendant's expert.

- The treating consultant agreed to review J and X-ray him. The X-ray revealed that, as previously suggested, the fracture had healed, but the plate was causing the ongoing pain, which would probably not improve much until it was removed.
- Subsequently, J continued to work with ongoing pain and some restrictions. However, he was able to increase his hours to full time. J previously worked night shifts, but, owing to lack of a co-worker and line-management support, he remained on day shifts for the time being.
- The VR case manager attended several RTW meetings with J, his line manager, HR and general manager, and also developed and adapted the GRTW plan, depending on the progress of J and the feedback from his consultant.
- The VR case manager also supported the employer and J with another Acess to Work claim, to help fund a support worker required for setting up the machine and fixing underneath the machine. J could do about 75–80 per cent of his role and needed to remain on these reduced duties until further surgery to remove the plate. After this surgery, J would need to embark on another medical rehabilitation programme, likely to consist of physiotherapy and work hardening, then a further GRTW plan.

Summary

The development of VR in the United Kingdom is following the pattern found elsewhere in the Western world, one of state provision driven by reducing benefits payments and addressing social exclusion, and insurance-driven private sector services aiming to reduce absenteeism and levels of compensation payments. Although some large Third Sector VR service providers operate in both the public and private sectors, such as the Shaw Trust and Remploy, smaller services tend to specialise in one arena or the other. As a means of cost-cutting, the public sector is being driven towards very large service providers whereas the private sector has fostered a growth in individual as well as corporate service providers. It remains to be seen how the final version of the Work Programme addresses the needs of people with health conditions and the extent to which specialist services are subcontracted.

Given the nature of Jobcentre Plus, there is an argument against maintaining internal specialist disability services (Chapter 8), and, for administrative purposes, they have been incorporated into mainstream activity. However, owing to the 'disability lobby', they are unlikely to disappear and they will continue to survive with a new Supported Employment programme. 'Joined-up', public sector, case-managed VR services ought to be delivered through the NHS and associated services (although much remains to be done), but the disappearance of Condition Management Programmes has weakened NHS services for a vulnerable section of the population.

Although individual VR practitioners in the private sector do not have all the resources of a limited company, the case studies illustrate how experienced personnel are able to pull together various threads in order to achieve positive outcomes. Despite differing disciplinary backgrounds, the modus operandi of VR practitioners is often remarkably similar, such as in the preparation of GRTW plans.

Student exercise

7.1 Common features of VR intervention strategies
Identify the common features and differences in the RTW process in the case studies provided by Chartis, the physiotherapist and the independent VR practitioner.

8   Jobcentre Plus
Employment and disability services

Key issues

- Changing face of services.
- Identifying 'the best' support available for a particular client.
- Role of DEAs.
- Job Introduction Scheme/Work Preparation/WORKSTEP: Work Choice.
- Residential training.
- Access to Work.
- Work psychology.

Learning objectives

- Awareness of where a particular service fits into the pattern of RTW provision for people with disabilities/health conditions.
- Ability to identify and access Jobcentre Plus services.

Introduction

Following the election of New Labour in 1997, the approach towards providing RTW services for people with health conditions began to incorporate both the specialist disability services, developed following the 1944 Disabled Persons (Employment) Act, and, more significantly, new services underpinned by experience developed from the National Disability Development Initiative (NDDI). NDDI contributed to a range of developments that can be categorised into five main types of employment and disability welfare-to-work strategy, three aimed at the individual and two at the work environment (Bambra *et al.*, 2005). Points 1, 2 and 5 of Box 8.1 contain aspects of the VR process.

In addition to the specialist disability services, Pathways to Work and the New Deal for Disabled People (NDDP) were introduced to deliver new services (see Table 8.1). Although the Conservative/Liberal Democrat coalition has begun the process of combining the major programmes, Pathways and New Deal, into the Work Programme, the specialist disability services are likely to remain within Jobcentre Plus; however, the Supported Employment programme has recently undergone radical changes.

In respect of internal Jobcentre Plus administration, the specialist services are now an integral part of mainstream provision. Although Pathways and New Deal will be

---

Box 8.1 Welfare-to-work strategies

1   Education training and work placements.
2   Vocational advice and support services.
3   In-work benefits for employees.
4   Employer incentives.
5   Improving accessibility of work environment.

(Bambra *et al.*, 2005)

Table 8.1 Jobcentre Plus disability services

Pathways to Work	*NDDP*	*Specialist disability services*
Pathways advisors	Job brokers	Disability employment advisors
Work-focused interviews (WFIs)	Personal Advisors (PAs)	(DEAs)
Condition Management		Work preparation
Programmes (CMPs)		Work psychology
		Job introduction scheme (JIS)*
		WORKSTEP*
		Access to Work*
		Choices
		Residential training

* Now integrated into work

replaced by the Work Programme, their development is important for a number of reasons. Not only will the nature of service delivery be continued, with a reliance on the private and third sectors with a network of job brokers, but, even more significantly, the final version of the Work Programme will reflect the extent to which the new government has taken on board the positive lessons from Pathways and NDDP, particularly with regards to maintaining working relationships between Jobcentre Plus and the NHS and serving the 'hard-to-place' population (which is often expensive to keep on benefits).

Of concern is the capacity of existing and new programmes to cope with the volume of potential customers arising from the changes being made to benefits payments and to offer a qualitative service to the 'hard to place'. The case advanced by Freud (Chapter 3) is that benefits savings will pay for the Work Programme, and weighted payments will ensure that programme participants with the greatest needs will receive support. Although the detail has yet to emerge, such reasoning appears to owe more to wishful thinking (or ideology) than any objective analysis of the market. *The Times* (11 October 2010) reported plans to move 500,000 people off IB on to JSA, which would produce estimated savings of around £2 billion. However, around 40 per cent of people are successfully appealing decisions.

Pathways to Work

Pathways refers to a package of reforms set up in October 2003 as a pilot project, delivered by Jobcentre Plus, to help people on IB return-to-work. By 2007, Pathways had been rolled out to cover the whole country. Jobcentre Plus run Pathways have operated in around 40 per cent of the United Kingdom, with provider-led (contracted) Pathways delivered in the remaining 60 per cent. The main elements have included the following:

* Support:
  - three mandatory WFIs for new customers;
  - PAs developing a RTW plan;
  - in-work benefit calculations and a RTW credit of £40 per week, payable for a maximum 52 weeks to those working 16 hours or more, but earning less than £15,000 per annum.
* Choices:
  - a choice of interventions, such as easier access to NDDP, Work Preparation, Work-Based Learning for Adults (Training for Work in Scotland) and CMPs delivered through local NHS trusts;
  - in-work support.

In addition, other existing support remained available, such as access to DEAs.

Work-focused interviews (WFIs) and Personal Advisors (PAs)

From October 2005, it became compulsory to attend a series of three (initially six) monthly work-related interviews with a PA, from 8 weeks after the benefit claim, and to complete an Action Plan.

Personal advisors

PAs became responsible for WFIs for all new benefits claimants. As one commentator noted,

> government has embraced the concept of personal advisors providing individually tailored advice and support to benefit claimants. Recent years have witnessed a move towards such personalised support, not just in its flagship New Deals but also in the mandatory work-focused interview regime.
>
> (Thornton, 2005)

As such, PAs began to have an important part to play in providing access to public sector VR services. Not all critics are enamoured of their role, accusing them of a failure to engage with customers, assuming that the customers are uninterested or unable to work, and lacking disability expertise. It has been reported that they are anxious about probing work issues, because their own lack of medical knowledge makes it hard for them to understand how certain conditions affect the customers. In particular, when customers have MH problems, there is a reluctance to probe into details (Goldstone and Douglas, 2003; Lissenburgh and Marsh, 2003; Taylor and Hartfree, 2003). On the other hand, during the roll-out of WFIs, participants found the work-related purposes of the meeting well communicated and the advice helpful; one in five customers said that the advice made them more motivated to find a job, and a similar proportion said that it increased their confidence. Take-up of voluntary further meetings was very limited (Coleman *et al.*, 2004).

IB PAs

The Jobcentre Plus response to reported shortcomings was a move towards specialist PAs working with IB (later ESA) customers. Thornton (2005) maintains that the move towards specialist advisors is at odds with the mainstreaming approach in New Deal and contrary to the government's Advisory Committee for Disabled People in Employment and Training (2001), which holds that specialist provision labels people as different and in need of special handling. On the other hand, the move towards specialist PAs was supported by 90 per cent of the eighty-seven organisations and individuals responding to the Green Paper *Pathways to Work* (DWP, 2002).

Condition Management Programmes (CMPs)

From the VR perspective, the most significant Pathway development was the roll-out of CMPs. CMPs were established in 2004 and represented a breakthrough in Jobcentre Plus–NHS collaboration, primarily to support three main health conditions:

• mild/moderate MH conditions, e.g. depression, anxiety and stress;
• coronary heart disease/respiratory problems;
• MSDs.

In practice, a generic programme with 'add-on' modules developed.

Jobcentre Plus emphasised that CMPs did not provide treatment, but were based on psycho-educational programmes using a cognitive behavioural/biopsychosocial model to provide education, advice and reassurance. These work-focused rehabilitation programmes became the largest public VR service available to sick/disabled people without access to private sector services. In general, CMP delivery was based on core modules of 2 days per week, delivered away from NHS premises (so as not to reinforce any sickness label), plus additional supporting modules (Table 8.2).

Although considered a 'success' by many participants and programme providers, CMPs have fallen victim to existing contracts not being renewed. This has occurred when a

Table 8.2 Core and supporting modules of CMPs

Core modules	Supporting modules
Understanding your health condition	Know your heart
Managing your condition at work	Breathlessness/breath easy
Pacing and goal setting	Coping with stress/anxiety
Healthy lifestyle and exercise	'Back' to work
Confidence building and communication skills	Managing pain
Stress and mood management	Alcohol/drug dependency
	Understanding and coping with depression
	Coping with fatigue/poor sleep

large number of hard-to-place IB/ESA claimants are being found fit for work. Although CMPs have rarely reported higher than 20 per cent employment placing rates, they have served a difficult population, with programme providers reporting a high percentage of service users with MH problems. It is regrettable that CMPs should find their contracts not being renewed after developing programme expertise and in view of the evidence regarding the need for such services. Closure has occurred in the absence of any cost–benefit analyses, including savings in benefit and demands on health services.

Example of a CMP

The Derbyshire CMP began to be administered from two NHS locations in Clay Cross and Derby, from spring 2004. By 2010, the budget, entirely funded by Jobcentre Plus, had grown to £1.4 million, and the programme served around 1,500 people a year. The contract with Jobcentre Plus was not renewed from December 2010. Around 68 per cent of the referrals were for people with MH problems, with MSDs forming the second-largest group of conditions at around 30–40 per cent. Other conditions, including cardiorespiratory, did not feature in any significant numbers. Around 70 per cent of referrals completed the course. A frustrating aspect for the programme managers was the lack of data on non-completions, particularly those who left because they found a job. Of those who completed the course, around 25 per cent found work, with a further 50 per cent having 'positive outcomes', such as voluntary work, education or training.

Although the programme was designed to take referrals from Jobcentre Plus, following a WCA, the WCAs took longer to administer and produce a decision on a benefits claim than the stipulated 8 weeks; hence, PAs made referrals without this process being completed. At interviews, it was found that customers (Jobcentre Plus terminology) not only made decisions on whether or not they considered the CMP could help them, but also decided which of two pathways were appropriate for them: a 'physical' or a MH programme. Although the former programme was run in-house by NHS staff, and the latter contracted to Trent CBT, there was some programme flexibility, so that someone receiving cognitive behavioural therapy could, if they desired, also attend one of the modules in the other stream (Figure 8.1). A fundamental aspect of the CMP programme was case management support, provided by an OT or physiotherapist.

The initial assessment, conducted by an OT or physiotherapist, relied on the CORE Outcome Measure (CORE-OM) and/or COTNAB. The Hospital Anxiety and Depression Scale was used, but it was found to be superfluous to customers' own self-assessments. The CORE-OM is a thirty-four-item questionnaire designed to measure clients' global distress, including subjective well-being, commonly experienced problems or symptoms and life/social functioning. The main purpose of the tool is to offer a global level of distress, expressed as the average mean score of the thirty-four items that can be compared with clinical thresholds before and after therapy, to help determine clinical and reliable change. The measure has been extensively validated and it has good psychometric properties.

New deal for disabled people (NDDP) and the introduction of job brokers

NDDP, part of a raft of New Deal programmes, became New Labour's main employment programme for people in receipt of a disability or incapacity-related benefit and an important part of the government's Welfare to Work strategy (Stafford, 2003). NDDP

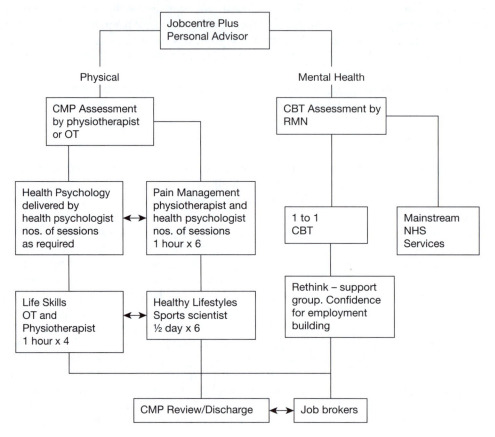

Figure 8.1 Derbyshire CMP

has been instrumental in building a network of job brokers around the country, from the private, voluntary and public sectors.

Although NDDP and Pathways to Work had factors in common, particularly the key role of PAs, NDDP was designed to be an enhanced support and placing service, delivered by not-for-profit private and public sector job brokers to volunteering Jobcentre Plus customers receiving a wide range of disability-related benefits. As such, its legacy can be seen in the proposals for the Work Programme.

Job brokers

Each job broker offered different services said to be tailored to individual needs (Box 8.2).

Some job brokers had a disability expertise, such as the Shaw Trust; others did not. Customers wanting to participate in the programme had to register with a job broker accessed through the NDDP Gateway at Jobcentre Plus offices. PAs informed their customer of local job-broking services, and the customer could choose their own. Job brokers received both a registration fee and outcome payment for job entries and sustained employment.

Box 8.2 Type of support offered by job brokers

Support said to include:

- the examination of skills and abilities to identify suitable job opportunities;
- help with filling in application forms;
- advice about writing CVs;
- help with preparing for interviews;
- identifying training needs and working with local training providers to find the training;
- information about local job vacancies;
- help through the process of applying for jobs;
- support during the first six months in work;
- benefits advice;
- extra support in the workplace, such as special equipment.

DEAs and Work Preparation

For over 60 years, many people have perceived DEAs (until 1994, known as disablement resettlement officers) as synonymous with public sector employment and disability services. The creation of Jobcentre Plus reduced the comparative significance of their role, although they continue to carry case-loads of around forty customers and maintain an advisory and support role for other staff. From the early 1990s, the main rehabilitation service available to DEAs was Work Preparation.

Work Preparation

Following the 1990s closure of Employment Rehabilitation Centres, Work Preparation courses were introduced to replace the rehabilitation element of the service, and PACTs were introduced to provide vocational assessments and implement action plans. Work Preparation continued to support around 7,500 people per annum until 2010, when the revised Supported Employment programme began to take shape.

Throughout their existence, different perceptions existed in relation to the overall remit of Work Preparation programmes (Banks *et al.*, 2002; Riddell, 2002). Riddell and Banks (2005) considered that,

> although relatively small-scale, the rationale for the programme was to help disabled people into employment, but . . . relatively small number of people progressed into the open labour market. Service users often saw Work Preparation as a stepping-stone into work and were disappointed when a paid job did not follow a work placement. By way of contrast, service providers and Employment Service professionals emphasised that work was only one valid outcome, deciding to work on a voluntary basis or not to work at all should be seen as equally valid options. Providers and Employment Service workers pointed out that, if achieving paid

employment was heavily 'incentivised' within funding regimes, then there was pressure on service providers to reject clients who need greater support for a longer period of time.

Work psychology

Occupational psychologists were first employed in IRUs during the 1950s. On the closure of ERCs, work psychologists (WPs) as they became known, became members of PACTs. Although practice varies, the WPs now predominantly support DEAs and PAs by accepting referrals from them. They do not carry their own case-loads.

There are four designated groups of Jobcentre Plus customers for whom WPs mainly, but not exclusively, provide an assessment service. These are for customers with MH problems, specific learning difficulties, for example dyslexia, brain injury and those requiring ergonomic considerations (known as 'work solutions').

The WPs have developed their own 'lead groups' covering these four areas. WPs can also receive retention referrals from DEAs and, in such a circumstance, can visit an employer and apply job-analysis skills. Following an assessment, a report will advise the DEA or PA on the appropriate course of action, such as conditions to avoid or a referral to Access to Work.

Supported Employment/WORKSTEP

The Supported Employment programme has recently been rolled into a rearranged package of work support known as Work Choice.

During the 1990s, the Employment Service adopted the title the Supported Employment programme (SEP) to describe what was previously called its sheltered programme. This change reflected a move away from segregated workshops to a reliance on employer placements through the Supported Placement Scheme (SPS), rebranded WORKSTEP from April 2001. This model required not only a host employer, in open employment, but a sponsor. The sponsor, the legal contractual employer, needed to be a local authority or a registered charity (unless an injured employee was retained, in which case the employer could be the sponsor). Major sponsors included the Shaw Trust, the RNIB and Scope.

Historically, the demand for supported placements always outstripped the supply of places, a matter exacerbated by the low throughput into open employment (Honey and Williams, 1998; Jackson *et al.*, undated).

Reform

A consultative document (DWP, 2007) pointed to NAO recommendations for the specialist disability services (NAO, 2005) stating that there should be more emphasis in WORKSTEP on progression to unsupported, open employment. Between April 2001 and October 2005, one-third of WORKSTEP providers did not progress a single person to open, unsupported employment. Fewer than one in ten people in the programme made annual progression into open employment. It was further considered that Work Preparation was too rigid in terms of what providers were expected to deliver, and 6 weeks were not enough for people with more profound disability-related barriers to employment.

In its response to the consultative document, the government proposed to:

1   tie the job introduction scheme to when an employer makes adjustments;
2   use Work Preparation as an assessment or job entry service in conjunction with WORKSTEP;
3   enhance the role of DEAs by developing a support package for customers;
4   reduce the number of WORKSTEP contractors and push up the quality. While acknowledging that it is hard to make progress towards open employment with the clients of some service providers, it was proposed to increase financial incentives in order to do this; and
5   develop a distance-travelled tool to assist providers and their customers in keeping track of their goals and progress in meeting them.

In order to ensure that only disabled people requiring specialist support enter the new programme, a points system of assessment has been developed. The programme proper starts with the DEA identifying a package of support covering one or more of the three main elements:

1	*2*	*3*
Work entry employment	Transitional supported employment	Longer-term supported

Transitional SE refers to when a customer is considered capable of progressing into open employment. Longer-term SE refers to when a customer is considered unlikely to progress into open employment.

The consultative document illustrates how the programme would work: for example, in looking at contract tenders and work entry, it would look towards the provision of vocational guidance and action planning, confidence building, personal- and job-skills support, job search advice and job matching, job application support and job-retention skills, working closely with employers and acting as a broker with an employer to explain adjustments and available support.

For all customers entering a job, the DWP expects service providers to check that the individual has settled into their work; ensure that transport arrangements are working and that the individual is receiving appropriate benefits advice; put in place an agreed support plan; help the employer make adjustments; and be available for advice and support.

An example of how the Work Choice programme operates for people with an acquired brain injury in north-west England is provided by Ways to Work (accessed at www. waystowork.co.uk), working in partnership with the Shaw Trust. A full list of providers can be found at www.dwp.gov.uk/supplying-dwp/what-we-buy/welfare-to-work-services/specialist-disability-employment/.

Access to Work

This programme is designed to help disabled employees, and employers, find solutions to practical obstacles at work. It can also help if a disabled person is about to start paid work (including self-employment). Both unemployed and employed disabled people who need the help of a communicator at a job interview can get assistance. To be eligible, the type of work undertaken by the disabled person has to be affected by a disability or health condition likely to last for 12 months or more. The scheme is administered by regional Access to Work Business Centres, accessed through DEAs in local Jobcentre Plus offices.

Access to Work can help pay for such matters as:

- communication support for hearing impaired people; this includes British Sign Language (BSL) interpreters, lipspeakers and note-takers;
- a reader at work for visually impaired people;
- special equipment (or alterations to existing equipment);
- help with the additional costs of travel to work for people who are unable to use public transport.

Access to Work can also pay for a support worker at work or getting to work. The type of support on offer might include someone to read or communicate or a specialist coach for a person with learning difficulties.

The application process

An Access to Work adviser will usually speak to the applicant and their employer to reach a decision about the most effective support. Sometimes, specialist advice may be needed, which the adviser will help to arrange. For example, the adviser may arrange for a specialist organisation, such as the RNIB, to complete an assessment and recommend appropriate support. Once the adviser has decided on the package of support, they will seek formal approval of their recommendations from Jobcentre Plus. The applicant and the employer will then receive a letter informing them of the approved level of support and the grant available.

The employer is usually responsible for arranging the agreed support and purchasing the necessary equipment. The employer can then claim back a grant towards approved costs from Access to Work. The amount of help received from Access to Work varies, depending on how long the applicant has been employed, what support they need and whether they are self-employed.

Access to Work can pay up to 100 per cent of the approved costs if the applicant is unemployed and starting a new job, self-employed or working for an employer and having been in the job for less than 6 weeks.

Whatever the employment status, Access to Work will also pay up to 100 per cent of the approved costs of help with support workers, fares to work and communication support at an interview.

Access to Work pays a proportion of the costs of support if the applicant has been working for an employer and has been in the job for 6 weeks or more.

The precise level of cost-sharing is agreed between the employer and the Access to Work adviser. All help provided is for a maximum period of 3 years, after which the Access to Work Business Centre will review a case.

Residential training for disabled adults

In view of educational establishments now having to observe disability legislation, many people may regard RTCs supported by Jobcentre Plus as anachronistic. However, the service is provided only when there are no suitable alternative programmes available locally, and a visit to any of the ten funded colleges will reveal expertise not always available elsewhere. Eligibility is based on:

- having a physical and/or sensory disability or learning difficulty;
- being aged 18 or over;
- being unable to access suitable local training; and
- being unemployed and having the potential to take up employment, including SE.

Courses vary from college to college, with over fifty courses of vocational training available, including administration, audio-visual technician, catering, construction trades, cycle mechanics, decorating, electronics, engineering, horticulture, information technology, leisure/tourism/travel, recording, retail, teleworking and vehicle refinishing. The lengths of courses vary but do not exceed 52 weeks. Some training programmes are specifically designed for people with a hearing or visual impairment.

The courses are run at:

- Doncaster College for the Deaf;
- Enham, Andover, Hampshire;
- Finchale Training College, Durham;
- Portland College, Mansfield;
- Queen Alexandra College, Birmingham;
- Queen Elizabeth's Foundation Training College, Leatherhead;
- Royal National College for the Blind, Hereford;
- Royal National Institute of the Blind (RNIB) College, Loughborough;
- St Loye's Foundation, Devon.

Employment services in Northern Ireland

In Northern Ireland, the Department for Employment and Learning (DEL) has a network of Job and Benefit Offices/Jobcentres, where jobseekers can access 'Jobpoints', providing vacancy information. The Disablement Advisory Service (DAS) is part of DEL and provides the same range of services as found in the rest of the United Kingdom, with programmes delivered largely by independent contractors. Workable is a programme that gives people with disabilities the opportunity of working in a wide variety of jobs. The person's disability must have a significant adverse impact on their ability to carry out the particular job they are currently doing, or the job they are applying for.

Summary

The specialist disability services within Jobcentre Plus have a long history. Although mainstream programmes serving people with disabilities will be incorporated into the Work Programme, the specialist services will continue to operate, through Work Choice and other services.

The extent to which a reduced number of Work Programme providers are able to offer a qualitative service to disabled referrals remains to be seen, as does the extent to which they subcontract their services. It is evident that the prime driving force behind change is one of reducing public expenditure, and, operating on an outcome-related basis, service providers may be inclined to keep as much job broking/placing activity in-house as possible. Whether or not people with significant health conditions receive an appropriate service is likely to depend upon the level of payment being high enough for contractors to invest their resources in providing sufficient support.

Changes to the nature of services and cuts in public expenditure are likely to create a great deal of uncertainty for the VR market. Although the devil is in the detail, evidence on barriers to employment suggests that funding differentiation alone will not significantly reduce the total number of benefits claimants with health problems (whether on IB or ESA). What it will do, without appropriate RTW programmes, is create a large number of unemployed people with health problems and a reduced benefits income. A large influx of people with health problems into the labour market is likely to make the market even more competitive, with the whole system of moving claimants from one benefit to another being clogged by appeals owing to a flawed assessment process, although this might be addressed (see Chapter 6). In turn, this will create extra demand and pressures on remaining specialist services.

Student exercise

8.1 VR Accountability

(a) What are the main issues to take into consideration when measuring a VR service user's distance from the labour market?
(b) How can 'distance travelled' through VR intervention be measured?

9 National Health Service

Key issues

- Department of Health initiatives following the Black report (DWP/DH, 2008).
- The role of primary care.
- The use of barrier flags.
- VR aspects of the NSFs for long-term neurological conditions (LTNCs) and mental health (MH).
- The Scottish NHS.

Learning outcomes

- Knowledge of Department of Health developments.
- Ability to identify the appropriate use of rehabilitation flags.
- Familiarity with the guidance on delivering VR services for people with LTNCs and MH conditions.
- Knowledge of the individual placement and support (IPS) model of Supported Employment (SE).

Introduction

It is claimed that GPs and the primary care team are the patient's main source of advice about work (Waddell and Burton, 2004). Arguably, the historical separation of clinical care from employment and the rise in the number of IB claimants suggest that GPs and primary care teams have rarely sought or had the opportunity to address employment issues. Dame Black's Health and Well-Being report recognises that the United Kingdom has difficulties in getting GPs to address the employment aspects of a patient's condition (and, related to this, in getting employers to take a proactive approach to sickness absence). The report has contributed to a number of developments, including 'Fit Notes', a Workplace Well-being Tool and Fit for Work pilot programmes.

Implementation of the VR components of the National Service Frameworks (NSFs) faces different issues. Short-sightedness has led to the loss of VR resources and skills within the NHS. Although commissioners have until 2015 to implement the NSFs outside the MH sector, the extent to which NHS trusts in England and Wales are demonstrating a commitment towards meeting the VR requirements of the NSFs is questionable.

This chapter addresses the outlined developments arising from the Black report, as well as the requirements of the two NSFs with the greatest implications for VR. In the

MH sector, there has been a 'policy wave', to the extent that it is an artifice considering NSF requirements in isolation from other initiatives. Services for people with MH conditions do not operate in a vacuum isolated from each other. Hence, the IPS model of SE and the role of Jobcentre Plus are developed with a view to illustrating how MH strategies are serving a diverse population. The chapter concludes with a brief review of NHS progress in Scotland, where the Scottish government has taken the lead in rolling out a centrally developed rehabilitation strategy.

Developments arising from the Health and Well-Being Strategy

GPs and sickness certification

Mowlam and Lewis (2005) interviewed twenty-four GPs and found they had a very limited knowledge of VR services, including the work of Jobcentre Plus. A related study with participants in the JRRP (Chapter 3) found that patients generally did not look towards their GPs for advice about when to return-to-work (Farrell *et al.*, 2006). GPs often took a cautious approach, and participants talked of having to '*convince*' their GP that they were fit enough to work. VR service providers were also of the view that GPs tended to be conservative in their advice. They perceived a lack of active case management, with clients making slow progress within the NHS, especially if waiting for treatment, with a lack of referral to suitable specialists and clients not being encouraged to take action to help themselves. Various attempts have been made to stimulate a commitment towards employment issues among GPs. One successful, experimental approach is to place employment advisors in GP surgeries (Sainsbury *et al.*, 2008). There is much that can be done by GPs, such as identifying when a health condition results in an employment problem by using barrier flags and making appropriate referrals (Ford *et al.*, 2008). In the circumstances, it is not surprising that the Black report made recommendations to facilitate such developments.

Fit notes

From October 2009, new benefits claimants unable to work owing to ill health or disability became eligible for the new ESA instead of IB. Under the new regime, within weeks of making a claim, claimants have their capability assessed. Although it is claimed by government that the assessment focuses on what the claimant can do, many VR professionals are likely to consider the assessment process flawed, being based on a 'snap-shot' medical assessment and not a functional one.

From March 2010, the old sick note (Form Med 3), issued by GPs when a person had an illness or injury and was unable to work, was replaced by a statement of fitness to work. The fit notes have three categories of ability to work:

- fit for work
- not fit for work, and
- 'may be fit for some work now'.

When a GP places a patient in the final category, he or she must then go on to describe the functional effects of the employee's condition. GPs are now able to suggest workplace adjustments that may enable a patient to return-to-work at an earlier stage in their recovery: for example, a phased return, altered hours, amended duties and workplace adaptations.

Writing fit notes requires some knowledge of workplace health. The British Society of Rehabilitation Medicine (BSRM, 2004) identified two specific gaps in the knowledge of health professionals: a lack of understanding of the relationship between health and work (both how work may affect health, and how illness or disability may or may not affect work) and a lack of awareness of alternatives to, or options to minimise, sickness absence, such as work adjustments, organisational and other supports available and rehabilitation services. Although a GP can give an accurate statement of an individual's symptoms, the extent of their incapacity and a prognosis for how long the condition is likely to last, he/she will often have little idea of the impact that these have on the employee's role. GPs rarely have access to enough information about an individual's work to be able to make an informed assessment of their work-related capabilities. In any event, it may be considered that such an analysis is more properly the task of an OH professional. Some efforts are being made to address GP training. In May 2009, the Royal College of General Practitioners announced a National Education Programme, consisting of workshops designed to help GPs increase their knowledge, skills and confidence in dealing with clinical issues relating to work and health.

Black does call for an 'expanded role for occupational health', stating that such a service should be available to all. However, nothing like the required improvement in access to OH services is in prospect, leaving the question as to whether fit notes could aggravate the health problems of some employees assessed as fit for work.

As well as the practical issues surrounding fit notes, there are legal concerns. A doctor's recommendation in a fit note is not binding. However, if the employee can satisfy the definition of 'disabled' set out in the DDA, he or she may be able to insist that proposals in a fit note are reasonable adjustments and should be implemented by the employer. A difficult situation might also arise if there is a disagreement between a GP and a patient about what they can do. Under the new system, if a GP certifies an employee capable of light duties, but the employee does not want to do such work, or feels unable to do so, the question is raised as to whether or not an employer can insist on the modified return-to-work, on pain of a disciplinary sanction.

The Workplace Well-being Tool

This tool (www.dep.gov.uk/health-work-well-being/) has been designed to help employers deal with absence. It is divided into four sections:

1 measuring the cost of poor health and well-being;
2 comparing the level of absenteeism and turnover rate against those of other organisations;
3 practical ideas to help reduce health and well-being costs; and
4 estimating the costs and benefits of investing in well-being.

Fit for Work service

In October 2009, the DH and DWP revealed the ten sites pilot-testing the Fit for Work service (www.workingforhealth.gov.uk), the primary focus being to reach out to SMEs without access to specialist OH support. The pilots were also given a remit to look at models of support to help people on sickness benefit and interventions designed to support employees at risk of losing their jobs because of ill health. An evaluation is due during 2011.

Barrier flags (Box 9.1)

A 'flag system' has been developed to enable primary carers to identify potential work barriers (Kendall *et al.*, 2009). The flags provide a key framework in primary care to facilitate the assessment of patients and plan their return-to-work. Two or more flags can co-exist. For example, someone with 'red flag' back pain may also have yellow flag or blue flag harmful health beliefs.

Red flags

Red flags are the conventional biomedical barriers to employment. For example, in back pain, a red flag may be due to nerve-root pressure symptoms or signs, such as weakness in the leg, alterations in sensation or bladder symptoms. Other examples of red flags are serious cardiac arrhythmias, joint/locomotor instability, possible cancers or, in MH, suicidal intent or thought disorder.

Dealing with red flags

Although the emphasis is on clinical intervention, it must not be assumed that in all cases such activity excludes work. For example, pending investigations or surgery, there might be a possibility of continuing to be employed. Redeployment might be possible using transferrable skills and/or experience, for example from a manual to a non-manual position. Adjustments might facilitate job continuity.

Yellow flags

Yellow flags are usually regarded as health beliefs unrelated to the workplace (as opposed to blue flags, which are related). In this respect, the influence of the medical profession and the choice of language are significant: for example, dramatic comments such as 'you have had a severe heart attack' or 'you will never be able to do that again (a job or task)' might lead a patient to believe that they are severely incapacitated for the foreseeable future.

Dealing with the yellow flags

It is difficult for VR personnel to deal with yellow flags if someone has it firmly established in their mind that they should not work as a consequence of a discussion

---

Box 9.1 Barrier flags

- **Red flags**: medical barriers.
- **Orange flags**: mental health.
- **Yellow flags**: psychosocial factors.
- **Blue flags**: health beliefs within the workplace.
- **Black flags**: financial barriers.
- **Chequered flags**: social barriers.

with a GP or a consultant. Although there are instances when someone should not attempt work, what might be required is a GRTW plan or even a change of job. The importance of primary carers establishing a positive attitude that is going to facilitate the VR process cannot be underestimated. Examples of measures that can be taken include preventing harmful beliefs from becoming persistent, for example by GPs limiting the period for which they issue sick notes; making the point that waiting for an investigation does not necessarily preclude work; and avoiding specialist language that might create the impression of chronic disability.

Blue flags

Blue flags are the workplace barriers to recovery. They are often accounted for by psychosocial interactions between the employee and workplace managers, supervisors or colleagues.

Dealing with blue flags

The blue flags could be the most difficult ones for primary carers to address, because of a lack of familiarity with the workplace. The first principle must be to do no harm to the patient. Appropriate strategies include commenting with caution: for example, it might be easy to attribute a problem to 'workplace stress', but stress is not a medical term and can imply all sorts of conditions. Unless anyone knows what is going on in the workplace, such a diagnosis can only be speculative. Provided there is some evidence, it is always possible to indirectly refer to workplace difficulties, for example suggesting workplace support; preparing a patient for RTW by encouraging workplace contact; and careful use of the expression '*light duties*'. In the workplace, such a description often results in frustration as to what this means. It needs to be stated what a patient can and cannot do.

Black flags

Black flags are the barriers to rehabilitation caused by financial circumstances, such as benefits, insurance payments and litigation.

Dealing with black flags

Black flags are often characterised by timing issues, such as the end of half pay/ full pay. As a patient approaches such periods, he/she may be more receptive to suggestions to help them return-to-work. It is often wrongly assumed that a person cannot be dismissed while 'on the sick'. The reality is that anyone can be dismissed on the grounds of capability (albeit, any employer presumptuously taking such action runs the risk of unfair dismissal).

Chequered flags

Chequered flags are social factors, including care responsibilities, retirement preparations, civic and social responsibilities and other commitments outside work.

Dealing with chequered flags

An example of an approach that can be used is keeping a focus on work, so that, for example, if it is known that other activities are taking precedence over work considerations, the subject of (re)employment is raised.

National Service Frameworks

The problem of a lack of attention to vocation is not restricted to GPs. It has been found that rheumatologists and hospital-based therapists focus on physical rehabilitation and appear not to recognise which patients could benefit from a referral to Jobcentre Plus or the support that can be offered to working patients (Gilworth *et al.*, 2001).

Although many clinicians may perceive that their own lack of training and workload limit their involvement in employment matters, it is hard to escape the impression that many continue to consider that employment issues are not a priority and have little to do with them. This is not altogether surprising, given that clinical care must take priority and the limitations on VR facilities. Beard (2007) draws attrention to both the decline in resources and what can be positively achieved. The Occupational Therapy Assessment and Rehabilitation Service, based at the Royal Cornwall Hospital (Treliske), Truro, has one of the few remaining NHS trust workshops in the United Kingdom enabling patients with a broad range of disabilities, such as head injury, stroke, cardiac problems, amputations and hand injuries, to attend for treatment for up to 4 days per week, while providing a safe environment in which to work and receive support with either a return-to-work, education or voluntary work. Patients' treatment goals take on board required attributes for employment, such as stamina building and memory and perceptual, cognitive, physical and psychological skills. There is also a therapy gym and a Work Hardening Programme, enabling cardiac patients, in particular, to improve their psychological well-being with increased cardiovascular exercise. Employment support is often provided in liaison with Action for Employment (A4E), a Pathways to Work private sector provider, DEAs and the voluntary sector. The service's OT conducts workplace assessments and, if necessary, liaises with employers about any possible alternative job role, condition management within the role, and a GRTW plan. The OT monitors the GRTW, which is reviewed at regular intervals, and adjustments are made if necessary. During the initial stages of the GRTW process, patients continue to attend treatment. As they begin to decrease the amount of time they attend treatment, they increase the number of hours at the workplace. Only when a successful reintegration has been achieved will the patient be discharged from the service. Although many NHS trusts have some comparable service, without the same facilities, it is also the case that, historically, there has been a considerable loss of employment focus, which the VR aspects of the NSFs seek to address.

It remains to be seen if trusts fulfil the requirements or, facing financial restrictions, there remains a gap between existing government policy aspirations and the capacity of trusts to meet them.

LTNCs

The course of a neurological disease differs according to the condition and personal circumstances. Some conditions, for example stroke and traumatic brain injury (TBI), come on suddenly. The former is often associated with ageing, whereas young males are more likely to sustain TBI than females or other age groups. Other conditions, such as epilepsy, can be intermittent and unpredictable. Some, such as MS, are progressive, whereas others, for example cerebral palsy, are stable but with changing needs due to ageing. People with different conditions require different types of VR at different times.

The provision of VR services for people with LTNCs in the United Kingdom is patchy, and services are poorly defined. Some are provided by existing NHS rehabilitation services, some are linked to Jobcentre Plus, and others operate within the private or voluntary sectors.

Quality Requirement 6 of the NSF for LT(N)Cs highlights the need for services enabling people with LTNCs to enter work, education or training, remain in or return to their existing job, or withdraw from work at an appropriate time. All adults of working age with a LTNC should have their vocational needs considered as a routine part of their rehabilitation (Section 34). All adults of working age with a LTNC who are considered to have potential to work in any capacity should have access to local or specialist VR services, in accordance with the complexity of their needs (Section 35). Clinicians should put patients in touch with the relevant agencies as part of routine planning and refer, where appropriate, to a specialist VR programme. Patients with a LTNC seeking a return to employment, education or training should be assessed by a professional or team trained in vocational needs (Section 36). Assessment should take place within 4–6 weeks of referral and should include the patient activities shown in Box 9.2.

Rehabilitation teams should work directly with the person's local DEA and/or employer to support arrangements to enable the person to return to, or remain in, their existing employment or to identify alternative employment, including any training requirements, or need for VR or other support. Patients who are unable to return to employment or training should be given advice and support with regard to taking medical retirement, alternative financial support and other purposeful activities (Section 37) or be provided with alternative occupational provision or adult education appropriate to their needs (Section 38).

Box 9.2 NSF for LTNCs and assessment

- Evaluation of their medical condition to address any effects that might impact on their ability to work or study, and also to anticipate possible future effects.
- Evaluation of their individual vocational and/or educational needs.
- Identification of difficulties likely to limit the prospects of a successful RTW/education and appropriate intervention (including environmental adaptation, provision of assistive technology etc.) to minimise them.
- Direct liaison with employers (including OH services when available) or education providers to discuss needs and the appropriate action in advance of any return.
- Verbal and written advice about their return, including arrangements for review and follow-up.

Box 9.3 Evidence–based markers of good practice (LTNCs)

1   Co-ordinated multi-agency VR is provided which takes account of agreed national guidance and best practice.
2   Local rehabilitation services are provided that:
   •   address vocational needs during review of a person's integrated care plan and as part of any rehabilitation programme;
   •   work with other agencies to provide:
      – vocational assessment;
      – support and guidance on returning to or remaining in work;
      – support and advice on withdrawing from work;
   •   refer people with more complex occupational needs to specialist vocational services.
3   Specialist vocational services are provided for people with neurological conditions to address more complex problems in remaining in or returning to work or alternative occupation including:
   •   specialist vocational assessment and guidance;
   •   interventions for job retention including workplace support;
   •   specific VR or 'work preparation' programmes;
   •   alternative occupational and educational opportunities;
   •   specialist resources for advice for local services.
4   Specialist VR services routinely evaluate and monitor long-term vocational outcomes, including the reasons for failure to remain in employment.

Quality Requirement 6 is accompanied by four evidence-based markers of good practice (Box 9.3).

Guidance on the delivery of VR services for LT(N)Cs

Existing guidelines for people with acquired brain injuries (BSRM *et al.*, 2004) call for partnership working between health and social services and statutory and voluntary services to bridge service gaps and ensure that people can access services when they need them. Following publication of the NSF, the DH/DWP recognised that new guidance was required, addressing a wider range of neurological conditions than brain injury, and they commissioned *Vocational assessment and rehabilitation for people with long-term neurological conditions: recommendations for best practice* (BSRM, 2010). This document contains a literature review of the four exemplar conditions serving to illustrate particular difficulties – SCI, MS, epilepsy and cerebral palsy; recommendations for best practice; and an implementation section to help put recommendations into action. This includes key messages for specific professional groups, such as medical practitioners, community therapy staff and Jobcentre Plus work psychologists. The recommendations are divided into nine different subsections to account for the diversity of vocational support needs of people with neurological conditions:

1   General issues such as disclosure, consent and capacity.
2   Identification of vocational need and provision of information.
3   Vocational and employment assessment.
4   Job-retention interventions.
5   Return to occupation.
6   Withdrawal from work on health grounds.
7   Preparation for alternative occupation.
8   Transition from education to employment or other occupation.
9   Occupational and educational provision.

Exemplars of good practice

The DH has published models of good practice designed to encourage VR take-up by NHS Trusts (http://webarchive.nationalarchives.gov.uk/+/www.dh.gov.uk/en/Health care/Longtermconditions/Bestpractice/index.htm). This guidance includes:

- The National Hospital for Neurology and Neurosurgery, London. The Vocational Rehabilitation Service was established in 2006, and aims to support work retention for people with MS. Intervention consists of assessment, workplace visit, work planning, advice about and referral to Access to Work scheme, fatigue management and, where necessary, psychological assessment and physiotherapy input.
- The Pre-vocational programme for Adults with Acquired Brain Injury at the Moor Green, West Midlands Rehabilitation Centre. The programme assists service users to move towards their goal of returning to work through formal and informal assessment, the teaching of specific strategies and skills as part of an individualised programme and opportunities to practise work skills in-house. Defining RTW as a meaningful occupation (including paid employment, voluntary work, further vocational training and education), the programme has a reported 70 per cent success rate.
- Working Life Service and Vocational Service, Neurosupport, Liverpool. The Working Life Service works with people affected by neurological conditions. It offers advice, guidance and counselling around future directions, including work and meaningful alternatives to work. The Vocational Service works closely with the Working Life Service but focuses exclusively on vocational outcomes, such as jobs, retention, vocational training and voluntary work.
- 'Working Out', Community Head Injury Service (CHIS), Vale of Aylesbury PCT. In the early 1990s, the DH established a number of specialist head-injury projects including 'Working Out'. The Employment Service later provided funding under the Work Preparation programme. Despite the success of Working Out, it has not been replicated elsewhere, although there was such a recommendation from the House of Commons Select Committee on Health in 2001. The service is provided by a rehabilitation team comprising clinical psychologists, medical practitioners, nursing staff, OTs, physiotherapists, social workers, speech therapists and administrative staff, working in conjunction with local acute and community services, including the specialist Regional Neuroscience Services and other agencies, particularly Social Services, Jobcentre Plus and the local Headways Group. The programme was established with the aims shown in Box 9.4.

Box 9.4 Working out programme aims

1   To assess the vocational impact and needs of persons with severe TBI.
2   To provide specialist rehabilitation programmes to clarify and enhance vocational potential.
3   To set up and evaluate voluntary work trials to prepare persons for a return to productive occupation.
4   To find, set up and support suitable long-term work placements for persons with severe TBI.

The aims are addressed through four interlinked phases of vocational assessment, work preparation, voluntary work trials and long-term/supported placements, as indicated. Each client activity is given the following time span:

Vocational programme	*Typical duration*
Initial assessment	Half-day
Vocational assessment	3 weeks
Work preparation	12 weeks +
Voluntary work trial	12 weeks +
Work placement	6 months +

Assessment

The initial approach to meeting the client's needs is based upon an assessment undertaken at the weekly Head Injury Clinic. The aim is to obtain a detailed social and clinical history and a profile of current problems, as perceived by the person and their family. Close family members are requested to accompany a new referral. An extended vocational assessment consists of a full 3 or 4 weeks of interviews, formal tests, group work and observation/ratings of work performance and behaviour, as well as the application of other assessment tools as required, for example functional capability and work personality (see Boxes 9.5 and 9.6).

Box 9.5 Functional assessment inventory

- task orientation
- social skills
- work motivation
- work conformance
- personal presentation

(Bolton and Roessler, 1986a,b)

Box 9.6 Work personality profile

- adaptive behaviour
- motor functioning
- cognition
- physical condition
- communication
- vocational qualifications
- vision

(Crewe and Athelstan, 1984)

Following the assessment, there is a feedback session with the client and family at which subject aims are addressed. Specific objectives are agreed with the referring agency as well, where appropriate.

Work preparation

Subjects referred within 12–24 months of injuries and others, who have had little or no specialist head-injury input are considered likely to require a period of VR/work preparation to prepare for a RTW. A reliance on voluntary work trials is accompanied by a continuing in-house placement support group and education/training. The aims of the rehabilitation programme are as indicated in Box 9.7.

Rehabilitation programmes consist of any combination of the following components:

1   work-preparation group
2   community-rehabilitation activities
3   individual project work
4   rehabilitation counselling
5   vocational counselling
6   psychological therapy
7   personal-issues group
8   cognitive-rehabilitation group
9   Brain injury educational programme.

Box 9.7 Working out rehabilitation aims

1   to facilitate further recovery and adaptation
2   to assess realistic work potential
3   to promote more accurate self-appraisal
4   to foster positive work attitudes and behaviour

In the final week of the programme, a formal review with the client, discussion with the Working Out team and liaison with the DEA and, where appropriate, other agencies, are conducted prior to a feedback/review meeting with the client and family in the Head Injury Clinic. Following rehabilitation, the client will usually progress to a voluntary work trial.

Voluntary work trials

A placement co-ordinator works with the client to find a suitable part-time, voluntary work trial, usually of up to 12 weeks, in a local service or business. These typically start with half a day per week, with a graded increase in line with progress. Voluntary work trials are usually run in parallel with a reducing rehabilitation programme, gradually replacing individual project work and community group activities. The trials serve a number of purposes, including independent assessment of work potential; identification of, and adaptation to, outstanding difficulties; the re-establishment of work routine and behaviours; supervised and graded rebuilding of self-confidence; and an independent reference for those applying for jobs. Trials are monitored by the placement co-ordinator (in some respects acting as a job coach, but not providing *in situ* work support). Any major difficulties highlighted in the trial are addressed within the rehabilitation programme. On completing the trial, a review with the person and supervisor and, as appropriate, liaison with the DEA are undertaken to agree further plans. This is usually a long-term placement, but, in some cases, a further voluntary trial will be required. Clients then graduate to one of a wide range of long-term placements, depending upon their potential.

Mapping VR services for people with LTNCs

The DH recognises that it is unclear as to what extent existing services fit with NSF recommendations or meet the differing needs of people with LTNCs. As a consequence, a project led by Dr Diane Playford, University College, London, and Dr Kate Radford, University of Central Lancashire, has been identifying VR services available in England and considering the extent to which they fit published recommendations. The project will provide:

- a directory of specialist VR services for use by those who provide or need a VR service;
- maps showing the location of specialist VR services in England;
- a guide to establishing VR services for both commissioners and providers;
- support for partnership development, with the potential to set up communities of VR providers;
- exemplars of good practice;
- a questionnaire that can be used to monitor the development of new VR services and the implementation of the NSF; and
- an online forum for sharing information about services, which will include examples of good VR services.

Mental health

Because of cross-government approaches to MH, the NSF needs to be considered in relation to broader developments in the sector. *Pathways to Work* (DWP, 2002) records

MH as the largest cause for claiming IBs (35 per cent). Commonly reported restrictions among people with less severe conditions are limitations in the type of job; the need for a support person; difficulty in changing jobs; and limitations on working hours. People with MH problems are particularly sensitive to the negative effects of unemployment and the loss of structure, purpose and identity it entails. Not only is work important in maintaining and promoting MH, it reduces the need to use health services. Work provides: (a) social identity and status, to the extent of being perceived by many as a yardstick of recovery; (b) social contacts and support; and (c) a means of structuring and occupying time and a sense of personal achievement (Evans and Repper, 2000).

Dame Black commissioned a report on MH from the Royal College of Psychiatrists, separate to her review of the health of Britain's working-age population (Lelliott *et al.*, 2008). This report describes two separate groups: those with symptoms of common mental disorders, who account for the majority of costs related to mental ill health, and people with severe mental illness (SMI). A recognition of the nature of the population is reflected in New Labour's response to the problem of unemployment, where the Social Exclusion Unit addresses issues cutting across government departments, with the DH taking the lead with regards to people with SMI, supported by social services at a local level, and DWP/Jobcentre Plus has responsibility for people with less-severe conditions, frequently undertaking this activity in conjunction with local NHS services (SEU, 2004). Although this division is simplistic, it helps to understand the nature of services. Vocational strategies need to reflect the client's history and distance from the labour market; hence, CMPs, accessed through Jobcentre Plus, began to receive service users with more commonly found conditions, whereas supported models of employment, accessed through health and social services, dealt with people with SMI.

The NSF primarily addresses the VR needs of people with SMI and requires action within the enhanced CPA to enable service users to seek paid employment 'as local circumstances allow'. Other significant policy papers are *Working our way to better mental health: a framework for action* (DWP, 2009) and *Realising ambition: better employment support for people with a mental health condition*, the 'Perkins Review' (Perkins *et al.*, 2009; see Box 9.8). The former paper provides the national MH and employment strategy and the vision of a society in which everyone can experience the benefits of employment.

Individual placement and support

Critical to the recommended VR approach for people with SMI, advanced in the NSF and by Perkins, is the development of the IPS model of SE. IPS does not rely on prevocational assessment and preparation – 'train and place'. Instead, there is an emphasis on rapid job placement combined with extensive support – 'place and train' (Stein and Cutler, 2002; Crowther *et al.*, 2004). The rationale for the 'place–train' approach is that, without knowing what type of job an individual will obtain, it is inefficient to train the person for the specific skills, including social skills, that will be needed in a particular job. Although 'place and train' reduces the need to transfer skills to a new environment, the process requires a considerable amount of client support. The mechanics of getting to work, learning the job and working flexible hours are all important (Cook and Razzano, 2000; Bustillo *et al.*, 2001; O'Flynn, 2001).

Although IPS is promoted as evidence-based practice, UK protagonists rely heavily on research findings from other countries, particularly the United States. Some evidence

---

Box 9.8 Main recommendation of the Perkins Review

1   Increasing capacity and dispelling myths:
    • Building links between DWP, health and social services.
    • Increasing the extent to which RTW services can accommodate the needs of people with a MH condition, for example by ensuring continuity.
    • Increasing extent to which support offered by DWP, health and social services meets the needs of people with MH conditions seeking work and their potential employers, for example by providing better information and assistance in managing MH conditions.
    • Supporting initiatives to address misunderstandings among employers, employees, and the services that support them.
2   Providing more support (this recommendation supports IPS for 'those who require more intensive specialised support'):
    • Health and social services to be responsible for those who need to be provided with the additional intensive support over and above that provided through welfare to work services. Employment specialists to be 'embedded' in primary care and secondary care MH teams.
    • DWP to be responsible for providing the resources necessary to provide the flexible, individually tailored assistance that some people need to sustain work through reformed Access to Work. Such support may be commissioned from a local agency with expertise in evidence-based SE.
    • To ease the transition from benefits to work, DWP to 'ensure the availability of time-limited internships in parallel with job search', gradually building up the hours for those needing work experience.
3   Effective monitoring and drivers for change:
    • Health and social services to routinely monitor employment outcomes for people they serve.
    • DWP to do likewise.
    • Service provision and employment outcomes for people with a MH condition to form part of core commissioning criteria, key performance indicators and inspection criteria for DWP, health and social services.

---

suggests 30–40 per cent job placement rates, compared with 10–12 per cent for other approaches, such as 'train and place'. VR clients placed through this approach are also said to work longer hours and have higher earnings and better job tenure (Dixon *et al.*, 2002; Lehman et al, 2002; Boardman *et al.*, 2003; Drake *et al.*, 2003; Crowther *et al.*, 2004). Bond *et al.* (2007) analysed the results of eleven randomised, controlled trials. One study, EQOLISE (Burns *et al.*, 2007), covered six European countries, including the United Kingdom. It found that IPS participants were twice as likely to gain employment compared with those experiencing traditional VR alternatives (Box 9.9). Although Burns found that employment outcomes are influenced by local employment rates and benefit levels, IPS was still more successful than standard interventions. There was no deterioration in MH as a result of taking up work. A proportion of IPS participants remained unmotivated or unable to maintain open employment, but it was not possible to identify these people when they first joined a programme. This is considered to show that a policy of zero exclusion is essential.

The principles of the IPS approach (Box 9.10) rely on the employment specialist rapidly engaging with clients to find a work placement, even if for only a few hours a week.

Box 9.9 Results from EQOLISE study

1 IPS participants are twice as likely to gain employment (55 per cent v. 28 per cent), compared with traditional VR alternatives.
2 IPS participants sustained jobs longer and earned more than those who were supported by the best local VR alternatives.
3 Better results were obtained by implementing IPS principles in full.
4 The quality of partnership working between health and employment providers is a critical success factor.

(Adapted from Burns *et al.*, 2007)

Box 9.10 The principles of the IPS model

1 Rehabilitation is considered an integral component of MH treatment rather than a separate service. Full-time employment specialists co-ordinate plans with the treatment/rehabilitation team.
2 The goal of IPS is competitive employment in integrated work settings, both part-time and full-time. The focus is on jobs anyone can apply for, paying at least the minimum wage.
3 People with SMI can succeed in open employment without pre-employment training. Job search starts soon after a client expresses an interest in working. There are no requirements for completing extensive pre-employment assessment and training, nor intermediate work experiences (such as prevocational work, transitional employment or sheltered work).
4 Vocational assessment is continuous and based in competitive work settings, rather than artificial or sheltered settings.
5 Follow-along support is continuous and maintained as long as client requires it.
6 Job finding, job preferences and supports are based on the client's preferences, rather than the provider's judgements.
7 Services are provided in the community.
8 A multidisciplinary team approach, rather than parallel interventions in separate agencies or systems, promotes the integration of vocational, clinical and support services.

(Becker and Drake, 2003)

Bond *et al.* (2008) reviewed evidence for the principles of SE, with the following findings:

- strong evidence that services focused on competitive employment are effective and more recovery-oriented than other kinds of employment;
- strong evidence that a wide range of consumers benefit with eligibility based only on desire to work;
- strong evidence that rapid job search for competitive employment rather than extensive preparation is more effective;
- moderate evidence for integration of SE with MH treatment;
- moderate evidence that attention to consumer preferences (tailoring the job) is effective;
- weak evidence that time-unlimited services and follow-along services are important (although this is a central tenet of the IPS model); and
- weak evidence that benefits counselling positively affects earnings.

Fidelity scales

Two available fidelity scales assess the extent to which VR agencies conform to the strict descriptors of the IPS model:

- IPS Fidelity Scale (Bond *et al.*, 2008). This scale appears to be preferred in the United Kingdom (Box 9.11).
- Quality of Supported Employment Implementation Scale (Bond *et al.*, 2000).

Box 9.11   IPS Fidelity-Scale items

Subscale	Item label	Item descriptor
Staffing	Case-load size	Employment specialists manage case-loads of up to 25 clients
	Exclusively vocational	Employment specialists provide only vocational services
	Generalist model	Each employment specialist carries out all phases of vocational services
Organisation	Contact with MH	Employment specialists are part of MH treatment team; routinely share MH team
	Vocational unit	Employment specialists work as a unit – have group supervision and shared case-loads
	Zero exclusion	No eligibility requirement (such as job readiness) for programme
Services	Continuous	Vocational assessment is ongoing and based on work experiences in competitive jobs
	Rapid search	Job search occurs rapidly after programme entry
	Client choice	Client preferences and needs determine employer contracts, not the job market
	Diversity of jobs	Jobs are diverse in type and setting
	Permanent jobs	Jobs are competitive and permanent
	Multiple jobs	Clients are assisted in finding new jobs after employment ends

These scales are similar, although the former is shorter and is easy to implement. Both scales have the capacity to distinguish high-fidelity from low-fidelity programmes. Scores have been shown to correlate with service users' success in obtaining competitive employment, and programmes with high fidelity achieve better outcomes (Gowdy *et al.*, 2003; Becker *et al.*, 2006).

The advantages of obtaining a high score on the Fidelity Scale are indicated in Box 9.12.

Although the advocates of IPS praise the resettlement figures, they are still low compared with VR resettlement figures in general. There remain questions in respect of job tenure. Anecdotal evidence from developments within the United Kingdom suggests that services often find it difficult to apply a true model of IPS, and that they have to rely on voluntary work placements. However, innovations in delivering the IPS model are nothing new, including using alternatives to competitive employment for clients and adding supported education to supported employment (Unger *et al.*, 2000).

In a literature review, Loveland *et al.* (2007) consider means to enhance IPS. This includes providing staff with access to model programmes and site visits, allowing flexibility when piloting the programme through incremental stages, and allowing staff a minimum of 12 months to implement a SE programme In addition, having a frontline clinician as the 'programme champion' and involving this person in the implementation process improve outcomes (*Ahrens et al.*, 1999). The 2009 Sainsbury Centre for Mental Health Briefing 37, *Doing what works* considers that,

> Implementation of IPS needs to be driven by senior managers in both commissioning bodies and provider organisations. They need a strong commitment to organisational change and capacity building as IPS requires changes in the thinking of many mental health teams and employment services and the will to make changes at every level.

The briefing adds that a lack of commissioning of IPS services is contributing to the holding up of developments in the United Kingdom, with employment still not being considered a priority for MH services, nor seen as a realistic goal for people who have

---

Box 9.12 Advantages of a high score on the Fidelity Scale

- People using services can be given a clear idea of what kind of service to expect, with a focus on their preferences and real jobs, good communication, with clinical teams and an assurance that quality standards will be maintained.
- Employment services can achieve the best outcomes possible, and their practice will be continually monitored and improved.
- Health services have a means of giving people's health attention within an integrated package of care, and this will lead to better clinical *and* vocational outcomes.
- Commissioners have a clear service specification that they can be confident will produce the best possible employment outcomes compared with any realistic alternative. IPS is also said to be cost-effective and have a built-in check on quality.

(Adapted from Rinaldi *et al.*, 2008)

experienced MH problems, a situation exacerbated by a lack of knowledge of, or belief in, the research evidence and a lack of IPS-trained practitioners, in both employment and health services.

It is difficult to establish the extent to which IPS and positive employment practices are being adopted within the United Kingdom. Standard 5 of the NSF requires that care plans for people with more serious MH problems include 'action needed for employment, education or training or another occupation'. Bertram and Howard (2006) found community mental health teams (CMHTs) a long way from achieving this aim, with only 8 per cent of case notes addressing vocational needs. Rinaldi and Perkins (2007B) discuss the implementation of the IPS model in eight CMHTs from two London boroughs, noting that, 'there is little evidence of such approaches in routine clinical settings in the UK'.

Implementing the IPS model

A principle of IPS involves co-locating employment services with MH teams. The benefits are said to be better communication; improved co-ordination and coherence in a client's journey through the 'system'; the process of seeking employment remains sensitive to a person's clinical needs; concerns of clinicians can be directly addressed; vocational information is incorporated into care plans; and first-hand observation can convince MH teams of the efficacy of the focus on employment, resulting in more effective engagement and retention and better outcomes for the individual (Drake *et al.*, 2003).

In establishing IPS, Rinaldi *et al.* (2008) stress the need to recognise the concerns of the care team: for example, there is no evidence that IPS increases the likelihood of relapse; the need to present a practical understanding of the evidence base, in particular the evidence on client characteristics and the likely predictors of success; and the need to encourage all clients to participate, regardless of their job readiness (Box 9.13).

An integral aspect of IPS is the full integration of a non-clinician in the care team. The role of employment specialists is described as:

•   case-managing clients' vocational needs, including assessment, help obtaining and retaining work/education, support and adjustments in the workplace and benefits advice;

Box 9.13 Fears and concerns of care co-ordinators and psychiatrists

1   Whether or not clients are able to work – not wanting to 'set them up to fail'.
2   The stress of working may lead to relapse and possible hospitalisation.
3   Work would interfere with the client's stability.
4   Welfare benefits would be jeopardised.
5   Employers would discriminate against people with MH problems.
6   Placing clients into positions of responsibility could increase the risk of harm to others.
7   Employment specialists are not clinicians, so they will not be able to judge whether someone is able to work.

(Rinaldi *et al.*, 2008)

- co-ordinating vocational plans with CMHT staff and ensuring vocational plans are given a high priority; and
- working with employers and other agencies, such as Jobcentre Plus, to develop opportunities and client support (Rinaldi and Perkins, 2007b).

In general, employment specialists work with up to twenty-five clients at a time. They are said to spend 70 per cent or more of their time in the community, carrying out vocational activities such as job finding, assessment and providing ongoing support (Rinaldi *et al.*, 2008). Although fully integrated as members of the clinical team, they do not carry out care responsibilities. The process of integration is not straightforward and can be accompanied by team members asking why more care co-ordinators have not been employed, rather than an employment specialist. Key competencies for an employment specialist are indicated in Box 9.14.

Does IPS spell the end for other VR models?

There is criticism of sheltered employment programmes for a failure to move participants into open employment (Rinaldi et al, 2008). The extent to which they have been designed and expected to fulfil a transitional role, or act as anything other than a worthwhile alternative to a lack of productive activity, is open to question. The comparison to sheltered employment for many people with MH problems is not the benefits of competitive employment but the downside of inactivity and social isolation. The extent to which sheltered employment may be supporting those people who cannot benefit from IPS is not known.

Although studies show that, when people with SMI are enrolled in specific employment-focused services, they achieve employment outcomes superior to standard services – such as day treatment – and results from controlled trials have demonstrated the effectiveness of IPS in placing participants into open employment, data point towards high drop-out rates and job placements that are typically part-time, low skilled, minimum wage and short lasting. Many clients of the IPS model are unable to benefit from it. Taking a broad view of the SE model, up to 50 per cent find work in the open labour

---

Box 9.14   Key competencies for an employment specialist

- Experience and knowledge of job development, job marketing and job securing.
- The ability to relate positively to employers.
- Knowledge of MH problems.
- The ability to identify an individual's interests, strengths, skills, abilities and coping styles and to match them with jobs.
- Knowledge about welfare benefits.
- The ability to advocate for people with other team members, employers and families.

(Rinaldi *et al.*, 2008)

market, but around half of these are unable to sustain a job beyond a very short period of time (Lehman *et al.*, 2002; Mueser *et al.*, 2004; Gold *et al.*, 2006, Latimer *et al.*, 2006; Macias *et al.*, 2006). IPS does not have alternatives to offer clients who do not succeed in finding or holding down jobs. Equally, the longer-term outcomes of IPS are not clear, as most studies end after 12–24 months. Although there are four studies with a time frame longer than 3 years, the findings are equivocal (McHugo *et al.*, 1998; Chandler *et al.*, 1999; Salyers *et al.*, 2004; Becker *et al.*, 2007). In the circumstances, including the requirement for organisational change and difficulties in finding 'real work' in a tightening labour market, it is not surprising to find some opposition to introducing IPS, although advocates continue to promote the benefits.

Integrating VR strategies

There are clear indications that different VR strategies are required for the two major groups of people identified with MH problems. IPS is just one of the various VR strategies for people with SMI that have been developed over the years (Table 9.1). Although the first clubhouse was established in 1991, the model, based on providing a base for recovery and transitional labour market participation, has not taken off in the United Kingdom.

People with more commonly found problems, such as anxiety and other neuroses, require a different approach to people with SMI. However, there are insufficient means of identifying into which group some VR referrals may fall, and there are insufficient guidelines (a lack of evidence-based practice) for matching job-retention strategies to individuals. In recognition of the multiplicity of factors influencing the employment prospects of people with a MH condition, Booth *et al.* (2007) outlined the principles for an effective employment strategy (Box 9.15).

The approach starts with an identification of the most relevant interventions for overcoming work-related barriers. Booth and colleagues describe a person's relationship to the labour market as a continuum (Figure 9.1). Movement along the continuum is often related to the severity of the condition, ranging from severe and enduring problems, such as psychosis, to more common and manageable conditions, such as anxiety and depression, through to those people who have always experienced good MH. An additional element is that many people have fluctuating conditions (one reason why there is no exact correlation between status and employment position). As a consequence, sustained employment interspersed with periods of worklessness is a common pattern. To make the transition to employment there is a need to build work capacity. Intervention requires recognition of the person's distance from the labour market in order to implement the key tasks (Figure 9.2).

Booth *et al.* accept that the absence of 'overarching local strategies', unifying health and other public and voluntary sector services, inhibits the delivery of a holistic approach

Table 9.1 Categories of employment support (after Crowther *et al.*, 2001; Schneider, 2005)

Sheltered work	*Prevocational training and education*	*Supported employment*
Sheltered workshops	Supported education	Individual placement and support
Work crews	Work rehabilitation	Transitional employment
Community businesses Clubhouse	Prevocational training	Workstep

---

Box 9.15 Key areas for a MH employment strategy

- Influencing the belief and aspirations of the client (self-efficacy is perceived to have a key function).
- Effecting cultural change by consistently enhancing the message that work is health enhancing for most people.
- Considering environmental factors and recognising the links between housing, health, educational attainment and employability to address unintentional consequences. (It is recognised that the Housing and Council Tax benefit tapers can be 'a stumbling block' for some trying work under the Permitted Work rules.)
- Responding to basic needs such as transport and mobility (particularly in rural areas).
- Building capacity for work.
- Supporting employers.

(Booth *et al.*, 2007)

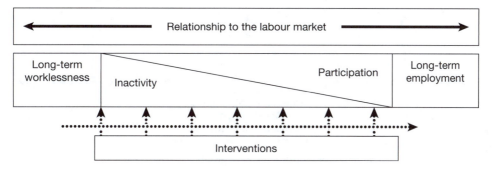

Figure 9.1 The employment continuum

Source: Booth *et al.* (2007).

to RTW needs. Nevertheless, they advance the capacity of VR stakeholders to support MH 'customers' through such measures as the use of CBT (Layard, 2005); awareness; and advocacy training, such as employment advisers believing they can deliver effective jobsearch support to people with MH issues and providing employment support. This may seem common sense, but it is observed that,

> whilst it is doubtless important to attempt to change the individual's beliefs about work, many of the barriers are systemic and many of the individual's current behaviours can be viewed as rationally based reaction to their perceptions about current chances of being helped to gain employment.

The need to increase and improve the skills and knowledge of current advisers is recognised.

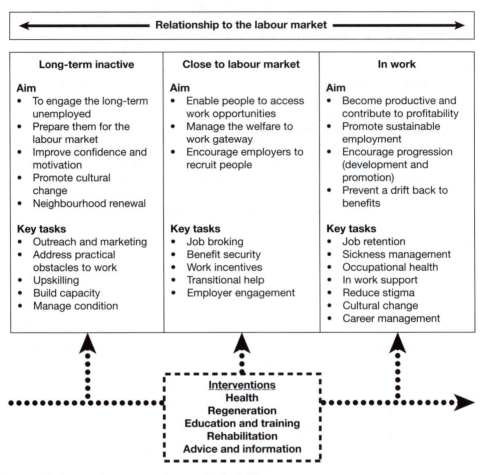

Figure 9.2 An employment continuum for the MH group
Source: Booth *et al.* (2007).

Process of keeping and finding a job

Booth *et al.* base their strategies on an analysis of effective work-related support, including:

1 Supporting the individual to prepare for jobsearch.
2 Supporting effective jobsearch activity. People with MH conditions have greater reason than other jobseekers to consider factors such as hours, travel and workplace conditions. Long-term dependency on the security of incapacity benefits (ESA) may also produce financial uncertainties.
3 Supporting successful job retention and career progression.

It will be apparent that an individual is likely to need different types of support at different stages of the RTW process, depending on their distance from the labour market. In respect of delivering work-related support to people with MH problems, Booth *et al.* propose an 'effective model' comprising:

- advice and information
- motivation and confidence building
- basic and employment skills
- job broking and advocacy support
- in-work provision
- OH services.

Although different elements of such services are provided in most areas, they are rarely combined into a holistic employment service, and, hence, a starting point is to 'compile a comprehensive map of appropriate services available in each vicinity with a view to identifying where there is duplication, overlap, sufficient provision or gaps, and to gauge their current suitability and effectiveness'. Organisations involved in providing RTW services, such as voluntary organisations, NHS, social services/social work departments, Jobcentre Plus, should agree:

1 an overall strategic framework to guide joint working;
2 a single entry point;
3 methods for deciding who is best placed to act as a case manager and co-ordinate activity between organisations;
4 specific roles for each organisation to ensure sufficient interventions are available;
5 funding flexibility to ensure that resources are directed to meeting individual need; and
6 a local skills audit identifying providers' need to increase skills base.

A number of 'core concepts' underpin the delivery of effective work-related support (Table 9.2).

Table 9.2 Core concepts for effective work-related support

1 Self-efficacy.
2 Medical model versus resources model. In contrast to the medical model, resulting in deficits that need to be treated being cited as a barrier to employment, the resources model encourages the individual to explore their own abilities and interests and to identify realistic job goals and development needs. The aim is to match personal resources to key job tasks and activities.
3 Managing the health condition.
4 Managing the jobsearch process, involving:
  – self-knowledge
  – labour market knowledge
  – decision-making
  – making the transition.
5 Job-keeping skills.
6 Managing retention.
7 Meeting individual needs.
8 Meeting employer needs.
9 Intermediary needs, relating to the case manager being able to demonstrate advanced skills in advocacy, negotiation, offering practical support to the client and employer and providing in-work support, such as job coaching and advice on work adjustments.

All of these concepts are very much part of the VR process addressed in Part 3 and equally applicable to VR service users with a wide range of health conditions. The skill of the VR service provider is in recognising, and being able to deliver, appropriate VR strategies for the unemployed who have MH problems but are close to the labour market and VR strategies for people in employment (Figure 9.3).

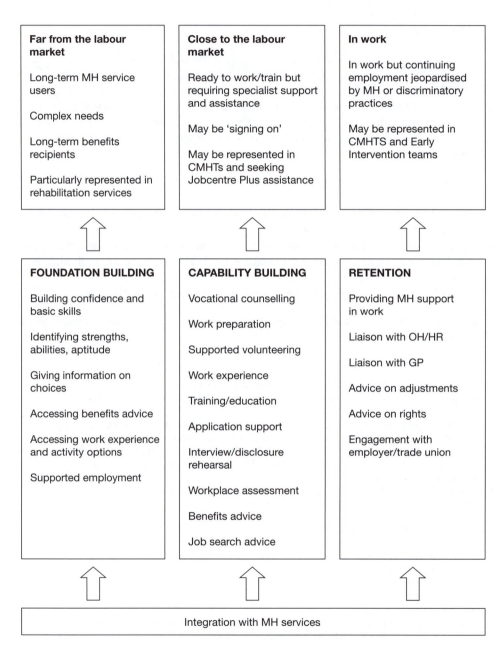

Figure 9.3 Matching support to VR service user's distance from the labour market

Scottish NHS VR model (see Chapter 3 for policy development)

In 2008, the Scottish government backed a pilot VR project based in Dundee. Owing to the success of this project, another two Working Health Service projects, based in NHS Lothian and NHS Borders, were launched, with funding from the Scottish government and DWP until 2011. These three projects consist of multidisciplinary teams and use a case management approach. An interim evaluation of the Dundee project gives strong indications that participants have benefited from the programme, with improved health and RTW. A greater proportion of men have been referred to the programme than might have been expected, based on employment levels (NHS Tayside, 2009).

The Dundee VR team

The Dundee VR team consists of a project manager, administrator, case manager (recruited on secondment from Jobcentre Plus), two physiotherapists, a part-time OT and a psychological therapist/counsellor. The team also has access to an OH advisor, OH physician and complementary therapies.

Location

As part of the ethos of developing community-based services, the team is based in an industrial estate, with staff running clinics in various community venues, including NHS and local-authority premises.

Referrals

The team promotes self-referrals. Referrals are also accepted from GPs and other health professionals, although the service user is encouraged to take the initiative in contacting the project. Although the service is promoted to employers, the role of managers is to highlight the service to their employees. This measure was taken to encourage the concept of self-referral and prevent employers from 'using' the project to 'offload' employees they no longer wished to employ. Subsequent to the launch of the service, there was a rush in numbers that levelled off (some 180 self-referrals during the first 6 months).

Use of technology

All information, including subsequent assessment results and the deliberations of the VR team at a weekly case conference, is entered onto an intranet programme, which is available only to the members and accessed by their password. Not only does this reduce the amount of paper records, but it also has the advantage of being accessible to the team members when out-stationed.

Team members and services

Administrator

The administrator is the first point of contact for the self-referral and records basic demographic details. The administrator also carries out follow-up interviews with all clients at 3 and 6 months post-discharge to determine health and employment status.

Case manager

Unless a problem has been identified, such as a speech impediment, hearing difficulty or any other challenges to the client, the initial assessment with the case manager also takes place over the telephone within 48 hours of the initial telephone contact with the project. In addition to developing the history and establishing the client's perspective on what they wish to get from the service, the case manager routinely administers the EQ-5D, addressing quality of life issues and the Canadian Occupational Performance Measure (COPM) (Chapter 12). The GHQ12 (General Health Questionnaire 12) is administered when a MH problem is identified. In contrast to the ease of administering EQ-5D and COPM, some of the questions on the GHQ12 may be considered too sensitive to ask over the telephone. The results of this preliminary assessment are used by the case manager to determine further intervention and referral within the team.

Psychological therapist/counsellor

The psychological therapist/counsellor is *not* a vocational counsellor (someone providing careers advice) but is an accredited counsellor trained in CBT. In addition, the counsellor has an OH background. This enables the team to address broader issues than just the immediate person–job fit. Following musculoskeletal conditions, people with MH issues such as stress, anxiety and depression form the second-largest group of referrals, although the process of encouraging early referrals, following an absence from work, has resulted in receiving some clients with more acute problems. With client consent, the counsellor may write to the GP to recommend referral to mainstream MH services.

Occupational therapist

Following initial assessment by the case manager, the OT may carry out a variety of specific assessments, including daily living activities, job analysis, work-site assessments and work–life balance. Work-site assessments are undertaken with the client's consent and permission from the employer. Not all clients require a work-site assessment, and not all clients want their employer to know that they are receiving support. If a work-site assessment is required and agreed, the employee is visited at work and observed carrying out the tasks required to do their job. Advice, education and use of different techniques and routines are discussed with the client. A written report is then sent to the client to highlight the recommendations and to assist with implementation. This information can then be disseminated to the employer. Display-screen-equipment assessments are common within the workplace. This takes into account not only the relationship of the person to the workstation but all the physical, organisational and environmental factors affecting their working day. There have been increasing numbers of referrals to the OT with stress-related problems. This is often a combination of life and work stressors.

Physiotherapists

Two physiotherapists work within the service. One therapist is part of the rotation scheme for staff within NHS Tayside. This enables more staff to gain experience in multi-disciplinary working within VR. Using standard physiotherapy tools and outcome measures, the physiotherapists assess clients presenting with any musculoskeletal problems. As this is a direct-access service to the working population, the physiotherapists also carry out appropriate screening to exclude any serious pathology prior to treatment, and may refer on as appropriate. The most common problems presenting to the service are low-back pain and neck pain. The physiotherapists also offer advice and support to other physiotherapists working within NHS Tayside regarding VR and work-related issues that may be affecting a client's recovery or RTW status.

Follow-up and evaluation

If a client fails to appear for an appointment, there is a follow-up procedure to establish the reason, but clients are under no obligation to participate. Clients completing the programme, of varying length according to circumstances, are followed up at 3 and 6 months to establish their status. Re-administering the COPM and EQ-5D forms part of the evaluation procedure.

Relationships with employers are critical to the success of the programme. There is a potential working difficulty not faced by private sector VR companies (instructed by insurance companies and employers). The OT and case manager are the only staff members likely to work directly with employers, but can only do so once client consent has been given. However, this does not guarantee that the employer will necessarily co-operate. Although no major problems are reported from 'the early days', the issues of approaching and negotiating with the employer have to be handled with tact.

Critical benefits advice is available from the case manager, and there is a working relationship with Dundee City Council's employment and disability services. There is also a link-up with Jobcentre Plus, so that clients who might require an assessment by a work psychologist may receive it, and those clients who are not going to return to their employment also receive appropriate support. It is recognised that there are clients who would benefit from a period of work hardening (WH) or conditioning (WC) as a stepping-stone back to their employment, and community links have been developed.

Summary

The provision of VR services within the NHS has suffered from historical neglect, with evidence of consequential high costs for employers, the state and, not least, the individuals concerned. Although pockets of excellence have continued to exist, the overall impression is that there is a low starting point for delivering the VR components of the NSFs. Although there is some modest progress in the delivery of MH services, elsewhere it can be difficult to identify significant developments in the NHS, England and Wales. VR is not high on the agenda of many NHS commissioners. This is in contrast to NHS Scotland, where the Scottish government has seized the initiative with regards to providing VR services for a section of the population not otherwise served and, in doing so, facilitating retention. It remains to be seen how the availability of funding affects the development of this innovative and successful venture.

It has taken 5 years from the publication of the NSF for LT(N)Cs to the BSRM detailed guidelines on how best to implement vocational assessments and rehabilitation. The detailed nature of these guidelines, in contrast to the limitations of Quality Requirement 6, raises questions as to the extent that the DH really understands and is committed to VR, as opposed to voicing a political orthodoxy. In the absence of an overarching, timetabled strategy, those wishing to continue to develop VR services, in the same piecemeal fashion, will continue to need to take the initiative and investigate local resources, including identifying and meeting their own training needs. Even in the MH sector, progress has been slow, particularly with regards to implementing IPS and developing local holistic services. As matters currently stand, the demise of CMPs, if they are left unreplaced, will reflect a considerable downturn in services for a difficult-to-place population. It is considered that further research is needed to clarify how best to implement the IPS approach to VR, particularly in areas of traditionally high unemployment, rural areas and small urban areas. Cost-effectiveness also needs to be evaluated.

Student exercises

9.1 Case study: AP and GP certification
AP is a 47-year-old, full-time process worker in a biscuit factory. Her job entails standing at the end of a conveyor belt, rejecting misshaped biscuits, keeping the packing machine loaded, ensuring boxes are wrapped correctly and stacking boxes on pallets. The jobs are routinely rotated to prevent boredom. AP has been off work for 3 months with a low-back injury, arguably sustained as a consequence of lifting and twisting the boxes. Her GP continues to write notes for 21 days stating, 'low back pain, unable to lift'. The company's OH advisor considers that any back problem is more likely to be a consequence of ageing and weight. She opined that, provided there is 'suitable adjustment for psychological concerns', there are no apparent reasons as to why AP should not return to work. However, the company will not insist on this because of the GP certification and the fear of any adverse consequences (both physical and legal), even though the shift manager has made his feelings clear about the inability to fill the post on a regular basis. Because of this impasse, AP has been referred to you. How would you advise all concerned?

9.2 Case study: JM and the role of barrier flags
JM is a 37-year-old care assistant in residential home for the elderly. She has visited her health centre four times over the last 6 months because of back pain and has been prescribed anti-inflammatory medication and analgesia. JM is overweight, but has no other medical problems. She states that low backache radiates to her buttocks and is made worse by stooping. JM wants time off work. Her job is 'heavy': many of the residents require assistance with bodily functions.

Assessment for 'red flags'
Age, trauma, progressive non-mechanical pain, thoracic pain, past medical history, structural deformity, restriction of lumbar flexion, widespread neurological symptoms.

Getting Jean back to work

The barriers:

- Jean's symptoms, her beliefs and fears, her understanding of the nature of back pain (yellow flags) and her relationship with her manager and colleagues (blue flags).
- Jean's mood and the possibility of moderate depression (orange flag).
- The availability of physiotherapy and other treatment options.
- The likelihood of short- or long-term adjustments to her work.
- GP's understanding of back pain and commitment towards encouraging Jean to work.
- Employer's beliefs about back pain and commitment to assisting resettlement when someone is not 100 per cent symptom-free.

List the roles of the following professionals in helping Jean to overcome the barriers to work and then suggest ways you would propose to case-manage this process:

- GP
- physiotherapist
- OHS.

You may add to this list as considered appropriate.

Part 3

The vocational rehabilitation process

The application of skills and knowledge

10 Vocational rehabilitation counselling, multidisciplinary working and client case management

Key issues

- The role of the vocational rehabilitation counsellor.
- Multidisciplinary teamwork.
- Case management and case recording.

Learning outcomes

- Understanding the work of VR counsellors.
- Developing an awareness of your own strengths as a VR counsellor and areas where you would like to improve your knowledge and skills.
- Development of case-recording practices.

Introduction

In Chapter 1, the distinction is made between the role of core and 'non-core' VR practitioners, the former's time being primarily allocated to providing VR services usually on a case-managed basis. Whatever discipline or training the core practitioner may have, they are likely to have some comparable professional and administrative tasks. They all undertake VR counselling. The United Kingdom does not have specifically accredited VR counsellors, and the term is used here generically to refer to practitioners with backgrounds such as specialist employment advisor, psychologist, physiotherapist or OT.

A key aspect of the role of any VR counsellor is case management. This may be delivered as part of a team input, either as a member of the team or team leader, or on a sole practitioner basis. Case management is critical to the success of any VR programme, not only as a means of checking the service user's progress but also as a means of providing accountability. At the present time, the United Kingdom has no agreed criteria for recording and reporting any service provider's delivery of services or even a service user's outcomes. However, the development of the UKRC and PAS 150 standards (Chapter 1) offers a means of facilitating this. Hence, this chapter addresses the common features of VR counselling and means of recording case details.

The role of the VR counsellor/case manager and the multidisciplinary approach to effective VR

Nobody knows how many people undertake VR counselling and case management in the United Kingdom, and, although there is no such accredited VR counsellor job title, many people working in the field are likely to identify with the one provided by the Rehabilitation Counselling Association of Australia:

> Rehabilitation Counsellor is an allied health and human service professional who works with individuals experiencing injury, disability and/or social disadvantage to achieve occupational, social and personal goals. To achieve this, Rehabilitation Counsellors work with individual strengths and facilitate change in both the person and their environment.
>
> (http://rcaa.org.au/)

There is an absence of data in the United Kingdom as to what VR counsellors do, such as undertaking assessments, tools used, the opportunities to arrange and monitor work trials and time spent liaising with other agencies. However, there are likely to be some common professional and administrative tasks, including determining client eligibility to the service and intake/initial interviewing; diagnosis of factors affecting VR process and resettlement; VR course planning and development; VR review; client and family support; placement and follow-up; employer liaison; and consultation with other professionals and employment services.

VR is recognised as a multidisciplinary process; Gobelet *et al.* (2007) noted that a rehabilitation team will be made up of professionals working in the disciplines of physiotherapy, occupational therapy, psychology, psychiatry, work counselling, work training, job teaching and, potentially, others. In some VR services, particularly small, single-disciplinary ones, all tasks are undertaken by one person, calling on other resources when the required level of expertise is not available.

Box 10.1 The role and task functions of the VR counsellor

Professional role	*Related task functions*
Initial assessment (based on psychological tests of interest, ability, aptitude etc.)	Case finding/taking referrals
	Eligibility determination
	Intake/initial documentation procedure
Transferable-skills analysis	
Diagnosis (barriers to employment)	Completion and maintenance of client records for both referring and funding agencies
Initial VR plan development	
Vocational assessment	
Labour market analysis	Service provision (in-house or external)
Rehabilitation counselling	
Job retention	Final report
RTW plans	
Placement and follow-up	
Post-employment services	

In most services, administrative staff are available, but this is not always the case. In any event, there is a relationship between professional and administrative duties, for example when determining eligibility/suitability for VR. Eligibility may be a simple matter of checking benefit receipt and funding, whereas suitability may involve professional skills in forming a judgement as to the referral's 'readiness'. Both tasks contribute to the same task function.

Agency and disciplinary co-operation

Within the United Kingdom, the historical separation of RTW services between the medical and employment sectors has contributed to some mutual distrust. This is a problem when a VR service user is being referred from one service to another, or advice from a particular source of expertise is required. This may dilute the quality of the VR service or even lead to a breakdown in working relationships. Criticisms tend to be of a stereotypical nature: Jobcentre Plus/non-clinically trained personnel:

- do not understand clinical conditions
- do not receive professional training
- are not interested in people with severe problems.

Clinically-trained personnel:

- are not co-operative
- do not understand the labour market
- have unrealistic expectations.

Although such developments as CMPs and the placement of employment advisors in GP surgeries have contributed to breaking down such misconceptions, the lack of multidisciplinary and multi-agency VR training appears to contribute to such division arising in the first place.

Skills of the VR counsellor

VR counsellors need both counselling and co-ordinating skills to be effective (Hershenson, 1990). VR counsellors use their *counselling* skills (Figure 10.1) to enable clients to re-examine their self-concepts and personal goals, and their *co-ordinator* skills (Figure 10.2) to monitor the wide variety of physical, social and vocational services that clients require to achieve their vocational goals.

A particularly significant aspect of the VR counsellor's role is the extent to which they use affective counselling skills. Affective counselling refers to dealing with client concerns, examples of which are psychological problems, for instance depression, coping with stress and the acceptance of limitations.

In the immediately foreseeable future within the United Kingdom, few graduates in VR-related disciplines seeking employment will be recruited by the public sector, other than the NHS. Most are likely to find work in not-for-profit organisations and the private sector. The issues that are likely to dominate discussion will relate to specialisation: not just a matter of developing expertise with a specific disability group, such as the brain-injured population or people with learning difficulties, but issues of exercising specialist

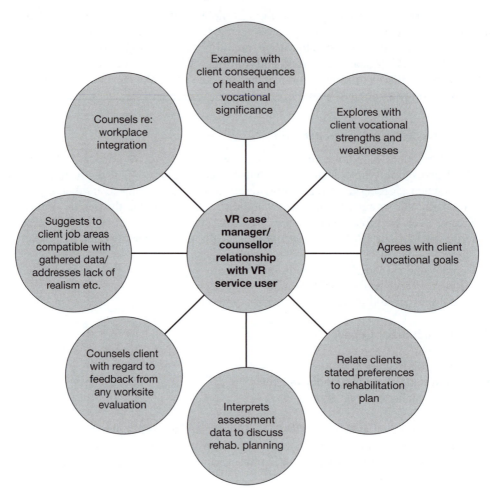

Figure 10.1 Vocational counselling skills

Box 10.2 VR counsellor activities

- counselling
- vocational counselling
- advocacy
- case management
- vocational assessment
- job development
- job placement counselling

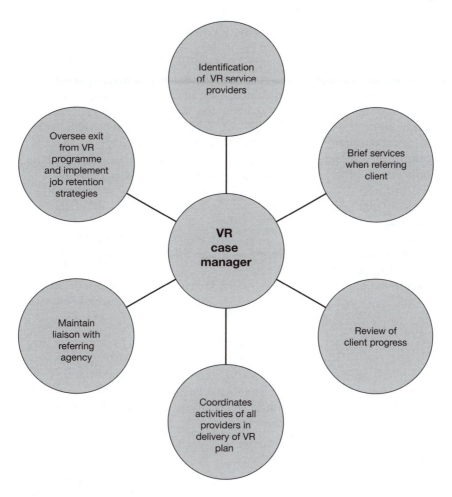

Figure 10.2 Service co-ordination tasks

functions, such as job development and placing or MH counselling. Such activity may involve the activities listed in Box 10.2.

Counselling

Common counselling skills and activities are likely to fall into the interrelated areas indicated in Box 10.3.

The specific attributes a VR counsellor is likely to require stem predominantly from the relationship with the service user and include client assurance; supporting a client by enabling him or her realistically to face obstacles that may initially seem insurmountable; achieving an emotional and intellectual acceptance of limitations imposed by a disability (and, with some VR clients, a realistic self-appraisal is one of the most significant issues affecting a positive outcome); assisting a client to understand or change their feelings about themselves or others; and discussing client's interpersonal

---

Box 10.3 Common counselling activities and skills

Example	*Description of counselling activities*
1 Information seeking	Client work/education history
2 Information giving – administrative	Course/support arrangements
3 Advice, opinions	Suggested course of action
4 Listening	When client input predominates
5 Information giving – occupational	Job requirements
6 Information giving – exploratory	Open-ended seeking information
7 Information giving – client based	Test scores, clinical advice
8 Clarification	Checking client has understood
9 Friendly discussion – rapport building	Chat so client can feel at ease
10 Supportive	Conveying willingness to assist
11 Information giving – structuring the relationship	Describing client/counsellor
12 Confrontation	Discrepancies between client's self-perception and actual behaviour/test scores etc.

---

relationships to facilitate appropriate behaviour. Separating domestic from employment issues, and determining how far one can intercede, can be difficult. The VR counsellor needs to recognise their own limitations and be aware of when and where to refer clients with problems outside their expertise.

Vocational counselling

Activities can involve feeding back test results and their implications; interpreting results of any work evaluation; examining the consequences of a disability/health condition and its vocational significance; exploring with the client his or her vocational strengths and weaknesses in order to reach a realistic understanding and acceptance of them; suggesting to the client occupational areas compatible with the gathered social, educational, psychological, clinical and vocational information; recommending to the client occupational/educational material for them to explore vocational alternatives; and consulting experts in a particular field, for example educational or clinical, and feeding back their advice. Highlighting the complexity of such activity is the fact that the counsellor may have to work with community-based agencies to augment the service user's rehabilitation. Such programme development and resource utilisation highlights the need for case management functions relating to service planning and co-ordination.

Advocacy

There are many occasions when a VR counsellor may have to intervene on behalf of a service user, including negotiating with Jobcentre Plus; making a case to continue supporting a client; and providing appropriate support when problems occur following a work placement.

Case management

Activities may involve developing a rehabilitation plan with the service user; monitoring client progress towards the specified goal; co-ordinating the activities of all the agencies involved in the rehabilitation plan; establishing timetables for various rehabilitation services; referring the client for a medical examination or psychological evaluation; referring the client to a training or educational facility; and explaining administrative arrangements.

The extent to which placement activity should be the role of the VR counsellor is a debatable issue. In some UK agencies, there are staff with this specific designated responsibility. However, there would appear to be common ground that the VR role may involve facilitating the following activities:

1   visiting employers to solicit jobs for particular clients;
2   discussing the client's capabilities with employers;
3   securing information in respect of the client's performance and any adjustments that may be required; and
4   arranging on-the-job training/induction programme for the client.

Vocational assessment

Tasks include arranging for, or undertaking, a functional assessment (of physical capability); a psychological assessment (of cognitive capability); an occupational assessment of client interests, skills and aptitude; an on-the-job evaluation; and co-ordinating assessment findings and writing an assessment report.

Job development

This refers to the process of developing the skills, and identifying appropriate job opportunities, for the client, for example by matching assessment findings against a labour market/job analysis. Successful job development is likely to entail:

1   addressing identified client weaknesses/building on strengths;
2   establishing a good knowledge of the local labour market;
3   being aware of companies with a good reputation for employing people with disabilities or offering work experience; and
4   being aware of adjustments and other support to facilitate a placement.

Placement counselling

Some VR counsellors are involved in 'job club' activity; others only see their clients on an individual basis. Hence, the extent to which they may undertake the following activities varies:

• using supportive techniques to encourage the client to undertake their own job search activity;
• informing clients how and where to look for jobs;
• interviewing a client seemingly lacking motivation to establish the reason(s) for their behaviour and to seek a way forward;

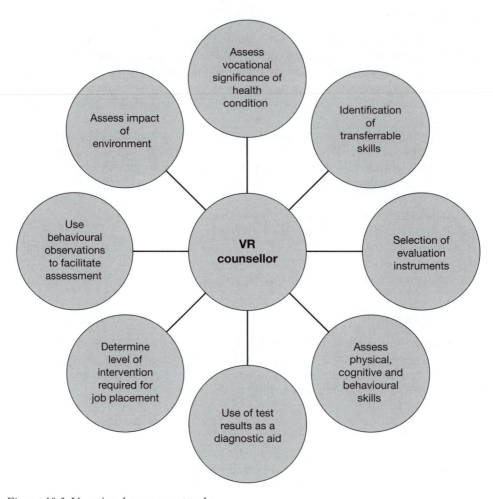

Figure 10.3 Vocational assessment tasks

- discussing with a client alternative ways to present themselves to an employer;
- role-playing job interviews.

All the above attributes require broad-based *knowledge* of the functional demands of relevant jobs in the labour market, available vocational training programmes and the variety of possible adjustments and supports, such as technological innovations, and the role of job coaching, as well as other support services, for example benefits advice and the Access to Work scheme. There is also a need for a range of related *skills*, including case management, counselling and advocacy, assessment, job analysis, marketing and networking.

Approaches to the management of VR

Generally speaking, the following approaches have emerged within the United Kingdom with regards to the management of vocational rehabilitation:

Self-management

The case-managed approach typifies private sector VR services. Such an approach can also be found in public sector programmes. However, self-efficacy involves the VR service user taking some responsibility for their own prospects. Self-management is a strategy generally regarded as effective for those with less complex needs.

Case-load management

Case-load management in UK VR practice receives little attention. The distinction between case and case-load management relates to areas of responsibility. In many large organisations, there is a person allocating and overseeing cases, the case-load manager, although they may have a range of job titles, whereas the person working directly with the client is the VR case manager. Grubbs *et al.* (2006) state that case-load management is there to ensure that VR activity is undertaken, although some case-load managers have their own clients. The key management functions are indicated in Box 10.4.

In addition to working with, or overseeing, more than one case at a time, other prominent activities of case-load management are directly related to the work of VR counsellors within line-management supervision (Box 10.5).

Many publicly funded VR agencies receive referrals from Jobcentre Plus and, funded on a per capita basis, invariably accept them. In such circumstances, it can be more difficult to identify the case-load manager than in a large private sector VR service

---

Box 10.4 Case-load management: key functions

- control
- decision-making
- data control
  - classification system
  - case flow
  - case recording/documentation
- client consideration
- organisational processes

Box 10.5 Case-load management tasks

1   Establishing a calendar of activities for a reasonably structured day or week for the most effective use of the VR counsellor's time.
2   Orchestrating a group of other professionals to rehabilitate clients through co-ordinating a group effort.
3   Initiating actions through a consistent decision-making style that keeps activities moving towards a targeted goal.

operating on a case management basis. This means that agencies delivering VR have to delineate staff *functions* to ensure that both the processes of case-load management and individual casework support are delivered, even if there is no staff with such designated job titles. Grubbs *et al.* conceptualise the essential elements of a case-load management model as shown in Figure 10.4.

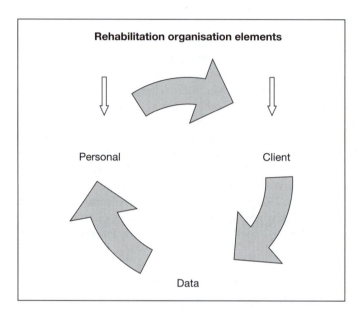

Figure 10.4 Essential elements of a case-load management model: rehabilitation organisation elements

Source: Adapted from Grubbs *et al.* (2006).

Personal elements

Without a firm level of personal control, effective case-load management will always be difficult to achieve. Decision-making and time management are also viewed as pivotal to the case-load management process and reliant upon how well control has been achieved.

To avoid the data managing the manager, there is a need to master (1) the basic classification system (and in public sector services, this often acts as the trigger to funding); (2) case flow (that is, where clients are 'in the system' at any one time); and (3) case recording and documentation (again, this is often a funding requirement).

Client elements

This aspect of case-load management relates to how the characteristics of the clients affect the delivery of services. These characteristics have been described as physical, emotional, financial, vocational and motivational (Kreider, 1983).

The final element of this conceptualisation of case-load management is the organisation or agency structural and procedural processes. This aspect is related to such matters as policies set by government, contractual obligations, guidelines, priorities and so on.

There is much that can be learned from the United States with regard to case-load management. A major problem in the United Kingdom with regard to assessing the efficacy of VR services is the lack of any common language and the ability to account for the client experience. When services are unable to report the progress of clients at any one time, or options they may be choosing, then, in addition to such matters probably not meeting audit requirements, they are not in a position to evaluate the cost–benefits of the services they are providing. As the United Kingdom moves towards a more professional VR counsellor case management model of service delivery, there is likely to be an increased need for monitoring and accounting for individual experiences. This makes both service delivery and the VR counsellor more accountable for their activity.

Case management

In VR practice, case management has been defined as 'a collaborative process which assesses, plans, implements, co-ordinates, monitors and evaluates the opinions and services required to meet an individual's health, care and employment needs, using communication and available resources to promote quality outcomes, with effective management of resource' (Hanson *et al.*, 2006). Internationally, the role of case management in VR is well established (Grubbs *et al.*, 2006). Countries such as Australia and the United States have their own education and accreditation bodies. The case manager is frequently not a health-care professional, although the education and training covers many subject areas that health professionals in the United Kingdom would regard as within their province. The model of a non-clinical case manager was followed by Healthy Working Lives when establishing the Scottish pilot VR programme (Chapter 9). In VR practice, case management generally involves the activities listed in Box 10.6.

Effective case managers:

- help to define a health or injury problem;
- arrange specific health-care;
- develop a clear plan for safe, sustainable RTW;

Box 10.6 Case management

1 moving clients from intake to closure
2 completing proper case documentation
3 delivering an identified evaluation and assessment strategy
4 delivering intervention and support services
5 monitoring of services
6 arranging placements and making follow-up arrangements
7 appropriate cost accountability

- manage resources effectively, proactively using resources to purchase interventions with known effectiveness at the most beneficial time;
- interact with other stakeholders and adopt appropriate roles when communicating, emphasising:
  - worker's needs to the employer;
  - employer's needs to the health-care provider;
  - early and sustainable RTW to employee.

Good communication skills (between bodies such as an employer, Jobcentre Plus, treating professionals, client and his/her family, insurer, service provider etc.) are essential to casework practice. In addition, the process requires the case manager to act as an individual support worker and advocate. The effectiveness of any case management service is likely to be dependent on a number of counsellor attributes, including their skills, knowledge and experience; the amount of time spent with the client (intensity of the service); and the duration of the service. In turn, the case manager/VR counsellor is likely to rely upon the circumstances considered in Box 10.7.

Nothing can be achieved without the VR process being carefully managed, in terms of VR counsellors both receiving appropriate case-load management supervision and accepting responsibility for their own case management activities, including completing appropriate documentation and accounting for their time. The process of case recording not only provides an aide-memoire but also evidence of activity and progress towards an agreed goal. It also serves to flag up any obstacles to resettlement, as well as enabling the counsellor to reflect on the strategies deployed to address them.

Case management does not necessarily involve the counsellor in delivering the service. Although good case management is crucial to the success of VR, the fragmented way services have developed in the United Kingdom means that VR counsellors may have to access other services, for example, if employed in the private sector, and, given a specific task of facilitating client retention by advising on accommodation adjustments, there may be a need to refer to the Access to Work scheme administered by Jobcentre Plus. The fact that RTW services do not neatly dovetail makes the co-ordination of services vitally important.

Hanson *et al*. (ibid.) provides evidence of how case management can be applied by employers and 'health-care providers' to help employees with MSDs stay at work. They note that the usual VR practice is to deploy a single case manager for an individual worker.

> The case manager can function as a) a 'broker' who passes on information and arranges referrals without direct contact; b) 'generalist' who provides both coordination and direct services such as advocacy, casework and support systems, or c) 'primary therapist' who supplements the therapeutic relationship with case management functions. It seems that the skill of the individual case managers is more important than their professional training or background.

The key components of cost-effective case management are indicated in Table 10.1.

Box 10.7 Circumstances contributing to effective case management

1 **Appropriately timed intervention**.
2 **Empowering the client** (encouraging self-efficacy).
3 **Access to information**: data systems need to be established and regularly updated.
4 **Confidentiality**: written authority should be obtained for personal information being passed to a third party, such as Jobcentre Plus or an employer. Likewise, case managers need to respect any information they are told in confidence, whether from the client, employer or any other source.
5 **The range and accessibility of support services**: a full case-management service will provide access to a range of specialists if required, e.g. a psychologist in stress cases. If an individual service provider lacks the necessary range of skills, the case manager needs to know where else to obtain such a service.
6 **Authority and autonomy**: case managers need the authority to determine and implement VR plans. Although autonomy is bounded by organisational considerations, trust is enhanced when the freedom to make decisions is set in the context of a defined reporting framework, so that information about activity is available to those who need it.
7 **Adequacy of service environment**: the case manager must be able efficiently to access assessment, rehabilitation and employment support services. Lengthy waits reduce their effectiveness, leading to a loss of confidence from service users.
8 **Control over resources**: although, in many cases, access to funding or equipment will be affected by the procedures of the employer, as long as the case manager's decisions meet organisational guidelines, they should be implemented without delay.
9 **Sequence of service delivery**: a sequential delivery of services is a key factor affecting successful rehabilitation programmes.
10 **Continuity**: regular contact with the service user and the employer (if there is one) is an important aspect of the VR process. Employers are particular concerned with absence from work, and they need to be kept informed regarding an anticipated return date and any adjustments that need to be made.
11 **Appropriate income arrangements for the client**.
12 **Monitoring and evaluation**: in an ideal situation, supervision should be maintained at least for a period following a permanent placement.

Case recording

Case recording provides the means for a supervisor to determine the quality of a VR counsellor's work and for the practitioner to keep a record of their VR plan and what they have covered with the client. Case recording and documentation cannot be standardised because of the different nature of VR services, but what is required is a

Table 10.1 Key components of case management (Hanson *et al.*, 2006)

---

1 Individual worker has his/her own case manager.
2 Case manager facilitates safe and sustainable RTW by recognising and addressing personal and occupational obstacles to securing RTW.
3 Case manager interfaces with health services but does not also provide the service.
4 Best clinical guidelines are followed.
5 Case manager monitors all aspects of intervention, including time and costs.
6 Case manager makes treatment-funding decisions.
7 Duration management techniques are available (using normative data on likely absence duration for conditions).
8 Case manager liaises directly with employer over RTW.
9 Case manager negotiates transitional work arrangements.
10 Early intervention focus.

---

structured framework by which the VR case-load manager can objectify the practice of case development. A case folder, therefore, serves a number of purposes, for the agency, VR counsellor and client (Box 10.8).

Styles of case recording

1 **Recording on established forms**: forms are useful when minimal amounts and types of information must be gathered uniformly in all cases.
2 **Summary recording**: this refers to a condensed account required, of transactions between the service user, counsellor, agency and so on. There may be a summary of what occurred at a given interview, or over a series of interviews, particularly recording anything impacting on the rehabilitation plan.
3 **Process or verbatim recording**: this refers to a highly detailed record that covers the events and emotions that occur in an interview. Such records are primarily used for psychological evaluation, content analysis and training purposes, to demonstrate interview and counselling techniques.
4 **Narrative recording**: this is commonly used and tells a story about the client, counsellor and agency. It should include factual data about the client. What is required is a dynamic description of what has happened and is happening to the client.

Box 10.8 Purposes of a case-load file

1 Means of bringing together all relevant data.
2 Visible description of case progression and direction (which can be examined by insurers and other funders, in a quality audit, solicitors etc.).
3 Means of providing a better service to the client by keeping track of progress, outstanding issues etc.
4 Record for the counsellor to ensure the continuity and consistency of support towards agreed targets (and a basis for assessing the effectiveness of their own intervention).
5 Basis for supervision by the agency.

Basic elements of case recording

There is a need to adopt systematic procedures (Box 10.9).

Use of formats

VR service providers need to devise or adapt their own. There are at least six critical areas in the VR process that can benefit from effective case recording and pre-prepared pro formas (Box 10.10).

It may be that some organisations need fewer or more forms. One report that is prepared by many VR counsellors is the 'final one'. It helps to prepare such a report if there is a case file to which the VR counsellor can refer and if they follow reporting guidelines.

Guidelines for report writing

The content of an intermediate or final report is obviously influenced by the nature of instructions. There is a need to keep a report to the point. Employers, insurers, lawyers and others do not want to read pages of description. They are interested in the conclusions. If unsure as to how they were reached, they will ask.

1   Preparation: there is a need to ensure that:
   • the instructions have been fully considered and addressed;
   • there is a clear idea as to who is likely to read the report;
   • reference is made to all the relevant documentation on which the report relies, such as medical reports and research references.

Box 10.9 Effective case recording

Step 1 Record information immediately, or as soon as possible
Step 2 Use a format for organisational assistance
Step 3 Separate objective and subjective data
Step 4 Record significant data only
Step 5 When in doubt, consult
Step 6 Data collection (counselling sessions etc.)

Box 10.10 Critical areas of case recording

A   Initial interview
B   Rehabilitation plan
C   Routine contacts
D   Assessment findings
E   Feedback from job-development activity
F   Follow-up, retention strategy and closure

2   Contents and structure:
- a front page is required, setting out:
  - client's name, address etc.;
  - for whom the report has been prepared;
  - your name/organisation;
  - date of report writing.
- there should follow a brief identification of the writer (in PI litigation, it is common to annex a CV);
- identification of the purpose of the report and the issues to be addressed;
- identification of everything on which the report relies, for example medical reports, employer visits, dates of any visit(s), assessments, others consulted etc.;
- a brief executive summary of the conclusions;
- an explanation of any assumptions or drawn inferences;
- if further information is required, an explanation as to what this is and why it is needed;
- an avoidance of opinion, unless this is required and the premise is clearly stated;
- annex any test data, charts as considered appropriate.

3   Layout:
- use of a well-sized font;
- double spacing;
- numbered paragraphs (for ease of reference);
- appropriate headings/subheadings;
- use of headers/footers.

Client confidentiality

Before a report is released to a third party, there is a need to establish the limits on confidentiality. The declaration shown in Box 10.11 distinguishes between service user and provider confidentiality.

Summary

VR service users need to be managed through the VR process, involving such practioner/counsellor activity as vocational counselling, advocacy, assessment, job development and job placing. Whether the service provider is an individual or an organisation, there is a need for data recording professional and related task functions as well as the client's progress. Effective case management is facilitated by good record-keeping. Records facilitate reporting on a client and establishing the benefits of the service. VR service providers in the United Kingdom are some way from using the same reporting criteria, although the developed standards (Chapter 1) provide a starting platform, ultimately enabling the efficacy and cost–benefits of service providers to be compared and contrasted.

Box 10.11 Client confidentiality

Client declaration
I have contributed to the information in this Vocational Report as a general guide to my skills, ability and potential. It also provides information on my aspirations and support needs. The contents have been discussed with me and the person acting as my advocate/advisor (if latter applicable).

I give .... permission to copy this report (as applicable) to:

* Jobcentre Plus
* supported employment agency
* employer
* insurer
* solicitor

Signed (client) .... Date ....

VR counsellor .... Date ....

Position ....

Service declaration
We will use the information given in this Vocational Report for the benefit of the client above and will liaise with him/her in an effort to find the best employment option. The release of information to a secondary party, such as an insurance company or solicitor, will only be done subject to a secondary signed agreement and (if applicable) that of your advocate/advisor.

Signed .... Position ....

Print name .... Date ....

Student exercise

10.1 Case study: SR
SR is a 47-year-old hairdresser. She has had no other job since leaving school aged 15 years. She has had controlled diabetes mellitus for 7 years, but has recently developed circulatory problems in her legs, with pain and limited mobility. She has been advised to avoid working standing and walking.

1   Identify the professional role of a VR counsellor.
2   Identify likely case-management service tasks.

11 The vocational rehabilitation process, stage 1

Initial evaluation, inclusion and rehabilitation planning

Key issues

- Models of disability.
- Theoretical models in vocational rehabilitation.
- Self-efficacy.
- The four-stage, twelve-step model of vocational rehabilitation.
- VR initial evaluation/engagement.
- Documenting demographic and clinical data.
- VR planning.
- Client contracts.

Learning objectives

- Understanding of the theoretical base on which social policy has developed and influenced VR practice.
- Awareness of a comprehensive model of the VR process.
- Understanding of what is required to initiate the VR process.
- Ability to formulate a client VR plan.

Introduction

The aim of any RTW intervention is to return the employee/service user to work. This need not necessarily involve a detailed, case-managed VR programme. In respect of 'what works', the 2004 National Framework document (DWP, 2004) notes that many RTW techniques are low cost and within the reach of small as well as large employers. In this respect, illustrated adjustments include reducing hours, offering light or transitional duties, carrying out RTW interviews and modifying the workplace, such as reducing the height of shelves. It is also recognised that, although such actions may facilitate the RTW in cases of minor injuries, a different approach may be required for more severe injuries.

Two significant issues emerge when considering the effectiveness of intervention:

- The range of strategies and techniques required to facilitate RTW 'requires a mix of competencies from providers' (DWP, op. cit.).

- 'Many RTW techniques can only be provided by the employer.' In other words, contracted VR service providers can only do so much, and any VR intervention that does not fully involve the employer and employee is less likely to be successful than one that does so.

The obvious problem for service providers working with unemployed people is that, unless involved in placing activity, they are unlikely to have the opportunity to negotiate a RTW plan with an employer and make an assessment of potential adjustments. Nevertheless, a systematic approach to the VR process will identify the strengths and weaknesses of a service user, enabling the best job match to be made, and result in the establishing of issues affecting resettlement and job retention for both the service user and any placement service provider.

This section of the book sets out a four-stage, twelve-step, model VR process. Although it is not necessary to take the steps sequentially, if 'skipping steps', then at least taking them in order, so that a higher one follows a lower one, will contribute to a more effective VR process.

Before setting out the model, this chapter considers theoretical frameworks for VR practice. Theoretical frameworks are important for providing the structure around which services are designed. VR has often lacked an underlying unifying perspective. The biopsychosocial approach is now strongly advocated within VR practice (Waddell and Burton, 2004). This perspective has been developed from various models of disability advanced over the years.

Theoretical models of disability

Moral model of disability

This model regards disability as the result of sin, and it is historically the oldest. There are many cultures that continue to associate disability with sin, and disability is often associated with feelings of guilt, even if such feelings are not overtly based in religious doctrine.

Medical model of disability

This model is based on the premise that disability is a defect or sickness that must be cured through medical intervention. The person with a disability is in the sick role, and they are excused from the normal obligations of society, including getting a job. Although a medical model of disability dominated the formulation of post-war disability policy, it did not achieve much by way of increasing the participation of disabled people in the labour market, although it is wrong to reject its therapeutic aspects. It needs to be recognised that the medical model may foster existing prejudices in the minds of employers. Because the condition is 'medical', a disabled person will *ipso facto* be prone to ill health and sick leave and will be less productive than work colleagues.

Rehabilitation model

This model is an offshoot of the medical model and regards disability as a deficiency that must be fixed by a rehabilitation professional. Historically, it gained acceptance after World War II, when many disabled veterans needed to be reintroduced into society, and underpins much early VR practice in the United Kingdom.

Social model

The social model of disability has taken hold as the disability rights movement has gained strength. The social model considers discrimination as the most significant problem experienced by persons with disabilities. In this model, 'the problem' is defined as a dominating attitude by professionals and others, inadequate support services, as well as attitudinal, architectural, sensory, cognitive and economic barriers, and the strong tendency for people to generalise about people with disabilities. The recent history of employment and disability policy in the United Kingdom reflects a gradual recognition of a social model of disability in preference to a medical model. However, the social model has proven difficult to implement in many employment-related circumstances (Danieli and Woodhams, 2005).

Biopsychosocial model

The biopsychosocial model, encompassing the interrelationship between the person and his/her environment, was first postulated as an OT model of practice (Mosey, 1974), but it is now recognised and accepted more by other professional groups (Silcox, 2006). In the VR field, it has been applied to work hardening (WH) (Fisher, 1999). In the United Kingdom it was given a boost by Waddell and Burton (ibid.) applying the model to a number of conditions, including MH and MSDs. The biopsychosocial model recognises that the cause of disability may include a substantial psychosocial aspect, in turn involving systemic factors affecting the worker, including the health-care system, the workplace and the compensation system (Loisel *et al.*, 2001). Two examples of the application of the biopsychosocial approach are the Canadian Model of Occupational Performance (CMOP) (Townsend, 2002) and the Model of Human Occupation (MOHO) (Kielhofner *et al.*, 2002).

Economic model of disability

This model is not well documented in VR literature, but it affects developments in the employment field, not least because it drives Treasury and government policy. In this model, disability is defined by a person's inability to participate in work. The model assesses the economic consequences for the individual, employer and the state, including loss of earnings, loss of tax revenue and potentially lower profit margins for the employer, and state benefit payments. The challenge facing the economic model is how to justify and support, in purely financial terms, a socially desirable policy of increasing participation in employment. Classic economic laws of supply and demand stipulate that an increase in the labour market supply results in decreased wages. Arguably, extending access to work through equal opportunities reduces an employer's labour costs. However the value of labour is based upon its contribution to marginal costs. Although most disabled employees are able to compete on equal terms, especially when given appropriate support, there are others who make a lower contribution than their work colleagues. This is not a popular thing to say, and there is a need for care when describing what is not a homogeneous population. Employers invariably hold the

Table 11.1 Perspectives on barriers and bridges to work

	Medical	*Social*	*Biopsychosocial*	*Economic*
Barriers/ problem focus	Disability results from impairment	Disability results from society's failure to adapt	Impairment, but also depends on psychosocial/social factors	Issue added value of employing disabled person v paying benefits
Bridges/ solutions	Medical treatment and rehabilitation	Society has to remove barriers	Combination of health care, rehabilitation, personal effort, adjustments	Increasing the value of the work, keeping down level of subsidy and benefits
Assumptions about work	Sick/disabled people are excluded from labour market	Disabled people are being excluded from work	More could work if individual and systems barriers removed	More could work if incentivised
Focus of intervention	Individual	Employer	Individuals, health-care professionals and employers	Reducing level of benefit payments

economic viability and operational effectiveness of their organisation as higher priorities than demonstrating social awareness. The economic option is to pay disabled employees less, or have the losses met through subsidy. The Workstep model of SE opts for the former practice, but this carries a stigma for the disabled person by underlining their inability to match the performance of work colleagues. The policymaker needs to balance the right of the individual to self-fulfillment and social participation through work with a need to protect the public purse.

Customer/empowering model

This model is gaining in popularity. The professional is viewed as a service provider to the disabled client and his or her family. The service user decides and selects what services they believe are appropriate, while the service provider acts as consultant, coach and resource provider. Recent operations of this model in the United States have placed financial resources under the control of the client, who may choose to purchase state or private care, or both.

From theoretical models of disability, the next step is one of developing VR models of practice with intervention strategies reflecting the models from which they are developed.

The way the biopsychosocial model has been adopted in VR practice is reflected in the Canadian Model of Occupational Performance and the MOHO.

Canadian Model of Occupational Performance (CMOP)

CMOP postulates that the *occupation*, *person* and *environment* interact to produce the occupational performance. An understanding of the occupation involves asking such questions as:

- What are the main work tasks?
- What are the demands of the work?
- Where, when and for how long are they performed?
- What is the skill level of the tasks?

The person, as a worker, has affective cognitive and physical components. An individual's beliefs and attitudes towards their condition and its consequences can present RTW barriers (Frank and Thurgood, 2006). Another element Ross (2007) discusses is 'spirituality', defined as *'the essence of self'*, what a person values and believes in.

The workplace, the 'environment', is conceived as having different 'levels': the physical environment; the social environment; the institutional environment, for example the impact of the DDA, economy and the availability of jobs; organisational influences, for example terms and conditions of employment, size of employer; and broader cultural influences.

Although job descriptions can form a starting point for addressing the points above, skills related to task and job analysis are necessary to refine the process. At the same time, there is a need to keep in mind the interests, abilities and aptitude of the worker, if there is to be a match and fit between the worker and the job, an essential aspect of any RTW process.

Although the CMOP is usually presented as a model of OT practice, there are no reasons as to why other VR practitioners cannot use it, provided they have sufficient expertise in assessing the physical and cognitive components. Many of the analytical activities are drawn from occupational and organisational psychology and will be familiar to human resource practitioners and employment advisers. Likewise, the MOHO can be used by other VR counsellors, subject to the same caveat.

Model of Human Occupation (MOHO)

The Model of Human Occupation (Kielhofner, 2002) is designed to facilitate an understanding of a person's work performance or dysfunction. Within the framework are interrelated core factors:

1   *person* considers
    - volition, and how this influences experiences and choices;
    - habituation: how a person's occupation is organised into habits and routines;
    - performance capacity, relating to physical and mental capabilities;
    and how these factors act upon
2   the *environment* (workplace).

By way of illustration as to how these factors work, many people feel that they have little choice but to continue to work in a job they do not like for financial reasons, resulting in occupational dissatisfaction. Likewise, disability might result in a person struggling to stay in an unsuitable position and having to reorganise their lives, such as rising earlier to get to work on time because it is taking an increasingly long time to get ready and travel. Performance capacity can be affected by changes in either an individual's volitional or habituational systems, or by their own subjective views of their capabilities.

The four-stage, twelve-step VR model (see Table 11.2)

This model encompasses most aspects of the VR process for most VR service users. Although guidelines exist providing model VR programmes for the main neurological conditions, the stages are either the same or similar (BSRM, 2010). Outside a limited number of specialists NHS centres, the financial viability of most VR services rests on serving a diverse population.

The VR process needs to conform to a set of principles (Box 11.1) requiring good management skills.

It will have been noted in Chapter 1 that there are very different views on what constitutes VR, ranging from any intervention that supports the RTW process to a detailed and structured, case-managed programme. Most core practitioners are likely to take the second view. Even if not in a position to deliver a complete VR service, core practitioners are likely to recognise the elements outlined in Figure 1.1.

The VR process (Table 11.2) systematically sets out a hypothetical model for ensuring that the elements of a comprehensive VR service identified in Figure 1.1 are delivered.

Client involvement and the value of self-efficacy

Self-efficacy is considered essential to the process of client involvement, to stop VR being something that is 'done to' the client. Bandura (1995) defined the term as 'context specific assessment of competence to perform a specific task or a range of tasks in a specific domain – an individual's judgment of his her capabilities to perform given actions'. With careful planning, self-efficacy can be built into the VR process, beginning at stage 1. Personal accomplishment is the strongest source of self-efficacy. Any VR client who has a belief in a particular course of action is more likely to take responsibility for their own position and follow that course of action than someone who feels they are being told what to do.

Table 11.2 The four-stages and twelve steps of the VR process

Stage 1	**Initial evaluation, inclusion and rehabilitation planning**
Step 1	Documenting demographic data, e.g. personal circumstances, educational history, employment history etc.
Step 2	Documenting clinical data, e.g. condition(s), restrictions, medication, activities etc.
Step 3	Intake/initial interview
Step 4	Formalising and operationalising referral questions and the rehabilitation plan
Stage 2	**Assessment and evaluation**
Step 5	Initiating the assessment process
Step 6	Assessing physical, psychomotor and cognitive abilities a) functional assessments b) cognitive assessments
Step 7	Assessing vocational interest, abilities and aptitudes
Step 8	Assessing worker traits, e.g. emotional stability, learning style
Stage 3	**Pre-placement rehabilitation and job development**
Step 9	Support and development services
Stage 4	**Placement, job retention and follow-up**
Step 10	Placement options and strategies
Step 11	Work-site evaluation and adjustments
Step 12	Job retention, follow-up and case closure

Box 11.1 VR principles (DWP, 2004)

- **Client-centred**: focus on the needs of the individual and set within their personal, family and social circumstances. Client is enabled to take responsibility for VR outcomes.
- **Flexible and re-accessible**: responsive to the changing needs of the individual.
- **Holistic**: addressing vocational needs in the context of the whole person, with provision for, or linked access to, other relevant services.
- **Employers**: needs of employers are '*key*'.
- **Barriers to work**: service delivery is designed to identify and eliminate the barriers to employment.
- **Health care**: health care should relieve symptoms and restore function, recognising the benefits of work. Work is generally therapeutic and an essential part of rehabilitation.
- **Timely**: delivered within an appropriate time frame for the individual. Early intervention is often key. VR should be critically linked, where appropriate, with medical rehabilitation.
- **Integrated**: VR services operate as part of an integrated network of services (NHS, Social Services, Jobcentre Plus, independent and voluntary organisations and employers) to ensure the needs of the individual are met. Communication between the stakeholders is vital.
- **Knowledge- and skills-based**: VR services have the knowledge and skills appropriate to the needs of service users. Professionals should keep their knowledge base and skills current. Educating and motivating the client are also important.
- **Informed**: practice should be grounded in an understanding of the needs of the individual gleaned from all relevant sources (e.g. individual, relatives, health professionals, Jobcentre Plus and employers).
- **Realistic and sustainable**: VR services seek to identify and achieve goals that are both realistic and sustainable.
- **Accessible**: VR services should be provided fairly and equitably, irrespective of ethnic origin, religious belief, gender, sexual orientation and geographical location, and delivered, where appropriate, in the community or workplace.
- **Voluntary**: individuals have a choice.
- **Confidential**: VR services respect and protect the confidentiality and other rights of people attending their programmes.
- **Standards**: professionals practise in a responsible and ethical manner according to standards of practice and a code of ethics.
- **Cost-effective**: consideration of approaches and interventions related to VR are cost-effective and can be seen by stakeholders as value for money.

Applying self-efficacy

In the first instance, there is a need to establish the client's position. What do they believe and what do they want to do? In some cases, there may be a need to challenge beliefs, but, in other cases, facilitation will be the VR counsellor's primary function.

It is easier for the VR counsellor to work in a structured fashion and make reference to checklists. In this way, items are less likely to be overlooked, and there is a record of responses. If, for example, the service user has an employer, the suggested steps are:

1 establish the client's expectations of what they want to do;
2 explore their perception of any limiting physical, cognitive and environmental circumstances; and
3 examine the client's specific job difficulties and any possible solutions.

Box 11.2 presents suggestions in respect of using self-efficacy in stage 1, step 3 of the VR process. Even if the client is unable to rank his or her choices, he/she will have a preferred option, and this is an area to be explored.

Stage 1: Initial evaluation, inclusion and rehabilitation planning

Although the four stages and twelve steps in the VR process (Table 11.2) appear sequentially, how the process is delivered varies from agency to agency, *and there should be available a return loop to earlier steps to be utilised if necessary.*

Box 11.2 Client expectations questionnaire

What you would like to happen is the foundation for our consultation.
What do you see as your options? Please tick the ones that apply to you. If you can rank them in order of preference, 1, 2, 3 etc., so much the better, but do not bother about this if you are undecided.

	Tick	*Rank in order of preference, 1, 2, 3 etc.*
Keep present job		
Part-time in present job		
More limited duties full-time		
Keep aspects of present job plus new duties		
New job with same employer		
Same kind of job with new employer		
Different job with new employer		
Retraining or education		
Medical retirement		
Other (please specify)		

Conducting an interview

The success or failure of the VR process can depend upon the relationship established between the VR counsellor and the service user. Conducting interviews requires an appropriate style and consideration of nonverbal and verbal behaviour, such as establishing an appropriate distance between the counsellor and client, squarely facing the client, maintaining eye contact and keeping an open, relaxed posture. In most circumstances, social chit-chat is not an appropriate gambit; something simple and professional is all that is required, such as, 'Would you like to tell me something about yourself so that we can begin to make vocational plans?'. Encouraging the client to speak, with the use of open-ended questions, can be encouraged with non-committal remarks such as, 'I see' or 'um-hmm'. Occasionally, the verbose client will need to be told that, 'I don't need any more information on that subject, that's sufficient thank you'. The client needs to be given regular feedback to check that he/she is being understood.

Answering referral questions

During the last decade, there has been a growth in private sector VR services, and this means that:

(a) VR service users in the private sector are more likely to have a job and employer to return to than clients of public sector services; and
(b) the reason for the absence of work is often a (relatively) recent illness or an injury severe enough to trigger a claim large enough for an insurance company to fund intervention.

VR agencies working with privately funded clients are likely to receive specific referral questions, such as:

> 'Is this person fit to return to their usual occupation?'
> 'If not, is there alternative employment within their capability?'
> 'What adjustments are required to facilitate their return-to-work?'

Even though VR agencies working with public sector clients rarely receive such specific questions, they should ask themselves the purpose of the client's attendance. Vague notions of preparing the client for the labour market are not going to focus the VR process, nor get the client a job and justify public expenditure.

Step 1: Gathering and documenting demographic data

Step 1 follows a referral, be it a self-referral or one from a clinical service, Jobcentre Plus, insurance company, solicitor or employer. Many organisations have developed their own forms for recording information. Typical demographic data that VR agencies are likely to require are listed in Box 11.3. Although information can be gathered without the client, this situation is not ideal.

Step 2: Gathering and documenting clinical data

At step 2, the VR counsellor is interested in the causes and consequences of injury/health conditions, with regard to such matters as:

Box 11.3 Recording demographic data

- address and contact details
- gender
- ethnic background
- birth date
- home circumstances
- education completed
- employment history, employer (if there is one) and nature of employment, contact details
- date of injury/nature of condition
- name and address of GP
- name and contact details of any other health-care provider, e.g. physiotherapist, district nurse
- current medication and dosage
- benefits received
- Jobcentre Plus office
- NI number
- referral agency/person
- any sources of support, e.g. brain injury case manager, social worker, support worker
- litigation pending; name and address of solicitor

- physical/sensory factors, e.g. seeing, sitting, standing;
- cognitive issues, e.g. memory, concentration, organisation;
- task completion, e.g. repetitive work, reading, arithmetic, using computer, using telephone, using machinery, following instructions;
- contact with others, e.g. working alone, working with others, working with customers/clients;
- working conditions, e.g. fixed hours, flexible hours, shift work, indoors, outdoors, noise, heat.

In keeping with the service user perspective, step 2 explores how clients perceive their condition affecting their work capabilities. A VR counsellor can prepare their own questionnaire based on what they know about the client. An approach for identifying job difficulties and solutions for an employed service user is illustrated in Box 11.4.

In such a fashion, the service user can be drawn into the VR process, with his or her aspirations, values and opinions being reflected in the VR plan. Documenting their responses can also serve as a useful reference for future counselling sessions.

The perspective needs to be interactionist and pragmatic. Although 'society' presents physical and social barriers to employment, there are occasions when the primary reason a disabled person is unable to pursue a particular activity is because of their disability, for instance when there are health and safety issues. For example, anyone who has had epilepsy may not be allowed to drive a large goods vehicle (LGV). As much as anything

---

Box 11.4 Job difficulties and solutions questionnaire

1   First, write down all the duties or tasks required.
2   Next, write down everything you feel you can't do. Take into consideration:
    •   your duties
    •   the equipment you use
    •   your work environment
    •   contact with others
    •   travel to work
    •   your work hours.
3   Go back over everything you have mentioned as being difficult and see if
    you can complete a sentence that begins, 'I could do this in my present
    circumstances provided that . . .'.

---

else, VR counsellors require clinical information addressing physical, cognitive and behavioural capabilities in order to make informed decisions on such matters as the client's capacity to benefit from a course and work situations to avoid. A failure to obtain and take into account medical advice can lead to a charge of negligence. Good clinical information can facilitate rehabilitation planning.

Two assessment tools that can be used to establish the service user's perspective are the worker role interview (WRI) and the work-environment impact scale (WEIS).

The WRI is based on MOHO and is designed to be used during an initial assessment to identify psychosocial or environmental factors positively or negatively influencing the RTW process. This includes such aspects as the worker's perception of their strengths and limitations; their view on how the disability has impacted on their role as a worker; the ability to change habitual patterns and their view of the workplace (Fisher, 1999). Different formats are available for use according to whether a worker has had a recent injury or has a long-term disability (Braveman *et al.*, 2005).

The WEIS includes a rating scale addressing how the worker with either a physical or psychosocial disability perceives their work environment. In order to produce a match between the worker, their skills and the work environment, this assessment identifies the environmental characteristics facilitating a successful RTW, plus other factors having a negative impact on the performance and satisfaction of the worker (Moore-Comer *et al.*, 1998).

Medical evaluations

The extent to which medical evaluations are included and considered in VR programmes in the United Kingdom varies considerably, invariably reflecting the nature of the service provider and when intervention occurs.

The position of clinicians is reflected by Chamberlain *et al.* (2009), namely, 'a complete medical history and full physical examination is an essential first step'. In this respect, it is considered that the International Classification of Functioning, Disability and Health (ICF) (WHO, 2001) is 'a useful tool to describe human functioning and the consequences of health problems on activities and participation'. The ICF is based on a biopsychosocial framework and provides recognised standards for describing how people with health-related conditions function in their day-to-day lives (Escorpizo *et al.*, 2010).

Problems in the United Kingdom relate not only to the number of physicians using the ICF but also to VR agencies understanding and using such information appropriately. Even when general medical reports can be obtained, there can be issues as to their usefulness. One has only to listen to expert medical evidence during High Court PI proceedings to recognise that the knowledge of disability, employment and the labour market among many clinicians is limited by their own labour market experience and the lack of occupational training. An example from brain injury is the oft-heard view that, 'this patient will not be able to return to his or her previous employment', on the grounds that the cognitive demands of the work are beyond the capabilities of the injured person. However, pre-injury skills and abilities are often well preserved, and, given a careful assessment, job analysis and supported job trial, the injured person might be able to undertake some, if not all, aspects of their former employment. This might be a better path to follow than the acquisition of new skills, in a new employment setting and with a new employer.

What VR counsellors require is guidance on the functional implications of a disability, so that, for example, the neurologist who defines the nature of epilepsy and provides information on the extent to which it is controlled by medication is proving invaluable assistance with placing and the observance of health and safety requirements.

If a VR counsellor is in a position to refer for medical advice, then they should specify the information they require and assist the examiner with vocational information, together with knowledge of the client's goals and what such work may entail. The examiner is then in a position to respond with the type of medical feedback that is required. A request for the following types of information can facilitate the VR process:

1   the client's general health;
2   a description of the extent, stability and prognosis of the present disability, as well as any recommended treatment;
3   information on the present and future implications of the disability/condition as it affects performance and essential job functions.

Collected data can be developed at the intake interview with the client, but the process of gathering data needs to begin at an earlier stage so that the counsellor knows what issues to address in the interview. There may be a need to further develop some issues emerging during the data gathering process. For example, when considering cognitive functions, the VR counsellor might wish to add a number of related matters, all likely to have some bearing on rehabilitation planning and future employment, as follows, for example:

Cognitive functions

• ability to learn
• memory for things to be done in the future
• ability to plan and carry out activities
• ability to self-evaluate

- initiative to start and finish tasks
- speed of thinking.

Social Skills

VR counsellors with brain-injured clients, ones with learning disabilities or with MH issues are likely to consider social skills of considerable significance:

- emotional status
- sensitivity
- social and interpersonal skills
- emotional tolerance to stress
- relationship to line managers.

In many cases, it is necessary to go into further detail in respect of establishing clinical factors to take into consideration when establishing intervention and placement strategies. In the absence of expert medical advice, simple questions at step 2 addressed to the client and/or family members/supporters, addressing physical, social/emotional and psychological issues, can be used for information gathering and identifying areas requiring consideration and further investigation; for example:

Health factors

1 How does the health condition impact upon employment potential?
2 Is the condition progressive or stable?
3 Is the client currently on medication with potential side-effects?
4 Do any recent medical reports clarify the extent of physical impairment?
5 Can the limitations imposed by the condition be reduced, by
   – modifying the worker?
   – modifying the work?
   – modifying the work environment?

Psychosocial factors

1 To what extent has the client adjusted to their condition (and is ready to 'move on?')
2 Is the family acting as a positive or negative influence?

Step 3: The evaluation-based intake (or initial) interview

An issue for VR services is the lack of evidence to identify clients only likely to return-to-work following VR. This is a matter of judgement that has to be made at some stage in the VR process. It is often based on a review of limited information from a referral agency completed on a pro forma (reason for referral, some medical and employment history, demographic data etc.). Step 3, the evaluation-based interview, is considered essential to supplement these data.

Integral aspects of step 3 are indicated in Box 11.5.

Box 11.5 Integral aspects of step 3: the evaluation-based intake interview

1 Engagement of the client/determining the reasons for seeking or participating in a VR programme.
2 Gathering, confirming and developing demographic and clinical data/giving agency information.
3 Decision on inclusion.
4 Obtaining consent/client contract/initiating the diagnostic process and rehabilitation planning.

Gathering and giving information can be divided into two main activities:

- Gathering information involves:
  - recording essential demographic and clinical data and giving the subject, and any supporter, an opportunity to discuss the impact the condition has had on their life and work. Although there may be a need to help the client better understand the range of his or her current and potential vocational functioning, this is not always possible at this stage, especially when the client has limited insight and/or refuses to recognise their limitations;
  - providing a structured means of assessing any client perceptions of changes in his/her behaviour, as well as a comparison of a significant other's response to the same items. This not always necessary, but in some cases essential.
- Giving information involves:
  - developing a rapport with the client (and any support worker or family member accompanying the client);
  - informing the client of medical, vocational and/or psychological evaluations he or she must complete and the reasons for them.

With regards to activities 3 and 4 (Box 11.5), during the intake interview it is suggested that the evaluator focuses on the referral issues and formulates an assessment hypothesis to determine the type of evaluation that will be pursued.

A typical intake interview procedure might need to cover the issues listed in Box 11.6 (the VR counsellor needs to use his or her judgement as to what is considered relevant). The interview is not intended to take the place of diagnostic reports but to summarise the viewpoint of the client and his/her family/support worker. The evaluator may wish to use a simple tick-list scale when collecting such information, e.g. no problem, some problem, significant problem. This will show up any discrepancies between the client's self-assessment and that of a significant other. In many cases, it will be necessary to have a reliable significant other person present. The essential issue is the attitude and response of the interviewee, in contrast to that of someone who knows them well.

Inclusion and client consent/contract

The giving of informed consent to participate in a VR programme can only follow the initial interview, and a client contract (supported by the subject and family) should be made on the basis of a VR plan (step 4). The client's capacity to understand exactly what they are consenting to clearly needs to be ascertained, and the family/any carers must be engaged in the process. There are circumstances when the client may not fully understand what they are being asked to agree to do. In such a circumstance, the VR counsellor must keep in mind that they have a common-law duty to act in the best interest of the client.

Box 11.6   Intake interview: employment and clinical issues to consider

Employment history and job goals:

- effects of the injury on employment potential
- pre-injury work skills, including educational status, that may assist in obtaining and maintaining a job
- immediate and long-term goals and alternatives
- potential for a job placement or return to a former job
- hobbies and spare-time activities related to work potential.

Activities of daily living:

- daily routine
- travelling means and skills.

Physical profile:

- physical capacity
- movement skills
- adroitness
- sensory perception
- sensory systems
- other issues.

Social–emotional profile:

- social adjustment
- emotional stability
- intrusiveness
- activity level.

Psychological profile:

- freedom from distractibility
- verbal factors
- performance factors
- immediate and delayed memory
- communication skills
- psycho-motor skills
- executive and higher-order skills.

Step 4: Formalising and operationalising referral questions and developing the VR (or graduated RTW plan)

Having gathered information from an interview and obtained (or arranged to obtain) any missing demographic/clinical information, including knowledge about the client's emotional reaction to their condition and values as they relate to work, the VR professional can then proceed with an initial VR plan. A VR plan is likely to be much more open ended than a GRTW plan (addressed in the next chapter), although, in some retention cases, it may be possible swiftly to move to this position. In general, at stage 1, the VR counsellor is only likely to be able to outline the general nature and intentions of the service (Box 11.7). This process needs to be undertaken with a clear expression of the client's rights (including the right to refuse or withdraw consent at any time), the responsibilities of the VR service and potential outcomes. The VR counsellor needs to address the issue of confidentiality and make it clear who has access to client information and to what purposes it is used.

The VR plan needs to be based around the perceived:

1   ability to work
2   preferences for different types of job and work activity
3   capacity to perform in a variety of vocational roles, and
4   need for training in specific and general skills.

The Plan also needs to involve finding answers to such questions as those posed in Box 11.8.

Service user/-provider contract

Although the service user/-provider contract at the end of stage 1 may not set out a detailed plan, the client needs to be given some indication of what is expected of him or her, and the VR counsellor needs to take into account any feedback. VR counsellors need to review the referral documentation and notes from this stage before deciding what test material needs to be used in the next assessment stage. In turn, this will not only influence the rest of the VR process, in terms of any in-house services and placement considerations, but will also lead to a more focused final report, addressing referral issues.

Box 11.7 The VR plan

The VR plan needs to make reference to:

1   objective(s)
2   duration of intensive support
3   responsibility of agency personnel
4   responsibility of client/family
5   how barriers to employment are to be addressed
6   review periods

Box 11.8 Rehabilitation plan: issues to consider

1   Are immediate and long-term goals likely to be realistic?
    If not, why not? If the job goals are realistic, there is a need to identify what may be done to remediate any identified problems that may cause work-related difficulties. If the problems are unable to be rectified or goals unrealistic, there is a need to consider alternative goals.
2   What type of employment position would appear to be of most benefit at present? There is a need to specify any support systems or special considerations that are needed. If specific questions regarding adaptability to a job exist because of behavioural problems, skill deficits or other reasons, there is a need to state the problem, estimate the likelihood of change and state the specific steps that could be taken to promote a positive change.
3   What areas of concern/doubt require clarification? What requires assessing? There is a need to specify the measures to be taken to answer these questions.
4   Would a referral to Jobcentre Plus for assessment/consideration for supported employment be beneficial?
5   Is a referral for further clinical treatment required?
6   Is a referral to other support services required?
7   What kind of support is required prior to placement:
    •   individual counselling?
    •   cognitive remediation?
    •   job club/work support group?
    •   benefits advice?
    •   basic/IT skills?
    •   other (specify)?
8   Prior to placement:
    •   will he/she observe safety regulations and other rules?
    •   is this client likely to be punctual?
    •   are his/her social skills likely to be adequate for the job?
    •   is he/she likely to require work induction supported by a job coach?
    •   what deficits are likely to be most problematic?
9   Measures to address any noted deficits.
10 Placement targets: these questions can be included in a documented plan and completed with a summary and answers to the questions:
    •   What is to be delivered?
    •   When is it to be delivered?
    •   By whom?
    •   Review dates.

Summary

Stage 1 of the VR process involves gathering and giving information in order to prepare a vocational plan. It provides an opportunity to draw the service user into the process and begin to make decisions affecting their own future.

Many VR service providers, particularly ones in the private sector, will have access to, or be able to refer a client for, a medical examination. Many will also be able to supplement this information with a functional assessment (in stage 2). Other service providers may have to rely on extrapolating information from a referral source, supplemented by the client and his or her family.

It is good practice to obtain a signed client consent form drawing attention to both their commitment and the limitations on confidentiality. In an ideal world, all participation in a VR programme would be voluntary. The reality is that there are service users who will feel pressured from one source or another to participate, and this can create difficulties that need to be worked through.

Student exercises

11.1 Requesting medical information

If the VR practitioner can be specific about the clinical information they require from a GP or consultant, they should focus their enquiries. For example, in respect of a client with diabetes, information to facilitate the VR process may include:

1   Can the client's diabetes be controlled at this time?
2   What work situations should be avoided, e.g. varying number of hours worked from day to day, shifts etc.
3   Can the client work for 8 hours per day/40 hours per week?
4   Should placing the client in a job be delayed until the diabetes is controlled?
5   Either consider your own clients with a specific condition or the following conditions; what information do you require?
    •   epilepsy
    •   multiple sclerosis.

11.2 Case study: TM

TM is a 34-year-old machine tool setter/operator. He left school aged 16 years with four modest GCSEs and subsequently undertook a 4-year apprenticeship as a capstan setter/operator, later receiving further training to work on CNC machines. (If you do not know what CNC machines are, then you need to find out.) He has remained with the same firm, a medium-sized engineering company. He is married, with two young children. His wife, Angie, works part-time as a school dinner lady. Four months ago, he was injured at work when a forklift truck backed into a step ladder on which he was standing while retrieving some tools from a rack. Although he received bruising to his back and a sprained wrist, the main injury occurred to his left kneecap as a consequence of landing heavily on a concrete floor. Possible cartilage damage was identified, and there has subsequently been a diagnosis of chondromalacia patella by the GP, although the term 'patellofemoral syndrome' was used by a consultant to whom he was referred by the company doctor.

Tony complains of pain in the knee and an inability to stand for long periods. However, the consultant's advice is to treat conservatively and that, with 'support', he ought to be capable of returning to work. This has not yet occurred, much to the frustration of Tony's line manager and human resources (HR). There is a reluctance to issue a deadline date because of Tony's service, but the issue is fast becoming intractable. Because of past good experience, the case has been referred to you.

Outline the issues to be considered before a VR plan can be drawn up. Remember this is a broad plan, which will gradually become a more focused graduated return-to-work plan (next chapter).

12 The vocational rehabilitation process, stage 2
Assessment and evaluation

Key issues

- Generic skills of diagnosis, information processing, job matching, client counselling and rehabilitation/placement planning.
- Assessment tools.
- Applying test results.

Learning objectives

- Understanding of what is involved in a VR evaluation and assessment.
- Awareness of assessment tools commonly used in the United Kingdom to establish a vocational profile.
- Ability to develop a GRTW plan and knowledge to make appropriate recommendations for any pre-placement work preparation.

Introduction

Many people use the terms vocational evaluation and vocational assessment synonymously, although assessment is only part of the evaluation process. Vocational evaluation combines several different assessment techniques and practices – for example, psychometric testing, work samples, job trials and analysing different types of data, for example behavioural observations, self-report and job analysis – in order to present a complete description of a person's vocational potential. Assessment strategies are only part of the evaluation process of identifying a client's strengths and weaknesses and, as such, tend to be focused on a particular aspect of an evaluation, for example physical limitations. At all times, it needs to be remembered that the evaluation and assessment process is undertaken to enable the client to find or maintain employment by meeting the aims in Box 12.1.

To achieve these aims, VR counsellors must have:

1. knowledge about the person
2. personal knowledge, including:
   - variety of possible supports and adjustments
   - available support services
   - knowledge of available job(s), and
   - available training programmes.

Box 12.1 Purposes of a vocational evaluation

It enables the client to:

- better understand the range of his/her vocational functioning and interests;
- become aware of the potential job opportunities compatible with such functional capacities and interests;
- learn about services and supports necessary to optimise such functioning.

Box 12.2 Factors influencing the nature of the VR evaluation process

Relevant factors may include:

- the nature of the disability or health condition;
- the client's education and employment history;
- the personal circumstances and the level of support available to the client;
- whether or not the client has an employer or job (assessment and rehabilitation can be focused if based upon a specific job analysis);
- the resources of the VR agency;
- the level of funding.

Stage 2: Assessment and evaluation

Goals

Both client and evaluator must set goals. These process goals should not be confused with the outcome goals arising from any referral questions. The three process goals for evaluators are indicated in Box 12.3.

When Employment Rehabilitation Centres operated (Chapter 1), every Monday morning the new intake was faced with a battery of the same psychometric tests examining basic skills, such as reasoning ability and interests. This was for ease of administration (group testing being more economical than individual testing) and because the referral agent, usually DEAs (or DROs as they were), rarely specified their

---

Box 12.3 Process goals for VR evaluators

1 Obtain the information needed to answer the referral questions.
2 Accurately determine the client's strengths and weaknesses.
3 Provide the opportunity for client self-assessment and exploration.

---

requirements. It was sufficient to refer someone to a VR course because the person was unemployed and had a disability. The test results were there for the case conference team to determine an appropriate course of action and make recommendations.

Such measures are no longer compatible with responding to any questions asked by the referral agency (particularly likely to occur in the private sector), individual planning and the involvement of the client in the VR process.

Even if it becomes evident during stage 1 that referral questions need to be rephrased, their existence means that they can be revisited during the evaluation process. Report writing can make reference to them and any developments that might have taken place. The more specific the questions referral agents ask, the more the VR evaluation and assessment strategies can be focused.

Examples of specific referral questions may include:

'Can Mrs Smith return to her usual work as an assembly line packer?'
'Taking into consideration her reported back problem, what adjustments may be required to enable her to return to this work?'
'Will she be reliable?'

Such questions begin to define the evaluation process. In contrast, questions facing an agency to which a long-term IB/ESA claimant with a brain injury has been referred may call for a different approach:

'Can Edward work part-time or full-time in open employment?'
'How does he best learn and retain a new task?'
'Does he maintain appropriate interpersonal skills?'
'What compensatory strategies can be introduced?'

Answering the first list of questions might start with a functional assessment of physical capabilities, leading to a comparison of the findings being made against a job analysis of a specific job. Answering the second list of questions might require an initial reliance on tests of cognitive ability, followed by more of an observational/situational approach.

Assessment practices aim to analyse a service user's:

* work skills, abilities and aptitude
* work behaviours, and
* work tolerances

and to

* identify the barriers to returning to work
* establish data/information to address the barriers.

Box 12.4 outlines assessment tasks.

Job identification/matching

The assessment process inevitably has a predictive element relating to a specific target job. For a VR service user with the prospect of returning to an existing employer, the job title will be known, although the precise physical and cognitive demands, or working

---

Box 12.4 Assessment tasks

- Selecting appropriate assessment tools.
- Using test results as a diagnostic aid in gaining an understanding of the client.
- Identifying client ability, aptitude and interests.
- Identifying transferrable work skills by analysing client's work history and functional strengths and limitations.
- Identifying client's work personality and social skills, observed and rated in an actual job or simulated work situation.
- Reviewing clinical information and assessing the vocational significance of the client's disability.
- Matching demographic and clinical data with vocational assessment findings in order to identify suitable work or training.
- Determining the level of intervention necessary for job placement, e.g. job club, supported work, on-the-job training.
- Determining the level and type of training that might be required.
- Making job, work area or adjustment recommendations.

---

circumstances, might not be clear. In such a circumstance, job, task and environmental analyses are advisable (Chapter 14) but not always possible. It is one thing recommending such activity, but getting access to standing on a factory floor, or in an office, and undertaking such activity may be considered intrusive by some employees and their representatives and requires consultation before proceeding. In many instances, it is possible to obtain a detailed job description from the employer.

When VR service users do not have an employer, or it appears that they need to change their job, then knowledge of the local labour market is invaluable. It is generally considered that around one-third of jobs in the economy are filled by word of mouth. This is a practice that has been declining for some years in large and medium-sized companies, so that they can avoid accusations of favouritism and discrimination; however, family and friends can still be an invaluable source of information and support. Around one-third of jobs are filled by Jobcentre Plus, and staff are likely to have an excellent knowledge of local labour market developments. Many local authorities also have employment units. An excellent example is provided in Dundee, where there is specific support for people with disabilities (www.dundeecity.gov.uk/employmentunit/). Since December 2006, public authorities have been subject to the Disability Equality Duty, which requires them to be proactive in promoting disability equality in their services and employment.

When considering alternative employment and analysing job titles, the British Standard Occupational Classification system has never provided the same level of detailed job information as the American Dictionary of Occupational Titles (DOT). From the DOT, the VR counsellor can learn about job functions in order to assess the appropriateness of a vocational goal. Although still in existence, DOT has been superceded by the O*Net classification and analysis system (http://online.onetcenter.org).

As suggested, when a VR service user has a job or employer to return to, the assessment can also include one of the work environment. The predictive aspect can be focused on the job and working environment, with the assessment data being used to match the findings against the identified criteria required to return-to-work and the identification of rehabilitation strategies to 'bridge the gap' between the findings and the job requirements. When the client does not have a job, there remains the task of using assessment data to identify rehabilitation strategies for suitable job opportunities in the open labour market.

Potentially, there are a large number of assessment tools. In the early stages of the RTW continuum, a number of tools have been developed for use by non-core VR practitioners, such as clinicians, to identify potential work-related problems. The application of work instability scales (Gilworth *et al.*, 2003, 2006) falls into this category. Further along the line there are assessment tools in which disciplinary expertise is an advantage if not an administrative requirement (although, as with all assessment tools, specific training is required to undertake administration and interpretation of the findings). Functional capacity evaluations (FCEs) and a large number of psychologically based assessments are in this category. Few assessment tools are restricted in their disciplinary usage. However, within the United Kingdom, the limitation on the availability of multidisciplinary VR training has resulted in the association of specific assessment approaches with particular disciplines. Although there are some signs that the market is becoming more enlightened, with private sector VR services broadening their recruitment criteria to include not only clinically trained personnel but non-clinically trained ones with specific VR expertise, until the United Kingdom follows other Western countries in requiring VR services and practitioners to have a set of identified skills, then the brakes are likely to remain on this development. There may be little incentive for a VR practitioner with a particular disciplinary background to broaden and deepen their expertise by acquiring skills associated with another discipline, or for an employer to contribute towards paying for this.

Collecting data is one matter. What the VR practitioner does with this information is something else. Too often it appears that assessment data are left dangling in the air and take resettlement no further forward, achieving little more than definition and clarification of problems that could be 'eye-balled' before the assessment started. When this occurs, it is almost always because the person undertaking the assessment has not had an end product in mind, a target occupation. Although it can be difficult to have a specific job in mind when a client is unemployed, few VR service users have no job history or aspiration that can be used to establish an objective for the assessment. The assessment data can then be used to refine the matching process and identify the types of VR rehabilitation service the client is likely to require.

Types of assessment

Service user assessments (as opposed to work-environment assessments) address issues specific to the client, such as their physical capability, cognitive abilities, work behaviours, skills and aptitude. There are various types and sources of assessment and data, including:

1   the interview;
2   transferrable skills analysis;

3   psychometric or standardised tests, such as work samples;
4   medical records and assessments;
5   functional assessments; and
6   situational analyses, including on-the-job evaluation (OJE); the difference between
     a situational assessment and an OJE is that the former takes place in a simulated
     setting, whereas the latter relies upon an actual workplace.

Generally, the data from these assessments – and data need to be regularly analysed
using a triangulation approach – can be grouped into five broad occupational areas
(Table 12.1) to facilitate both the next stage of the VR process, job development, and
job matching.

The examples following the headings in Table 12.1 are not exhaustive. For example,
the potential list of aptitudes may cover such factors as general learning ability, verbal,
numerical, spatial, form perception, clerical perception, motor co-ordination, finger
dexterity, manual dexterity, eye–hand–foot co-ordination and colour discrimination.

Table 12.1 Stage 2 of the VR process steps: areas for assessment

1   **Transferrable skills**: e.g. managing others, managing time, financial skills etc.
2   **Physical and cognitive capability**: e.g. work tolerance/stamina, work speed/productivity, dexterity, memory, concentration, capacity to follow instructions.
3   **General work interests, abilities and aptitudes**: e.g. work interests basic skills, e.g. literacy, numeracy, tool handling, mechanical aptitude, clerical skills, computer skills, potential for retraining.
4   **General worker traits**: e.g. motivation (interests and attitudes), work habits (behaviour) e.g. reliability, social skills, punctuality, personal presentation, work competence (skills).
5   **Occupation-specific skills**: in order to answer occupation-specific questions such as, 'Can this person return to work as a car mechanic/sales assistant/receptionist etc.?', most likely to arise in retention cases, an assessment of the workplace is likely to be required.

Step 5: Initiating the assessment process

Assessment based on matching psychological skills with potential employment has been
overshadowed by an increased interest in assessing functionality during the growth in
both NHS and private sector VR services. Function-based assessments provide a baseline
of client abilities in carrying out actual work tasks. Austin (cited in Reiman and Manske,
2009) defines function as 'any movement at the level of the person that is task related,
goal oriented, environmentally germane and involves the integration of multiple body
systems and structures'. 'Testing' is defined as using a set of problems to assess abilities.
Hence, 'functional performance testing' is the use of a set of tests to determine
performance abilities or functional limitations.

VR counsellor activity may involve carrying out, or arranging for, an assessment of
work tolerance, a FCE and job matching, and subsequently combining the physical,
psychological and behavioural aspects of the client's capabilities with knowledge of the
working environment.

Ideally, all assessment needs should be guided by the actual or potential tasks that
the client is likely to be doing. Unless they have a MH problem, the service users of

NHS and private sector VR services are more likely to have recently experienced illness/injury than the clients of services historically accessed through Jobcentres. In addition, the clients of private sector services are more likely to have a job or an employer to return to. When the service user has a job or an employer, the focus of the assessment can be on the match between the client's capabilities and the requirements of a specific job (as opposed to potential labour market capability in general), with the aim of assessing whether or not a good 'fit' can be achieved, and, if not, what can be done to improve the fit by changing the job or introducing strategies to enable the client to undertake the work more effectively. In such a case, there is a need to keep in mind that placement is more likely to be successful when the client can meet the job demands, than when the demands of the job have to be changed to meet the client's capabilities. If these approaches do not produce a positive result, then the VR counsellor (and client) is in a comparable position to when there is no employer (but with the added advantage of there possibly being alternative suitable employment). This assessment approach is indicated in Figure 12.1.

Location of assessments

Although there is some movement towards assessments being carried out in the workplace because they are more realistic (Gibson and Strong, 2003; Sandqvist and Henriksson, 2004), opportunities to do this are often restricted, not least for health and safety reasons.

Timing of an assessment

In line with the development of the biopsychosocial model, the United Kingdom has begun to develop interventions aimed at returning people to work that promote the message that many injured/sick workers do not have to have made a full recovery. In respect of MSDs, Frank *et al.* (1998) considered the disability process could be divided into acute, sub-acute and chronic phases, identifying the sub-acute phase as the 'golden hour' to address the disability problem, avoiding unnecessary health care but targeting those at high risk of prolonged disability and providing the optimum time for RTW intervention. At this juncture, a reasonable question might be, 'What is the point in

	Assessment		
	Job		**Client**
NO EMPLOYER			general physical cognitive and vocational skills and interests
EMPLOYER	job analysis task analysis environment analysis	⟹ **match** ⟸	specific physical and cognitive vocational skills and interests

Figure 12.1 Assessment considerations

undertaking an assessment, with a view to returning to work, if optimum recovery has not been achieved?'. The answers are that:

•   the assessment provides the baseline against which presenting capabilities can be matched against a specific job or the demands of the labour market in general; and
•   the assessment identifies barriers to work and where issues need to be faced or improvements addressed.

The assessment process needs to be structured (Figure 12.2). Getting to know the client before starting any evaluation is always a good idea. This helps in the anticipation of any safety issues, learning style and interpersonal skills.

When planning an assessment, the evaluator has to decide what techniques to use. The three major variables – costs, time and perceived relationship to 'real' work – and how they interact are illustrated in Figure 12.3.

If the assessor has to complete the assessment in a limited amount of time, this reduces the number of options as to the techniques to be used. Simply, there will not be time to arrange and undertake a situational or job-site assessment. However, there are some tests that give large amounts of specific information in a given time. For example, the

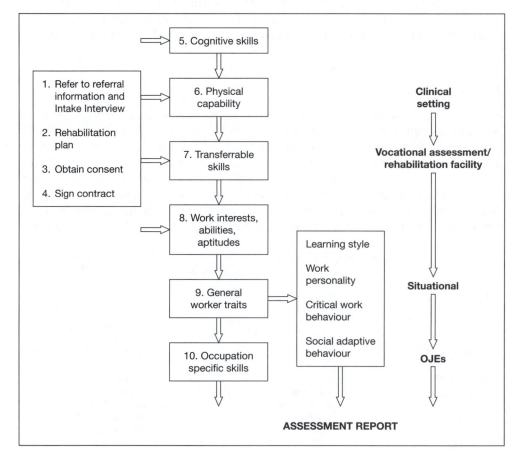

Figure 12.2 Client assessment flowchart

Techniques

Review of case history

Interview

Psychological testing

Work samples

Functional assessment

Situational assessment

Job site evaluation

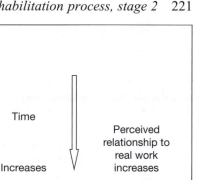

Cost

Increases

Time

Increases

Perceived
relationship to
real work
increases

Figure 12.3 Choice of assessment techniques: interrelationship between time, costs and relationship to 'real' work

Differential Aptitude Test provides several vocational aptitude scores and takes less than 3 hours to administer (see www.articlesnatch/Article/All-You-Need-to-Know-About-Differential-Aptitude-Test/666253).

A controlled situation is required to undertake most vocational assessments. In some instances, it is difficult to obtain a controlled situation, for example having to undertake an assessment on a home visit or when a suitable work placement cannot be found for an observational assessment. Ideally, the circumstances shown in Box 12.5 should appertain.

Assessment tools tend to be drawn from four different disciplinary perspectives:

1 clinical practice
2 psychology
3 industrial/commercial practice, including HR methodologies
4 VR practice itself.

VR practice in the United Kingdom is a broad church, and the specific choice of an assessment tool to measure a particular trait may only reflect disciplinary training. For example, OTs may be used to using a particular manual dexterity test, and psychologists/

Box 12.5 Ideal test circumstances

Nature of test	**Environment**
Clinical	Controlled clinical
Psychometric	Controlled distraction free
Work samples	Controlled rehabilitation
Situational/observational	Workstation

HR specialists another one. The assessment tools that VR practitioners use are likely to be influenced by:

- the training they have undertaken
- the client's condition, and
- the nature of the instructions received/reasons for the assessment.

A picture is emerging of current UK VR assessment practice, reflecting earlier intervention and a greater reliance on clinical assessment tools. Although this means that clinical training is a necessary prerequisite for administering certain tests, this is not always the case, provided the administrator has received appropriate test training. For example, although it is a significant advantage to have a clinical background to administer and interpret FCEs, some FCEs have been designed for use by non-clinical VR practitioners.

Responsibility for the governance of psychological tests in the United Kingdom rests with the British Psychological Society (BPS). It has established a hierarchy of qualifications required to administer tests. One need not be a trained psychologist to administer all vocationally relevant tests; for example, DEAs are trained to BPS Certificate of Competence in Occupational Testing Level A standard. This covers many routine tests of interest, ability and aptitude. Level B covers personality testing and, although this is generally not highly relevant to VR practice, the work personality profiling test is discussed later in this chapter.

Whatever the reasons for an assessment, it is useful to remember some basic rules (Box 12.6).

Organisations and VR counsellors can develop their own assessment tools, as long as they establish their reliability and validity and they avoid any potentially unlawful bias.

Identifying transferrable skills

Starting the assessment process by identifying transferrable skills from past employment or other activity provides a means of identifying salient issues to be addressed in the assessment process. It is also a process with which many service users are likely to identify, giving them the opportunity to talk about what they like to do and their strengths, although this may have to be drawn from them. Many VR service users unable

---

Box 12.6 Rules of assessment

1 The client must understand the purpose of whatever assessment tool is being used.
2 If recent accurate information is available on the client, use it to avoid duplication.
3 Use the technique that produces the most accurate data in the shortest time.
4 Use data collected from different sources whenever possible.
5 Use group-administered tests whenever possible.

to return to their usual work are likely to have developed a number of skills transferable to another position, even though they might not at first recognise this for themselves (Marchington and Wilkinson 2003; Japp, 2005). It is useful to have a structured approach to assessing such matters.

    Examples of transferrable skills include assessing and evaluating one's own work; assessing and evaluating the work of others; coaching; dealing with obstacles and crises; delegating responsibility; keeping records; motivating others; managing time; planning and arranging events and activities; presenting written and oral material; repairing equipment or machinery; handling complaints; managing finances; using computer software; and training or teaching others. There are many other skills that are not in this list. Worksheets can be used to identify transferrable skills.

Completing a transferrable skills worksheet

There is a need to complete a separate worksheet for each job or activity (see Figure 12.4):

1   In the Tasks column, ask the client to list each function of their (past) job or activity.
2   In the Skills column, they need to list the skills used to complete the task (see the examples list of transferable skills at: http://careerplanning.about.com/od/career choicechan/a/trans_skills_ex.htm).
3   In the Skill level column, the client rates him/herself according to their level of competency (1 = highly skilled; 2 = moderately skilled; 3 = needs improvement).
4   After the client has completed all the worksheets, they need to write a list of those skills they both enjoy using and in which they are highly skilled (1).
5   This is followed by listing those skills they both enjoy using and in which they are moderately skilled (2).
6   They can also keep a separate list of those skills in which they need improvement (3) but enjoy using. This list can be set aside.

Job or Activity		
Tasks	Skills	Skill level

Figure 12.4 Transferrable-skills worksheet

Step 6: (A) Assessing physical functioning

There are a number of tools for assessing physical capability, mainly, but not exclusively, associated with OT and physiotherapy practice. FCEs have been principally used in Australia and the United States to assess the physical activities associated with work, for example walking, sitting or bending (Table 12.2), and there are a number of models on the market, although the Matheson system appears to be receiving the most attention in the United Kingdom, where the use of FCEs has slowly grown in private practice (Matheson, 2003). The evaluation of various functional capacity tests is discussed by Gobelet *et al.* (2007) and Olivieri (2006). Chamberlain *et al.* (2009) report that, in the EU, the most frequently used tests are progressive isoinertial lifting evaluations (PILEs) (Mayer *et al.*, 1988), Isernhagen's FCE (Isernhagen *et al.*, 1999) and the ERGOS work simulator (Kaiser and Kersting, 2000). At whatever stage functional assessment is introduced, Holmes (2007) states that the assessor 'should be able to have the job demands of your client's work listed or at least in your mind when carrying out physical functioning assessments to ensure that you are targeting your assessments appropriately'.

Functional capacity evaluations

Mitchell (2008) considers that a routine medical examination can omit objective information and fail accurately to assess critical aspects relating to a patient's job. One claim put forward to support the use of FCEs – that they provide courts with objective data on capability (Mitchell, op. cit.) – has yet to be subject to legal examination in the UK High Court.

In contrast, in a number of countries, such as the United States, insurers, social security administration and the legal community frequently use FCEs in making decisions regarding:

*   identification of what the client can safely physically do (Raptosh, 2005);
*   identification of the capacity to return-to-work;
*   determination of work tolerance and endurance;
*   provision of an objective baseline for RTW planning, including rehabilitation needs (Allen *et al.*, 2004);
*   establishing of safe physical demand levels for future work physical capacity.

Predominantly owing to the influence of overseas private sector practice, FCEs are becoming more used in the United Kingdom, although there is no known evidence evaluating their applicability, reliability and validity in the United Kingdom. Holmes

Table 12.2 Physical demands characteristic of work (Matheson, 2003)

Physical demand level	Occasional: 0–33% of the workday	Frequent: 34–66% of the workday	Constant: 67–100% of the workday	Typical energy required (METS)
Sedentary	10 lbs	Negligible	Negligible	1.5–2.1
Light	20 lbs	10 lbs and/or walk/stand/ arm/leg controls	and/or push/pull of arm/leg controls while seated	2.2–3.5
Medium	20–50 lbs	10–25 lbs	10 lbs	3.6–6.3
Heavy	50–100 lbs	25–50 lbs	10–20 lbs	6.4–7.5
Very heavy	+100 lbs	+50 lbs	+20 lbs	+7.5

(2007) notes that, 'whilst there are quite a number of providers . . . FCEs have not entered into the language of our largest healthcare provider, the NHS', although a small number of NHS hospitals in Scotland now use them. It may be the case that evidence on the efficacy of FCEs in UK VR practice will only accumulate once the systems are being extensively used.

What does an FCE involve?

An FCE is an assessment of a person's physical capacity to work on a safe and dependable basis. There are three different types of FCE.

Baseline capacity evaluation

If there is no specific job in mind, a general FCE can identify the worker's capacity to undertake such activities as sitting, standing, walking, balancing, climbing, kneeling, stooping, crouching, kneeling lifting, carrying, pushing, pulling, motor co-ordination, fine finger dexterity, grasping and pinching.

Job capacity evaluation

If there is a specific identified job and a functional job description, or a job analysis has identified the critical job demands, these can be tested in a job capacity evaluation.

Work capacity evaluation

When there is a need to determine the potential of an individual to withstand the competitive demands of employment, such as a full-day's work tolerance and daily attendance, a work capacity evaluation is appropriate, with the results added to the baseline capacity evaluation or job capacity evaluation.

Procedurally, an FCE involves:

1   taking a history
2   performing a pre-evaluation screening examination
3   performing functional testing
4   interpreting results
5   preparing a report.

Short-form FCE

Gross *et al.* (2007) make the point that using FCEs is a burdensome clinical tool in terms of time and cost because of the extensive protocols, maintaining there is evidence that all or most of the important functional information can be obtained from shorter versions. For example, Cutler *et al.* (2003) studied the association between components of a twenty-item DOT FCE and RTW following chronic pain treatment. They found that only a crouching test was an independent predictor of short- and long-term employment outcomes.

Previously, Gross *et al.* (2004) identified that one item within the Isernhagen FCE (floor-to-waist lifting) was reported to predict back-injury claims outcomes, a finding consistent with Matheson *et al.* (2002), who found floor-to-waist lifting to be the most predictive item when the Isernhagen FCE lifting, carrying and handgrip tests were added simultaneously to a multivariate model predicting RTW at 6 months, in a cohort of individuals with MSDs.

Gross *et al.* (2006) describe the development of a short-term FCE for back-injury claimants, by excluding items from a more comprehensive FCE that did not provide meaningful prognostic information, but maintaining comparable predictive ability.

Who is qualified to undertake an FCE?

In the United States, FCEs have been undertaken for many years by various physical therapists, such as OTs and physiotherapists, although psychologists and vocational evaluators of various descriptions also use them. Although a clinical background is an advantage, some FCEs have been devised for non-clinicians. However, specific training in the administration of an FCE is required. Particular issues for non-clinicians relate to awareness of medical factors contraindicating testing, for example cardiac or psychological difficulties. There are currently few training opportunities in the United Kingdom, and anyone interested in FCE training is advised to contact the specialist work section of COT. A note of caution to anyone using, or planning to use, an FCE is to remember that RTW following injury or illness is a complicated, multidimensional human behaviour requiring the assessment, or at least the consideration, of multiple factors beyond functional ability and work demands.

Equipment and facilities

Appropriate facilities and equipment are required to undertake FCEs. Observation is an important assessment tool. This requires not only the availability of the range of assessment tools ordinarily found in VR evaluations, such as work samples and aptitude tests, but also tests designed to assess specific aspects of physical functioning, such as the use of a hand dynamometer designed to give accurate grip-force readings (available from www.promedics.co.uk) and equipment widely available from fitness suppliers, such as a heart-rate monitor and treadmill. Roy Matheson (www.roymatheson.com) supplies lifting equipment (EPIC lift capacity and PILE lift box) and the Matheson bench, a positional tolerance device. Casillas *et al.* (2006) describe the use of bicycle spiro-ergometry for the evaluation of work capacity.

Work instability scales

The Department of Rehabilitation Medicine at Leeds University has developed scales to measure work instability (WI), a state in which the consequences of a mismatch between an individual's functional abilities and the demands of his or her job could threaten continuing employment if not resolved. These scales address such matters as how much work a person can undertake and the number of hours they can work. Although initially applied to people with rheumatoid arthritis, they have been extended to cover ankylosing spondylitis, brain injury, two occupational groups – nursing and office workers – epilepsy and MS (the latter two scales are not yet published) (Gilworth *et al.*, 2003, 2006, 2007, 2008, 2009).

Pain

A common symptom of a physical problem is pain a matter that can have a debilitating impact on RTW prospects. The extent to which any screening for pain occurs in VR programmes has not been established. Among the tools that OTs, physiotherapists and other clinicians use for pain assessment are the McGill Pain Questionnaire (Melzack, 1975), Oswestry Low Back Disability Questionnaire (Fairbank *et al.*, 1980) and the Dallas Pain Questionnaire (Lawlis *et al.*, 1989). Watson *et al.* (2004) consider the role of pain management in returning to work unemployed subjects with low back pain.

Step 6: (B) Assessing cognitive skills

Specialist brain injury VR services, such as Rehab UK, employ their own neuro-psychologists. However, such specialist VR service providers are not always available, and generic service providers need to make arrangements to obtain a neuropsychological assessment (in addition to any other medical reports). Obtaining medical information from the NHS is often fraught with delay and objections, even after VR service users have consented to have such information released. A simple expedient is to ask the client to obtain this information him/herself.

The aim is to assess the degree of impairment in terms of cognition, mood and behaviour, and the implications for work. If requesting a neuropsychological assessment, the VR counsellor should enable the assessor to focus on the aims of the VR programme, even if only able to do this in a proscribed fashion. For example, a client with left-hemisphere damage seeking to return to a clerical position and not reporting visuo-spatial difficulties does not need an in-depth analysis of his/her visuo-spatial skills, and there is no need for an assessment to include such activity.

Neuropsychological assessments of cognitive function are invariably based on or around the administration of the Wechsler Adult Intelligence Scale- Revised (WAIS-R) (Wechsler, 2008) and generally include measures of memory, attention and concentration, speed of information processing, verbal and nonverbal reasoning, overall intelligence and executive functions.

Another test battery one finds commonly used is the Halstead–Reitan neuro-psychological testing battery (HRNTB). This was developed for use with adults by Halstead (1947) and later revised and extended. The revised battery for adults includes the category test (a measure of concept formation); tactual performance test (a measure of various sensorimotor functions); tactile form perception test (a measure of spatial organisation and kinaesthesis); seashore rhythm test (a measure of sustained attention and nonverbal auditory discrimination); speech sounds perception test (a measure of attention and verbal–auditory visual discrimination); and the finger oscillation test (a measure of finger tapping speed). The resulting battery (HRNTB) generates an index of possible brain damage, the 'impairment index', as well as other specific data useful in differential diagnosis of location, chronicity and the nature of the suspected lesion.

The HRNTB is generally supplemented with various measures of intelligence, achievement, sensory perception, sensorimotor functions and/or emotional–personality inventories. The wide range achievement test (Jastak and Jastak, 1965) and the Minnesota multiphasic personality inventory (MMPI) (Hathaway and McKinlay, 1967) have been frequently incorporated into the battery as measures of achievement and emotional–personality factors, respectively. The assessment of perceptual and sensorimotor functions has often been augmented by the trial making test for adults (Hathaway and McKinlay, 1967), also considered to have a cognitive component, grip strength using a hand dynamometer, tactile finger recognition, finger-tip number writing and tactile coin recognition. Certain speech, language and visual–constructional abilities have ordinarily been evaluated using the Alphasia screening test (Wheeler and Reitan, 1962).

In addition to the WAIS-R and HRNTB, the behavioural assessment of dysexective syndrome (BADS) should be noted (Wilson *et al.*, 2003). This is a self-complete questionnaire that can also be completed by a 'significant other', such as a partner or employer, to identify the degree of insight or self-awareness a client may have.

Although relating neuropsychological test scores to prediction of future employment status is frequently misunderstood, VR agencies need to be aware of client strengths and deficits, particularly when this may include such matters as disinhibition and anti-social behaviour. In general, there appears to be some consensus that, although such test scores are unreliable predictors of employment, neuropsychological disability is a major factor reducing successful labour market integration. This appears to be a contradictory statement. It needs to be remembered that neuropsychological tests are measures of highly defined and narrow aspects of human performance, designed to assess brain function rather than to reflect the many demands of 'real-life' activities.

VR counsellors are likely to find that neuropsychologists and clinical psychologists are very interested in the vocational rehabilitation of their patients, and that they will offer helpful advice in respect of such matters as the introduction of compensatory strategies. The obvious problems are that not all VR service users with psychological problems are offered clinical rehabilitation or referred to psychologists, and the demands on the time of such experts.

There is an obvious relationship between cognitive skills and vocational ones. Psychological evaluations are also useful when clients have conditions other than brain injury, such as MS, and work psychologists within Jobcentre Plus will provide appropriate advice.

Step 7: Assessing vocational interests, abilities and aptitudes

The emphasis on functional assessments in private sector VR and the fact that public sector VR service users no longer automatically receive a psychological evaluation have probably contributed to a lack of interest in, and/or awareness of, the value of such assessments in recent years. Their importance should not be underestimated. For many VR clients, a psychological assessment of their skills, abilities and aptitudes will be the most important part of the VR process, and, provided the VR counsellor has undertaken specific test administration training, there are no reasons as to why they should not administer such assessments when required to do so.

Psychological tests provide a standardised task, that is everyone taking the test is given the same standard set of instructions and the same test to do, and not only do the tests give individual data, but the results also show how groups of individuals have performed and how to compare the scores of the tested person against these – for example, a group of clerical or assembly-line workers.

Because tests have these properties, they allow the assessor to make objective, statistically based judgements about the client's prospects of:

1   succeeding in certain types of job
2   successfully undertaking a training course, and
3   behaving in a certain way.

Specific training is required to administer and interpret test scores; normally, the BPS Certificate of Competence in Occupational Testing (Level A) will suffice for most vocational tests. Level B is required to administer personality tests. There is a need for additional training to administer and interpret clinical tests of cognitive functioning.

Understanding test scores

Types of test score are as follows:

Raw score

This is the absolute number of correct answers on a test.

Scale score

For some tests, all the correct answers are added together to produce one scale score. To give an example, an ability test might contain twenty items designed to measure vocabulary and twenty to measure accuracy of spelling:

1   If the items are all mixed together, there is a single test that produces two scale scores, one for vocabulary and one for spelling.
2   If the two items are presented separately, there is a test battery (containing two tests: vocabulary and spelling).
3   The test might be used to provide a measure of general verbal ability. In this case, all forty items would be used to produce a single scale score.

In general, measures of maximum performance (test of how well a person can do) tend to keep the items for each scale in separate tests, whereas measures of personality and interests tend to mix up all the items together in one test, which produces lots of scale scores.

Norm-referenced score

A norm-referenced score defines where a person's score lies in relation to the scores of other people, the norm group. Such scores are relative measures, and results are often expressed in such a fashion; hence, a given ability score might be 'low' when compared with a university-graduate norm group, but 'high' compared with a sample drawn from the general population. More typically, norm-referenced scores are expressed as percentiles.

To make judgements about suitability for a job or a training course from the test scores, the assessor has to relate the scores to the potential performance in a job or training course. This is usually done in one of two ways:

1   There has to be an expert judgement as to what minimum test scores are required to be able to do the job or course. This is usually based on an examination of the

contents of a test item and the requirements of the job or course. The process is referred to as domain or content referencing.

2   The second method makes predictions of future performance from a person's test scores. This uses actual data about the relationship between the test scores and a job/course. This method is known as criterion-referencing.

Appropriate use of psychometric tests

The appropriateness of using psychometric tests with people with disabilities has been attacked on the grounds of poor predictive validity (Rogan and Hagner, 1990). Menchetti (1991) considered that they do not consider the influence of the actual work setting, and the ability to complete many standardised tests is adversely affected by the presence of a disability. More accurate prediction of a person's work adjustment requires assessment of the physical, intellectual and/or social demand characteristics of specific work environments.

Proponents maintain that tests are quick and easy to administer and produce standardised results, enabling clients to focus on realistic areas of work interest, although it needs to be remembered that testing takes place in an 'ideal', distraction-free environment, and, as such, the results may only reflect potential and not actual work performance. Ideally, they should be 'checked out' in a 'real' setting.

Examples of tests used in UK VR practice are as follows:

*   vocational interests:
    –   General Occupational Interest Inventory;
*   skills tests (Level A standard required):
    –   Basic Skills: Literacy and Numeracy (ASE/NFER-Nelson);
    –   General Clerical Test (Revised) (Harcourt Assessment);
    –   Modern Occupational Skills Test Series (ASE/NFER-Nelson);
    –   Watson Glaser Critical Thinking (Psychological Corporation), for employees working in managerial or supervisory type roles;
*   aptitude:
    –   Crawford Small Parts Dexterity Test (Harcourt Assessment);
    –   Differential Aptitude Battery (Psychological Corporation);
    –   General Aptitude Test Battery;
    –   Non-reading Aptitude Test Battery;
    –   Bennett Hand Tool Dexterity Test (Harcourt Assessment).

The use of work samples

The purpose of the work sample test is to allow the comparison of a person's performance on a vocational task with relevant performance standards, usually referred to as competitive norms or industrial or commercial standards.

Advantages

1   A work sample tends to look like a real job task and will hold the subject's interest.
2   Actual work behaviour can be observed.

3   The client may gain some insight into their capability.
4   A large number of areas can be evaluated: skills, interests, physical capabilities and work behaviours.
5   Additional medical information may be discovered, e.g. capacity to use a prosthesis.
6   They provide an alternative to paper-and-pencil tests when such measures are inappropriate because a person has verbal or reading deficiencies.

Disadvantages

1   They can be expensive to buy and they are usually not portable.
2   They can be time consuming.
3   Technical obsolescence is a problem in reflecting actual jobs.
4   They can only provide a 'snap-shot' of performance. Someone who tires may perform well over a short period but not over a longer one.
5   They can be used to assess actual performance but not potential capability.
6   Because they are designed for easy use, work samples might be used or conducted by individuals with little background or training in vocational evaluation, leading to questionable results.

The most commonly found work samples in UK VR practice are produced by the Valpar Corporation (www.valparint.com/); see Box 12.7.

The Valpar range has been around for some time, although some VR programmes continue to find the samples useful.

Box 12.7 Examples of Valpar work samples

- Small Tools (mechanical) assesses the ability to make precise finger and hand movements and to work with small tools in tight or awkward places.
- Size Discrimination assesses the ability to perform work tasks involving size discrimination, manual dexterity and finger dexterity.
- Numerical Sorting assesses the ability to perform work tasks involving sorting, categorising and filing by number arrangement and using numbers and numerical series.
- Clerical Comprehension and Aptitude assesses a variety of clerical-work skills.
- Multi-Level Sorting assesses ability to make rapid sorting decisions, involving several levels of visual discrimination of colour, numbers and letters.
- Simulated Assembly assesses the ability to perform repetitive assembly work requiring manipulation and bilateral use of the upper extremities.
- Tri-Level Measurement assesses work skills related to inspection and measurement tasks, ranging from simple to precise.
- Soldering and Inspection (electronic) assesses the ability to use small tools and to make precise hand and finger movements in close co-ordination.

---

232 The vocational rehabilitation process

Step 8: Assessing worker traits

- learning style
- work personality
- critical work behaviour
- social adaptive behaviour

Learning style

Although an assessment of learning style is more commonly associated with brain-injured clients, there are other conditions where such an assessment is helpful, such as learning disability and MS. Wheatley and Rein (1990) describe the learning style assessment, a method to identify the environmental and interpersonal characteristics to support optimal functioning, including employment, of the client with TBI. The learning style assessment is not, itself, a standardised instrument, but a way of interpreting the quantitative and qualitative results of tests to provide more effective intervention. For example, a person who was a verbal learner but is now aphasic as a result of a head injury must rely more heavily upon his or her visual processing systems, which are relatively less impaired. The learning style assessment involves identifying information outlined in Table 12.3.

The value of a learning style assessment is illustrated by reference to the problem of generalisation among clients with a brain injury. The traditional sequence of services in VR follows a process of evaluation, job development/training, job placement – the 'train then place' model. The model requires a client to be capable of generalising from a training programme/trial placement to a job site, in the process demonstrating the carry-over learning of new skills and a capacity for modification in response to work variations.

Table 12.3 Information to be identified in the learning style assessment (Wheatley and Rein, 1990)

Optimal method of presentation	Modality Visual Verbal Motor Rate of presentation Repetition required
Retention strategy	Internal External
Optimal environment	Physical Psychological characteristics Distraction Stimulation
Metacognitive capacity	Level of dependence on structure Capacity to generalise Capacity to respond to unanticipated events Level of awareness of cognitive characteristics Ability to resist distractors Motivation to maximise capacity Self-hindering characteristics Level of self-control

Recognition of how a VR service user best learns and retains new material facilitates any pre-placement rehabilitation activity, such as the development of commonly found IT skills, as well as induction and in-service training and supervision when in a job. With the use of domain-specific learning, that is the learning of skills particular to a task – for example, word processing with a certain program on a given type of computer – VR service users with severe memory impairments have been able to acquire sufficient skills for employment.

Work personality profiling

VR clients must either possess job-maintenance skills or develop them as a result of work adjustment intervention. Such skills include interpersonal, task performance and team working. To facilitate job-maintenance skills, one particular assessment tool used by the Working Out project at Aylesbury (Chapter 9) is an assessment instrument designed to measure vocational functioning, isolating those skills central to meeting the demands of the work role or maintaining the job, known as the work personality profile (WPP) (Roessler and Bolton, 1983, 1985).

Fundamental work capabilities (referred to collectively as the work personality of the client) consist of fifty-eight specific work behaviours organised into eleven categories of work performance and five high-order factor scales. The five factor scales are identified as task orientation, social skills, work motivation, work conformance and personal presentation.

Hooper (2003) concluded that,

> there is evidence for this instrument predicting success at key stages of returning to work. Among the factors derived from the items is one large one that consists of 21 of the 58 items representing 6 of the 11 rationally derived scales. These items describe essentially work performance including both cognitive skills and good work habits. High scorers in this factor would be initiating, performing independently, asking questions only when needed and having a capacity for self-direction. The other four factors are more narrowly defined and behaviourally orientated. These four factors cover interaction with co-workers, holding appropriate motivational attitudes, displaying conformance to rules and responsiveness to supervisors.
>
> The range of statements is such that it would take a number of days to have the opportunity to observe how someone would behave in most instances described. Thus this instrument would appear to be more suited to rehabilitation environments where raters have the opportunity to observe work behaviour at least over a week. Its reliability depends on trained and experienced raters. It would appear useful for some clients to self-rate.

The use of situational assessments for assessing worker traits

When they can be arranged, situational assessments often fail to provide detailed information on work skills because of the unskilled nature of much activity, for example basic clerical work or packing/shelf-filling. Nevertheless, there are many disabilities/ conditions where the work experience and the focus of such assessments can provide invaluable information, on such matters as accepting supervision; getting along with co-workers; sustaining productivity throughout the working day; tolerating frustration;

following instructions; initiating work; and observing work behaviours, for example, punctuality and safety.

There are limitations, and these need to be realised. Although a placement may help a former executive to get back into a work routine, they may not be motivated by tasks below their perceived level of capability. In addition, a simulated setting cannot provide the same variety of work and interpersonal demands as an actual job. Unless the VR counsellor is in a position to observe the work being undertaken, then he or she is likely to be reliant on a third party for feedback, and this can undermine a situational assessment. Not only can feedback be impressionistic and unreliable, but unhelpful 'allowances' might be made by supervisors.

On-the-job evaluation

On-the-job evaluations (OJEs) provide an assessment of the functioning of clients in actual work settings, where they are involved in activities considered compatible with their vocational interests and skills. Focusing on a variety of variables, such as personality, attitudes, aptitudes, work traits, work skills and physical capacities, OJEs can occur in any work setting. Although an evaluation usually takes between one and two weeks, the time period can range from 1 day to 1 month, or more (Genskow, 1973).

Historically, OJEs have been arranged towards the end of the VR process, with the placement based on earlier assessment outcomes. However, the growth in interest in the place–train model of VR has established a case for much earlier consideration. A job analysis and a general job-site inventory prior to placement are recommended. The job-site inventory provides information about the size of the company, types of work performed and the nature of the work. The job analysis profiles jobs in respect of (a) vocational aptitudes such as manual dexterity, (b) physical demands characteristic of the job and (c) interpersonal skills.

There are advantages and disadvantages to OJEs.

Advantages

1   They provide the opportunity to assess the client under natural conditions.
2   The OJE experience gives the individual an opportunity for self-evaluation of his/her performance in respect of such matters as producing work at specific rates of quantity and quality, reporting to work on time and responding to supervision.
3   On-site supervisors can supplement the evaluator's judgements with information from their perspectives regarding the client's suitability.
4   An OJE site has equipment for the job and eliminates potential costs to the evaluation programme.
5   A positive recommendation from a supervisor might facilitate a permanent placement.

Disadvantages

1   Opportunities for OJEs can be difficult to find.
2   Supervisors might be reluctant to devote their time to evaluation and simply regard the client as inexpensive help.
3   It can be difficult to apply standardised assessment procedures.

4   Premature placement might exacerbate the client's fears about the RTW process.
5   An OJE can be a time-consuming evaluation technique.

Situational assessments and OJEs need to be monitored. This is easier said than done when relying on a third party. Hence, the easier and shorter one can make this process, the better the prospect of obtaining a completed assessment. This means that there is a need to produce a specific assessment form for every client, as a standard pro forma might contain irrelevant items. In an ideal world, two assessors should carry out the task of completing the form, so that the results can be compared. It is easy to produce a focused form if one maintains a list of items that are likely to require addressing. These are likely to fall into two areas, critical work behaviours (Box 12. 8) and social adaptive behaviours (Box 12.9).

One can add specific job skills to this list or prepare another form – for example, in respect of answering the telephone appropriately and the acquisition of computer skills. Ideally, two supervisors should also rate social adaptive behaviour (Box 12.9).

It is important for any form to be completed in as standardised and informed a fashion as possible, if the results are going to be used with the service user to improve his/her performance, or as the basis for considering future placement options. For example, if

---

Box 12.8 Critical work behaviours

- Observes rules and regulations, including safety.
- Demonstrates knowledge of the job.
- Follows supervisor's instructions accurately.
- Works independently of supervisor after initial training.
- Reads instructions, memos etc.
- Remembers work instructions.
- Quality of work is acceptable/unacceptable.
- Has required dexterity for job tasks.
- Performs any required calculation, e.g. adding, measuring, and documentation.
- Work productivity/pace is satisfactory.
- Follows tasks through to completion.
- Attends work every day, satisfactorily explaining any absence.
- Punctual at start of the day and after breaks.
- Demonstrates a practical approach to problem-solving.
- Organises his/her own work and materials.
- Looks for things to do during slack periods.
- Requests assistance when needed.
- Has required stamina.
- Displays awareness of surroundings and activities in the immediate vicinity.
- Expresses self clearly and efficiently.
- Is appropriately assertive.
- Shows interest and enthusiasm for the work.
- Is appropriately dressed and groomed.

Box 12.9 Social adaptive behaviours

- Co-operates with supervisors.
- Refrains from complaining about supervisors, co-workers or work tasks.
- Profits from instruction or criticism.
- Works well with co-workers.
- Is accepted by co-workers.
- Maintains proper distance and posture from others during conversations.
- Demonstrates appropriate volume of voice.
- Displays appropriate expressions of emotion.
- Displays acceptable morals and ethics on the job.
- Maintains a realistic opinion of achievements and abilities.
- Handles minor work stress and frustrations on the job.
- Demonstrates swings in mood or unpredictable behaviour.
- Boldness presents a problem in social situations.
- Makes others feel uncomfortable because of actions, e.g. staring.
- Makes others feel uncomfortable because of inappropriate comments.
- Demonstrates an awareness and sensitivity to the feelings of others, e.g. knows when to end a conversation or not to interrupt others.
- Displays facial expressions appropriate to the situation.
- Distracts or disturbs others at work.
- Offers acceptable excuses for inappropriate behaviour if necessary.
- Attitudes of family or parents interfere with employment efforts.

---

the client is not punctual, there is a need to specify when this occurs, such as in the morning or after breaks. Such observations might help determine if the lack of punctuality is due to not giving him/her sufficient time to get ready in the morning, transport problems, socialising or the onset of fatigue during the day, thereby determining an appropriate response. Supervisors need clear guidance:

1 Each supervisor should be informed as the purpose of the evaluation. Each item on the assessment forms should be discussed before the assessment begins, in order to clarify requirements.
2 It is important that the supervisors rate the client in the same work setting as where the type of work is performed, as the setting can affect behaviour.
3 Each item requires some predetermined scoring, even if only a 'yes/no' tick list, with space for observations (particularly for 'nos').
4 If the supervisor is unable to complete an item, the reason(s) for this need to be clarified, and, if appropriate and possible, the evaluator might need to observe the described behaviour in the item not rated.

An example of how to develop a form is given in Figure 12.5. One can have one form combining critical and social adaptive behaviour or two separate forms. It is a matter of selecting items that the evaluator considers relate both to the client and work situation.

Worker

Supervisor

Observed and rated job tasks

Time and date of form

Employee work behaviours   Compared to other employees

	Currently a problem area	No longer a problem	Never was a problem	Unable to say

Compared to other workers does this worker have problems in any of these work behaviours (circle one number after each statement)

	Currently a problem area	No longer a problem	Never was a problem	Unable to say
1. Punctuality and attendance	1	2	3	0
2. Reliability as a worker	1	2	3	0
3. Stamina at job	1	2	3	0
4. Work productivity	1	2	3	0
5. Quality of work	1	2	3	0
6. Overall adjustment to their job	1	2	3	0
7. Relationships with co-workers	1	2	3	0
8. Relationships with supervisor	1	2	3	0
9. Amount of supervision required	1	2	3	0

Comments and specific problems identified:

....

....

Figure 12.5 Example of a supervisor rating form

Drawing assessment data together

Before moving on to stage 3 of the VR process, pre-placement support and job development, it is good practice to draw together all the assessment data. An example of an assessment summary form is given in Table 12.4. VR counsellors can draw up their own to meet their organisational and client needs.

Table 12.4 Example of an assessment summary form

Vocational goal	Rating	Comment
Physical strengths and limitations *(relating to client capacity to do the job)* Endurance Hand and finger dexterity Mobility Upper-body strength Lower-body strength Speech, hearing, sight		
Psychosocial strengths and limitations Adjustment to disability Emotional stability Effects of family and social environment		
Cognitive and behavioural strengths and limitations		
Educational/vocational strengths and limitations Education skills (basic literacy/numeracy) Vocational skill level Vocational interests Working with people Level of personal responsibility Work setting Opportunity for creativity Routine or variety Hours Pay Amount of physical energy expended Opportunities for advancement		
Additional considerations On-the-job coping demands Access Financial Transport Housing Childcare		

The resettlement issues then become ones of addressing deficits and identifying the services to meet the goal of returning to work. For a VR service user with an employer, this requires the drawing up of a GRTW plan (Figure 12.6).

In the example shown in Figure 12.6, the VR client was involved in a RTA, sustaining various musculoskeletal injuries including whiplash. She was said to have made a virtually full physical recovery but had developed an anxiety phobia, particularly over the journey to work and dealing with the unexpected. Even before the GRTW plan was introduced, a number of accompanied and, later, solo trial runs to and from work had to be made. Attached to the GRTW plan were:

1   an agreement signed by the client, employer and counsellor to support the GRTW; it is sensible planning to include other parties who might have an interest, such as OH;
2   an appendix listing expected duties; this was prepared with the assistance of the line manager and a job description; in the first instance, all routine tasks that needed to be undertaken in the office were identified; this included photocopying, filing, retrieving and putting away files, dealing with the post,including logging incoming mail and directing it to the appropriate person, and providing other routine clerical support to the planning officers; the client indicated that she would be happy doing this.

Responsibilities were gradually increased to involve answering external telephone calls, taking planning files down to a reception area to members of the public, making appointments for planning officers, and paginating files for planning hearings, necessitating some discussion with the concerned parties as to what to include. A co-worker with whom the client had a friendly relationship volunteered to accompany the client to any meetings with members of the public, as occasionally frustration with planning applications and decisions was vented on any available staff.

Every GRTW plan needs to be related to the employment circumstances of the individual and involve the employer, particularly when costs might be involved. When the VR service user does not have a job in order to establish a job goal, there is often the need to match the assessment findings against potentially suitable jobs. The GRTW plan is still a useful tool in any job trials/placements.

Summary

A vocational assessment is part of the evaluation process. The aim of the process is to identify an appropriate vocational goal, taking into consideration the service user's strengths and deficits. The more this process can be focused on a specific job or jobs, the more the assessment approach can reflect the service user's particular resettlement needs. Assessment tools are drawn from a wide range of disciplines, including work psychology, occupational therapy and human resources. There is rarely any disciplinary restriction on test usage, provided the administrator has undertaken appropriate training for the assessment in question. An exception relates to certain clinical tests, particularly of cognitive function. An issue for many UK VR practitioners is obtaining appropriate training. Although some universities and private sector organisations run short courses, often circulated by the VRA to its membership and/or put on the VRA website, there

Name:		Job title:	

Place of work:

Line manager:

Employment goal: to return to work full-time as a clerical officer in the local authority Planning Department (36 hours with flexi-time arrangements, core hours between 10.00am and 4.00pm and a 30-minute lunch break, 5-day week)

Start date:

Week	Objective(s)	Responsible persons	Review
1	Work 4 hours Monday, Wednesday, Friday undertaking modified duties	Client VR counsellor HR/line manager	Meeting of responsible persons at 2pm Friday VR counsellor contactable on phone by client and/or employer during the week
2	To work as week 1	As week 1	As week 1 (by phone or PC if need be)
3	To attend every day	As week 1	Meeting of client, counsellor, line manager
4	To increase hours to full-time	Clinet VR counsellor	Friday telephone consultation, client, line manager, counsellor
5	To increase responsibilities	Client VR counsellor HR/line Co-worker	Full review meeting to discuss progress and revise plan if necessary
6	As week 5	As week 5	Friday telephone discussion client, line manager, counsellor
7	Full-time hours and normal duties resumed	HR/line manager	VR counsellor available by phone/email

Figure 12.6 Graduated return-to-work plan

are limitations on availability. The United Kingdom is some way from developing the multi-skilled VR counsellor, and, hence, the VR practitioner relying on assessment tools, which they perhaps learned as an undergraduate or during in-service training, must be aware that, in order to obtain a holistic assessment of service user needs and prospects, it is necessary to take on board other disciplinary perspectives. There is no point or merit in gathering data for the sake of it. The information needs to be applied to identifying intervention programmes or strategies addressing the identified limitations/ barriers to employment and measures to build on strengths, in order to progress towards the vocational goal(s).

Student exercises

12.1 Assessment practice
Vocational evaluation relying on psychometric tests, work samples and in-house situational assessments for the purpose of diagnosis, placement or prediction is largely artificial and simulated, bearing little resemblance to actual community jobs. Discuss.

12.2 Case study: JJ
JJ is a 34-year-old aerial and satellite dish-fitter, working on a self-employed basis for one company. Ten months prior to referral he incurred serious injuries in a freak accident. The owner of a property on which JJ was working used her remote control to open a garage door on returning from a shopping trip. At the same time, JJ had begun to descend a ladder located over the garage door. On hearing and seeing the door open, JJ could not get down the ladder quick enough and jumped, breaking an ankle and severely injuring his back as he landed on the drive. JJ was hospitalised for 8 weeks, primarily to stabilise back problems caused by the accident. An orthopaedic report indicates that JJ was unable to stand for a prolonged periods and could not perform the physical demands of climbing, stooping and bending required in his job. In the initial interview, JJ explained that he had 'almost constant back pain', realised that he would not be able to return to his job and that he was learning to live with his pain. He had consulted a solicitor over the accident, but 'I don't know what is going on'. There are issues relating to the homeowner's household insurance cover and the fact that JJ did not lash the ladder. JJ has been referred to you by the solicitor for the insurer of the employer to whom he was contracted.

JJ left school aged 16 years, with four low-level GCSEs. On leaving school, he joined the Army and served in the Royal Corps of Signals for 9 years, having trained as a communication systems engineer and obtaining NVQs. JJ married Adele when he was 22 years old. The arrival of the first child coincided with the decision to leave the Army. They now have three children, aged 10, 8 and 5 years. On leaving the Army, JJ found employment through a family friend setting up video-conferencing facilities, fitting aerials, satellite dishes etc., initially 'on the books', but latterly he found he could earn more on a self-employed basis. JJ considered that he earned a 'good living'. Nonetheless, his wife had recently returned to work on a part-time basis as a school secretary because 'she wanted to get out of the house'. During the first interview, JJ stated that he had little time for hobbies, 'what with three children and 50 hours a week work'. He also said that he was keen to get back to work:

> At the moment my money is being made up but not to the level I was earning before the accident and I know it's not going to go on for ever. I need to do something but I honestly havn't a clue what to do. I've talked about self-employment with my wife . . . but what? I've only ever done outdoor manual work.

1   Identify potential vocational goals.
2   Identify what is to be assessed and how.
3   Identify how this information is to be used.

12.4 Case study: PM

PM has cerebral palsy, resulting in some loss of right-sided mobility and grip. He did not do well in his GCSEs and for the last 2 years he has been at college on a pre-vocational basic skills course. His dad is a long-established driver for T W Smith's, manufacturers and distributors of industrial fasteners such as nuts, washers, bolts, screws etc. PM's dad has suggested to you that the firm's personnel manager will consider offering his son a job 'if anything suitable can be found'. You ring the company and speak to Mrs Jordan, the HR manager. She says that PM's dad is a 'good worker' and that she has met PM. He is a 'nice lad' but, 'considering the nature of the work', she did not think there would be anything suitable for him, but 'you are welcome to come and have a look around'. On visiting T W Smith's, you are surprised by the number of employees, around sixty, housed in what you consider to be Victorian conditions. The company supplies major UK manufacturing companies with a range of fastening equipment. A lot of the material is bought in from abroad, but there is a workshop where various machine workers produce specialist fittings for employers. The personnel are as follows:

1	2	3	4	5+
Director/chairman				
Secretary				
Sales manager	On the road sales	Office sales		
	Sales clerks			
Accounts manager				Accounts
Personnel manager				
Reception				
Security				
General administrator				
Workshop manager				
Workshop supervisor				Skilled and
Stores manager				semi-skilled
Stores supervisor	Stores labourers			machinists (12)
				Stores clerks (8)
FLT driver	Assistant drivers/			Drivers (6)
	labourers			
Vehicle/maintenance	General labourers			
fitter	Cleaners			
	Quality control			

It is apparent that the company is tightly run: for example, when necessary, the receptionist is expected to undertake any required typing, including invoicing, and other office staff are required to cover for her when she is away. The hub of activity is around the workshop and the adjacent large stores. A racking system is in operation. Maintaining the correct level of stock is essential to the company's operations. Insufficient stock, and customers cannot be supplied. Too much stock, and there is wastage, with no income from goods standing on shelves. All the stores staff, except the labourers, use a computer system designed for stock-control purposes. Two of the stores clerks regularly deal with orders from the shop floor. Sometimes, it is a simple matter of collecting an item for a machinist; at other times, the FLT driver may be required to access a high shelf. A lot of time is spent on sorting incoming stock and making up orders, placed into either boxes or pallets on the stores floor, near the dispatch area. Sales staff are responsible for handing orders to the stores manager, and he then allocates the work. There is a staff restaurant, but no food is provided, although there are facilities for making a drink.

1   Identify potential vocational goals.
2   Identify what is to be assessed and how.
3   Identify how this information is to be used.

13 The vocational rehabilitation process, stage 3

Pre-placement support and job development

Key issues

- Rehabilitation support.
- Developing job search activity and interview skills.
- Job coaching.
- Shaping work behaviours.

Learning objectives

- Knowledge of interventions provided or arranged by VR agencies.
- Development of job search and interview skills training.
- Awareness of the pre-placement job coaching.

Introduction

The expression 'job development' means different things to different people. In the United States, it is often used to reflect an approach to supported employment based on the premise that everyone is 'work ready', and that it is a matter of finding the right opportunities and supports to enable each person to work successfully. In the United Kingdom, the term is used more generally to refer to pre-placement support and activity; usage is not restricted to supported employment.

The extent to which VR agencies provide or arrange support between the assessment and placement stages of the VR process varies considerably in the United Kingdom, reflecting:

- the modus operandi
- funding
- in-house resources.

In general, private sector VR counsellors tend to work on a peripatetic basis, and, hence, they have to access or buy into whatever additional services are considered necessary. Public and Third Sector-funded VR services are likely to have to have some specific support services in place in order to attract funding.

Table 13.1 Matching identified needs to interventions

Need	Intervention	Potential service provider
Work preparation		
'Checking out' assessment findings	Work trial(s) Job placement	Usual employer Other employer Jobcentre Plus agency Training organisation
Employment advice	Careers/job counselling	Connexions Jobcentre Plus PA Jobcentre Plus DEA Jobcentre Plus work psychologist VR agency Job broker Insurance-provided VR service
Basic skills, e.g. literacy, numeracy, computer awareness	Training/education	Jobcentre Plus agency Residential training college Education authority Training organisation
Increasing stamina	Work conditioning/work hardening	NHS PCT rehabilitation teams
Financial guidance	Benefits advice	Welfare Rights service Citizens Advice Bureau Jobcentre Plus
Change of lifestyle	Self-management	NHS PCT rehabilitation teams Replacement for CMPs
Transitional arrangement		
Long-term work support/transition to open employment placement	Supported employment Sheltered employment Rehabilitation work preparation	CMHTs Jobcentre Plus Remploy VR agency Community voluntary services
Acquisition of qualifications/ skills	Education/training	Local education authority Residential training college Private/third sector training agency
Job search skills		
Self-matching CV preparation Interview skills Disclosure rehearsal	Job club	Jobcentre Plus agency Job broker Residential training college Education authority Training organisation Local authority and voluntary organisations VR agency
Placement preparation		
Check out suitability of the workplace	Job and tasks analyses Environmental analysis	Access to Work NHS PCT rehabilitation teams Occupational health Insurance-provided VR service

Stage 3: Pre-placement support and job development

Step 9: Support and development services

Work hardening and work conditioning

Both WH and WC may be considered to be VR approaches cutting across assessment, job development and placing activity. Although much WH and WC activity can be found at the (early) clinical intervention end of a theoretical VR continuum, other intervention is closer to the placement and retention end. They are included in stage 3 because the aim is to 'bridge the gap' between initial assessment findings and placement activity.

PURPOSES

The American Commission for the Accreditation of Rehabilitation Facilities (CARF, 1988) describes WH as 'a highly structured goal-oriented individualised treatment program designed to maximise the ability to return-to-work, addressing the issues of productivity, safety, physical tolerances and work behaviours'. WH programmes involve clients in simulated or actual work tasks, endeavouring to provide the link between a client's residual physical functioning and the requirements of a particular job by focusing on physical (biomechanical, neuromuscular, cardiovascular), functional, behavioural and vocational needs. The tasks are structured and graded to progressively improve physical and psychosocial functions. In the event of a participant being unable to return to a previous role, the aim of the programme is to equip them for any other suitable occupation. A WH programme is recommended 6–12 weeks after the onset of acute symptoms (Mayer *et al.*, 1988; Krause and Ragland, 1994; Nachemson and Jonsson, 2000; Waddell and Burton, 2001). A psychosocial dysfunction, such as abnormal illness behaviour, fear and depression, is often present, but significant mental disorders should be excluded.

In order to overcome the multiple barriers to RTW, WH is not only based on work-oriented physical training (gym and work simulation); it also emphasises education and psychosocial interventions. Important issues are goal-setting, self-efficacy and the self-management of pain. There is a need to also include the optimisation of working techniques, tools, equipment and work organisation.

WC is a programme with an emphasis on physical conditioning that addresses the issues of strength, endurance, flexibility, motor control and cardiopulmonary function. WC has been applied by the American Physical Therapy Association (1992) to describe a less comprehensive programme than WH, a 'work-related, goal oriented treatment program for subjects with less complex conditions', provided by a single discipline and up to 4 hours a day. WC is limited to function- and work-related physical conditioning and does not include behavioural and psychological components.

The main goal of WC and WH programmes is to return injured or disabled workers to work, or to improve the work status for workers performing modified duties. The programmes either simulate or duplicate work, functional tasks, or both, in a safe, supervised environment. These tasks are structured and progressively graded to increase psychological, physical and emotional tolerance and improve endurance. Disabled workers learn appropriate job-performance skills in addition to improving their physical condition, through an exercise programme aimed at increasing strength, endurance, flexibility and cardiovascular fitness.

WH and WC can be labour intensive and, therefore, expensive, and should only be used with service users unlikely to return-to-work through other approaches. They can be particularly helpful when RTW after illness or injury is expected, but usual care has not resulted in this goal (possibly because there are factors listed by the yellow and black rehabilitation flags).

STAFFING

WH requires a co-ordinated interdisciplinary team, although not every member is likely to be required in every case. Members can include physiotherapist, OT, psychologist, vocational counsellor and other rehabilitation specialists.

FACILITIES

WH and WC require a gym for exercise and work simulation, as well as rooms for counselling and additional treatments. For out-patients, return to part-time work might be implemented during the programme, and on-site work evaluation can be added. WH activities are likely to include any combination of the following, carried out up to 8 hours a day, 5 days a week:

- physical conditioning
- simulated work activities
- education
- psychosocial interventions.

ASSESSMENT

A work-related baseline assessment should consider:

- the physical and psychosocial factors affecting the person's ability to participate in the programme and later return-to-work; the main part is a FCE;
- neuromusculoskeletal and cardiovascular status;
- work-related functional capacity;
- vocational status, including work demands; a job description from the client or company is the first step for compiling data on the worker's job tasks, physical, functional and psychological demands of the job and the use of specific equipment, tools and materials (Demers, 1992);
- incentives for a RTW;
- behavioural issues (including coping strategies and motivation to improve function, symptom-magnification tendencies, abnormal pain behaviours and work motivation);
- other psychosocial or financial factors.

Characteristics of WH and WC

(a) Use of goal-setting and self-efficacy: Goal-setting assists the client in listing their concerns and acquiring some responsibility for addressing them. Goals can be based on a specific activity level, for example walking a certain distance, or, more widely, a return-to-work. Negotiated personal and job-related goals also help to develop a basis for planning and monitoring the interventions. There is a questionnaire that can be used for assessing clients' beliefs about their work-related abilities and deficits, which can differ from results of an FCE (Matheson and Matheson, 1996)

(b) Structured information and education on coping with pain: This includes overcoming fear and avoidance behaviour (Waddell, 1998; Main and Spanswick, 2000; Vlaeyen and Linton, 2000).

(c) Symptom-negotiation training: Many prospective VR clients with chronic back pain feel unable to exert control over their pain, themselves and their environment. This, in turn, increases the lack of self-efficacy. Symptom-negotiation training is therefore an important aspect of a WH programme (Matheson, 1995). It is based on the following principles:
   • graded activity;
   • gradual exposure to feared movements (Vlaeyen and Linton, 2000; Vlaeyen *et al.*, 2001; Vlaeyen *et al.*, 2002);
   • pacing;
   • modification of working techniques, tools or workplace;
   • coping with exacerbated pain (Harding *et al.*, 1998).

(d) Physical conditioning and functional restoration: This is aimed at increasing strength (Saal and Saal, 1991), flexibility and cardiovascular endurance through such methods as circuit weight training (Gunnari *et al.*, 1984).

(e) Work simulation training: A work sample may address a single work trait, for example, manual dexterity, a collection of tasks common to various jobs, for example a mixture of strength, endurance, range of motion and so on, the common critical factors of a job, or all the key tasks of an actual job, for example electronic assembly.

(f) Other psychosocial interventions: This includes stress and pain-management counselling, as well as vocational counselling.

(g) Ergonomic interventions: Biomechanical analysis is the basic means of identifying matters requiring intervention (Armstrong, 2000). Modifications tend to fall into one of two areas, tool modification and job-site modification.

EVIDENCE

A Cochrane review (2004) concluded that work-related physical conditioning, including a cognitive–behavioural approach plus intensive physical training, seems to be effective in reducing the number of sick days for workers with chronic low-back pain, when compared with usual care (Schonstein *et al.*, 2002). A more recent review produces more equivocal findings (Schaafsma *et al.*, 2010). Based on twenty-three studies, eight comparisons of physical conditioning programmes were compared with other types of intervention, such as standard exercise therapy, for different durations of back pain and follow-up times. Physical conditioning programmes were further divided into 'light' or 'intense', depending upon intensity and duration. Results showed that light physical conditioning programmes had no significant effect on sickness-absence duration for workers with subacute or chronic back pain. Conflicting results were found for intense physical conditioning programmes for workers with subacute back pain. Further analysis suggested a positive effect on sick leave when the workplace was involved in the intervention. It was concluded that physical conditioning programmes probably have a small effect on RTW for workers with chronic back pain. No difference in effect was found between a 'light' or an 'intense' physical conditioning programme. CBT was of no significance.

Developing job search activity and interview skills

A common feature of many VR agencies is a job club. The person-centred approach (Box 13.1) starts with a focus on what the person wants to do now, rather than what he or she has to change to be job-ready (Hoff *et al.*, 2000). Understanding the preferences and needs of the individual also includes understanding the culture and values of the person, the family and community.

There is much that can be practised during the job search process, and activities requiring support can be assessed. For example, job-seeking normally encompasses the use of a telephone, completion of an application form and interview skills. VR counsellors can devise their own checklists for recording essential issues and arrange role-playing activity. Table 13.2 illustrates one such checklist.

Disclosure

Rehearsal is an important feature of the approach. One question frequently asked is, 'How do I present my disability/condition?' There is a need to remember that no one is covered by the DDA unless their employer is aware of the disability/condition; an employer is not obliged to create a job for a disabled applicant/employee; and employers are entitled to ask questions about a health condition, although the 2010 Equality Act prevents employers from asking candidates questions unrelated to the job role. This means that anyone with health conditions or a disability is not forced to disclose their condition prior to an offer of employment, unless it hinders their ability to do the job. There are guidelines for good disclosure that can be practised (Box 13.2).

Job coaching

Deal and James-Brown (1997) define a job coach as 'an employment specialist who facilitates disabled people in accessing and functioning and integrating in work settings

---

Box 13.1 Developing job search activity

- **Brainstorming**, generating ideas about work directions and the job search process.
- **Identifying personal networks**, and when there is no usable network.
- **Labour market analysis**, identifying:
  - major local employers;
  - types of employment;
  - organisations known to have a good track record in recruiting people with disabilities.
- **Market survey** of advertised vacancies.
- **Placement plan** setting out:
  - job goal;
  - skills, experience and qualities for the job;
  - contact strategy.

Table 13.2 Recording job search and interview skills

	X Not observed	1 Unaccept- able or poor	2 Adequate Marginal	3 Average	4 Above average	5 Very good
Job search skills						
Displays ability to identify realistic jobs						
Can produce correspondence or has assistance						
Can complete application forms or has assistance						
Demonstrates knowledge of how to independently make employer contacts						
Can supply references						
Demonstrates ability to describe health in a functional and non-stigmatising way						
Interview skills						
Uses telephone appropriately						
Arrives on time, presents adequately						
Enters interview appropriately, good initial impression						
Answers questions precisely						
Positively relates background training and work experience						
Explains employment difficulties appropriately, e.g. gaps in history						
Deals with sensitive issues in a positive manner						
Thanks interviewer for their time						
General rating of interview skills						
Comment						

Box 13.2 Guidelines for good disclosure

1 Scripting responses to anticipated questions such as:
   • 'How does your disability/condition affect you?'
   • 'Are there any accommodation arrangements you require?'
2 Rehearsing the answers until the applicant is comfortable with them.
3 Avoiding being too clinical or too detailed. The interviewer needs to know only four things:
   • Will the applicant be reliable?
   • Can they do the job as well as, or better than, anyone else?
   • Will they be of any value to the company?
   • Is there a need to make any 'reasonable adjustments'?
4 Being positive about skills and abilities.

---

through training, development and support within the employers' environment'. Support needs to commence before a work placement in order to prepare the VR service user for it. To be effective, information is required on the type of work the client is likely to undertake.

The development of job coaching in the United Kingdom mirrors the early use of employment specialists/job coaches in the United States, where they were initially employed to assist the placement of people with learning or psychiatric disabilities, later moving into the brain injury sector. Such initiatives were first recognised in the United Kingdom by public and Third Sector organisations that saw the value of moving clients from segregated, sheltered workshops into integrated, open employment. Changes to the nature of the SEP (Chapter 8) and the funding mechanism for the Work Programme are likely to increase the number of job coaches employed in the United Kingdom. The work of job coaches is indicated in Boxes 13.3 and 13.4.

Box 13.3 Job coach functions

(a) Identifying and analysing national and local labour market trends.
(b) Identifying job vacancies suitable for client group.
(c) Obtaining/creating profile of client.
(d) Making contact with employer.
(e) Learning and analysing jobs and identifying appropriate training method in line with company culture.
(f) Training and coaching clients using 'natural supports' where possible.
(g) Supporting the client to become integrated into the workforce.
(h) Giving feedback to client and employer.
(i) Producing appropriate documentation.
(j) Monitoring client progress long term in a manner acceptable to client, employer and Supported Employment/VR agency.

Box 13.4 Job coaching process

(a) Identifying potential employment opportunities.
(b) Creating profile of client.
(c) Making contact with potential employer.
(d) Learning job.
(e) Performing skills/task analysis.
(f) Learning company culture.
(g) Planning most appropriate method of training and development utilising natural supports.
(h) Delivering training to client and/or facilitating access to company training.
(i) Assisting co-workers to give support.
(j) Providing monitoring and feedback.
(k) Providing long-term support to client and employer.

(After Deal and James-Brown, 1997)

Within the workplace, traditionally job coaches in the United States have worked with clients in low-skilled occupations, although Brantner (1992) describes job coaching for TBI subjects employed in professional and technical occupations. The skill of the coach is not so much in respect of being able to learn the tasks of the job but being able to use a number of specialised instructional techniques to teach the job to the VR service user in the workplace. They may spend a number of weeks or months doing this and, over a period of time, often work with the same client in a number of different jobs with different employers. Cognitive and interpersonal training occurs on the job, as the client learns the job tasks. The amount and type of intervention are based on the requirements of the job and the needs of the client. This may range from continuous presence on-site during the initial stages, to a gradual, complete fading from the job site once the client is able to perform the job independently, according to standards set and agreed with the employer. 'Follow-along' monitoring and intervention occur, which can be increased or decreased as problems are encountered and resolved. It is apparent that a rationale for the development of the *in vivo* approach relates to criticism in respect of the transferability and retention of remediated skills acquired in a clinical setting.

Within the United Kingdom, Morrit and Clark (1997) noted that clients on their programmes tended to go into 'medium to high skilled jobs', involving tasks that cannot be performed by a person untrained in that job. They suggest that it is unreasonable to expect anyone quickly to acquire a working knowledge of such activity, and, as a consequence, they were rarely called upon to do *in situ* job coaching. They further note that, once a VR programme was completed, they would rarely see the clients again. They describe their role as being primarily one that places the emphasis on coaching clients *into* jobs (Box 13.5), starting with an advisory role and moving on to facilitating placement.

Other activity, not directly working with the clients, involved approaching employers, arranging work-experience placements, soliciting information about job vacancies, arranging outside placements (involving access and job analyses), preparing clients for

---

Box 13.5 Into job coaching

Activity:

(a) helping clients enhance existing skills and acquire new ones;
(b) helping clients relearn their employability skills;
(c) discussing changes in the labour market and how they could affect the type of work the client is aiming for;
(d) training in job search skills;
(e) training in job application skills.

(Morrit and Clark, 1997)

---

placements, monitoring, evaluating and record-keeping. They also added that they were frequently asked about benefits and legislation.

Deal and James-Brown (ibid.) recognised a need to take a pragmatic approach to the level of job coaching to be provided, noting that

> whilst in the ideal world, job coaches should provide ongoing support to the client in the work setting, in a manner appropriate to the individual, with daily contact of a one-to-one nature (if that is right for the client), the reality is often very different to this. Most (Supported Employment) agencies will simply not have the funding to provide intensive, permanent support and will therefore expect, after an initial time-limited period, the client in the workplace to take on a degree of autonomy.

They added, 'Natural supports from the client's workplace are vital to this process and must therefore be included as soon as possible in the process of support for the client.' They suggest that the role of the job coach is basically to support the client's work placement through a process of learning about how best to work with the client, and, second, to identify what natural supports are easily accessed and can be used long term, a role encompassing both pre-placement and placement activity.

Not everyone favours using job coaches. Fabian and Luecking (1991) considered that the reliance on a job coach might create problems for both employer and employee as a consequence of intrusiveness, a presence that is said to raise the issue of stigma in the workplace and questions the eventual attainment of integration; fading the job coach from the work environment and the related issue of dependency; retraining and subsequent promotional opportunities when the job coach has to re-enter the site and the issues of intrusiveness and fading emerge again; and job coaching possibly being a high-cost means of facilitating employment opportunities.

Such problems have given rise to alternative models of support incorporating the use of natural workplace supports, such as co-workers as job trainers, promoting mentoring relationships between the supported employee and others in the work environment (Nisbet and Hagner 1988) and using environmental cues as a means of sustaining new behaviours in the supported employee. The employment of job coaches and the use of such methods need not be exclusive activities. Job coaches working *in situ* may deploy such approaches. Indeed, job coaching in the United Kingdom has developed primarily from the need to provide additional support to VR service users with specific conditions, such as learning disability and acquired brain injury. These conditions, and others, can present challenges best addressed in the workplace (simulated or actual).

Obtaining job-coach training can be difficult. The British Association for Supported Employment (http://base-uk.org/) periodically runs related courses, and Ways to Work (www.waystowork.co.uk) runs a 2-day foundation course and a number of 1-day courses leading to certification by Lancaster University. The emphasis is on providing pre-placement support.

Behaviour (work adjustment training)

The application of behaviour management strategies in employment settings presents a number of challenges:

1   First, individuals are generally in the work environment for prolonged periods of time. Hence, strategies must be developed that do not rely on the continuing presence of a support worker.
2   Interventions must occur in situations where there might be a large number of co-workers, supervisors and members of the public, limiting the range of procedures possible without stigmatising the worker.
3   In some situations, a single occurrence of an inappropriate behaviour may lead to immediate and permanent exclusion from the job.

Examples of inappropriate support

One VR service user working in a florist's shop was asked to work with some young trainees on an arrangement, but swore and refused to co-operate each time this occurred. She was then re-assigned to work independently. The swearing and unco-operative behaviour were being maintained (negatively reinforced) by removing her from the undesirable group situation. Similarly, a proofreader in a newsroom repeatedly asked his job coach for assistance with tasks he was capable of performing independently. Each request was followed by a supportive response from the job coach. Although the job coach did not actually assist with the task, the high rate of unnecessary requests was being maintained (reinforced) by the supportive response. There are issues in respect of implementing appropriate responses. It might be practically impossible to apply any work adjustment training *in situ* and, if undertaken in any other setting, such as a rehabilitation facility, the issue of generalisation is raised.

Functional analysis of work behaviour

In the first place, there is a need to identify the causes of a problem by considering both the conditions under which the problem occurs and the consequences that follow. Behaviour can be challenged by altering the antecedents and/or consequential events.

Experienced, clinically trained professionals often use such terms as impulsive, emotionally immature, irresponsible, inattentive and so on to describe behavioural problems. Although they signify potential work problems, they lack an objectivity needed to assess required change. It is much more difficult to assess how often a person is 'irresponsible' than it is to determine the frequency of being late for work or failing to complete an assigned task. To implement appropriate intervention, there must be a specific knowledge of the inappropriate behaviour, such as:

- frequency;
- duration;
- the conditions in which it is most and least likely to occur;
- whether it is unacceptable behaviour or a performance or skill deficit.

The work adjustment problem needs to be objectively defined. There are few guidelines for doing this, and there is a need to develop appropriate responses to problem situations.

Types of behavioural problem

Behavioural issues at work are likely to fall into one of two categories:

1 a failure to meet minimal performance standards required in a given situation; and/or
2 inappropriate behaviour.

Skill deficits require interventions to teach the subject to have the desired strategies to compensate for the loss.

Performance deficits refer to those behaviours for which the subject has the requisite skills yet fails adequately to perform, for example refusing to do a task. Remediation of performance deficits involves modification of environmental circumstances to increase the probability that the desired behaviour will occur.

The reduction of inappropriate behaviour typically involves programming, not only to reduce the behaviour but increase appropriate alternative responses. Assessment begins with a baseline period, in which the target behaviour is measured as it occurs naturally in the work setting, without specialised intervention. These data are analysed to determine whether a discrepancy exists between the subject's performance and employer expectations. If a discrepancy exists, the significance is assessed by asking, 'What would happen if the behaviour remained unchanged?' If no significant negative consequences would result, then intervention is not necessary.

Antecedent and consequential analyses can be used to identify environmental events that precipitate and follow inappropriate behaviour. There are a large number of antecedent events that can evoke problems in the workplace, such as supervisor demands, interruptions, overstimulation caused by working in a noisy or crowded area, presence of specific co-workers or customers, unstructured break periods and changes in job tasks. Internal events such as fatigue from working continuously without a break, confusion and frustration from not understanding work assignments, and boredom caused by monotonous, repetitive work can also lead to problem behaviour. The premise for observation is that identification can lead to reducing antecedent conditions that lead to inappropriate behaviours.

Reinforcers and punishers can be used to address the consequences that follow inappropriate behaviour. Reinforcement involves receiving something of value (positive reinforcement) or escaping an unpleasant event (negative reinforcement) contingent upon the performance of a behaviour. Punishers are unpleasant events that cause a decrease in frequency of the behaviour they follow. If a stimulus event is reinforced, it will increase the likelihood that the behaviour it follows will reoccur.

Positive reinforcement is a process that results in an increase in the probability of a desired behaviour. A number of stimuli or events can serve as reinforcers, such as attention, positive feedback, performance and money. Praise is a common reinforcer, but, for some subjects, verbal praise might not work. Cognitive impairments, such as receptive aphasia, can interfere with the comprehension of spoken communication. In such a circumstance, verbal praise might be a source of confusion. A 'thumbs-up' gesture might suffice.

Subjects denying any performance deficits might view praise as condescending. Older subjects with years of pre-injury supervisory experience might resent praise from a younger person whom they perceive as less qualified and knowledgeable than themselves. In such situations, strategies such as self-monitoring and self-reinforcement, which place control with the subject, can be used.

The following steps can help maximise the effectiveness of reinforcement:

1   Reinforcers and the behaviours upon which they are contingent should be specified. For example, telling the client 'You may take a break after you have cleared up' is not as informative as saying 'You may take a break after all the tools have been returned to the store and the floor has been swept'.
2   Reinforcers need to be delivered immediately after the response to the inappropriate behaviour.
3   There is a need to speak slowly and pause frequently when specifying reinforcers and behaviours to subjects with attention deficits.
4   After giving instructions, the subject needs to be asked to repeat them and reinforce correct responses.
5   There is a need to use a variety of reinforcers.

The generalisation and maintenance of appropriate behaviours are crucial issues. There is clearly no guarantee that reinforcers begun in a rehabilitation trial will be generalised and maintained in a real job. Hence, subject to circumstances, it is recognised that a critical component is generalisation programming. This can involve teaching supervisors, peers and family members to identify and reinforce adaptive behaviour. A significant problem is in respect of what is known as stimulus-bound behaviour. Even small changes can result in a failure to show the desired response: for example, a change in a keyboard or a new part in the assembly order can provoke anxieties. The issue can be addressed by introducing variations of the critical discriminant stimuli, once the client has mastered the job – for example, a different keyboard. Generalising and maintaining reinforcers can be achieved by the job coach gradually moving from reinforcers after each occurrence to reinforcers after a variable number of occurrences. Reinforcement can gradually be reduced after a set number of tasks (known as variable ratio) or time (known as variable interval).

Shaping is another means of reinforcing appropriate behaviour. Lewis and Bitter (1991) cite the case of a 34-year-old male construction worker who could not meet the physical demands of his job but exhibited severe aphonia, a condition in which the voice volume and intensity are so low that speech is barely audible. The condition interfered with his ability to communicate at work and threatened his employment. The terminal target behaviour was to speak in a voice with normal intensity and volume. The shaping procedure began by having the subject read aloud scripts and vignettes of conversations among his co-workers while on breaks and at meetings. Initially, he was reinforced for any inaudible word. On subsequent trials, he was prompted to read loudly. Each time he read louder, he was given enthusiastic praise by his job coach. If his voice dropped to a lower volume, reinforcement was withheld. The procedure continued until he was reading the scripts in a clear, audible voice. In the next phase, the job coach and the subject role-played social and instructional situations at work. The shaping process was repeated in this context until the subject was speaking at normal level. In the final phase, the job coach arranged for conversations to occur between the subject and his co-workers at the job site. Audible speech was maintained by positive responses from the subject's co-workers and others. Lewis and Bitter maintain that the effectiveness of shaping can be maximised by following these steps:

1   defining the terminal behaviour;
2   defining the current performance level;
3   reinforcing a behaviour in the subject's repertoire that approximates the terminal behaviour, or withholding reinforcement for behaviours that are incompatible or do not approximate the terminal behaviour;
4   after a step in the sequence is mastered, increasing the criterion for reinforcement to a response that represents a closer approximation to determine a behaviour; no longer reinforcing behaviour occurring earlier in the sequence;
5   reinforcing the terminal behaviour on a continuous schedule;
6   fading intermittent schedule reinforcement to one where terminal behaviour is occurring consistently.

Further means of dealing with behaviour problems include:

•   contingency contracts; and
•   social-skills training.

The contingency contract is a formal agreement between the job coach and the client. This specifies the behaviours expected from the client and the reinforcements that the client can aim for by performing those behaviours. Contracts may be written or otherwise recorded.

Social-skills training programmes are typically conducted in control settings where the client receives high-density reinforcement and has a safe context in which to rehearse and develop target social responses. The specific training methods include: (a) instruction, (b) modelling, (c) role-play, (d) feedback and positive reinforcement and (e) homework.

Summary

The nature of services offered by VR providers between the assessment and placement stages of the VR process varies considerably within the United Kingdom (as the service provider examples in Chapter 7 illustrate). Some VR service users require support addressing their physical conditioning, although activities such as WC and WH are not commonly found. The emphasis at stage 3 of the VR process tends to be on both the management and presentation of the health condition in the workplace. Public sector services are more likely to have unemployed clients than private sector ones and, therefore, a greater focus on job search activity.

Although job coaching has been undertaken for a number of years within the United Kingdom, particularly within SE and brain injury programmes, the emphasis has often been on pre-placement support. Within many services, there is scope for more *in situ* support, although this can be intrusive, and the use of 'natural supports' has been suggested as an alternative to job coaching. The new arrangements for SE in the United Kingdom (Chapter 7) are likely to increase the demand for job coaches.

Student exercises

13.1 Preparing for labour market re-entry
How can a VR service user expressing anxiety over returning to work be prepared for labour market re-entry?

13.2 Disclosure
A VR service user is adamant that she does not want to reveal her medical history of depression to an employer. How do you respond?

13.3 Case study: problem behaviour
Following a traumatic brain injury, GP has generally made a good recovery and has retained his pre-injury skills, enabling him to return to work on a trial basis in a unisex hairdressing salon, washing hair, sweeping up etc. However, there is some disinhibition, and GP keeps making inappropriate remarks to female clients. The proprietor says that this is costing her business and the salon's reputation, and that she is going to have to 'let GP go'.
    How can GP's behaviour be appropriately shaped and managed?

14 The vocational rehabilitation process, stage 4

Placement, job retention and case closure

Key issues

- Timing of a placement; awareness of work-related ill health.
- Working with employers, placement options and strategies.
- Matching a client's capabilities to a job.
- A conceptual framework for job retention and vocational rehabilitation.
- Strategies to enhance retention:
  - workplace adjustments
  - self-management
  - natural supports
  - use of job coaches.
- Follow-up and case closure.

Learning objectives

- Awareness of the issues surrounding different placement options.
- Understanding of job and task analyses.
- Ability to achieve a 'good fit' between the client and a targeted job.
- Insight into the application of compensatory strategies in the workplace.
- Awareness of how to utilise natural supports.
- Understanding of the issues affecting job retention strategies.

Introduction

In view of the rise in the number of IB claimants over the last 25 years, remarkably little attention has been paid to how employers approach the retention of sick/disabled employees. Howard and Thornton (2000) highlight why this is the case historically:

- the first weeks of sickness absence (after self-certification) being verified by a GP with no brief to do more;
- the employer having little or nothing to do with the employee until no longer sick;
- the benefits system not being conducive to rehabilitation; and
- the private insurance sector not being motivated to intervene at an early stage (the insurance sector would disagree with this point, maintaining the problem is the late notification of a potential problem by employers).

Circumstances have changed in recent years as a consequence of the government-led drive to reduce the number of benefit claimants, the increase in health insurance policies providing payments when an employee is off work sick and the development of a so-called litigation culture.

However, the availability of a VR service to a sick or disabled employee, or unemployed person with a health problem, still depends on such random factors as the geographical location, the disposition of an employer and insurer and the priorities of health-service commissioners. In the absence of mandatory accreditation, standards remain voluntary and implicit. Nowhere in the VR process is the lack of uniform standards more apparent than in the job-placement process. There is no universal agreement on what constitutes a successful placement (for example, the number of hours or weeks worked) and frequently little reference as to the mechanics of how this was achieved. Chapter 14 aims to fill a void in UK literature in focusing on placement, adjustment and retention strategies.

Timing of a placement: awareness of work-related ill-health

Although work in general is good for health (Royal College of Psychiatrists, 2002; Aylward, 2004), there is a need to be aware of the relationship between health and employment. Despite work often being the best rehabilitation for many people, it needs to be recognised that this approach predominantly applies to people with commonly found conditions. There are many VR service users, such as those with an acquired brain injury, for whom the relationship between the demands of everyday living and employment needs to be carefully assessed and managed. In such cases, premature RTW may be injurious to their health and prospects. Many VR service users require at least one work trial, and, with some clients, work trials need to be of an extended nature.

Work-related ill health can arise when there is a mismatch between the capabilities of the employee and the physical demands of the work and/or social/emotional demands of the work. The importance of sickness-absence policies (HSE, 2004) and the development of a proactive approach to health management in the workplace cannot be overstressed. However, most employers in the United Kingdom, particularly SMEs, do not provide access to an OH service, and, even when they do, employees can be reluctant to have any problem exposed. (NHS Plus is always available to SMEs on a commercial basis, but there is little evidence as to the extent this service is consulted.)

Most work-related musculoskeletal issues relate to the relationship between the body, including posture and manual handling, and the demands made on it (Frank and Thurgood, 2006). A lack of control over the work situation and long hours can both exacerbate the situation. When the nature of the work, or working environment, is the problem, successful rehabilitation cannot be accomplished without an analysis of the workstation and environment.

The largest growth in occupation-related ill health in recent years is in the field of MH, where stress (a matter largely incapable of objective scientific definition), anxiety and depression are now the most common reasons for sickness absence (DWP, 2002). The causes are almost always multifactorial and may be difficult to pinpoint (DWP, 2002).

When the VR service user needs to find a new job, a work trial, approximating the final target occupation as much as possible, is likely to alert the VR counsellor to any unanticipated problems. As well as situational assessments based on 'real' work, travel and other non-work-related factors are actively managed in the job-placement process.

Even for a situational assessment/work trial, job-site training and advocacy might be essential for some clients. In the first instance, if not returning to the usual employer, placements need to be identified.

Stage 4: Placement, job retention and case closure

Step 10: Placement options and strategies

In the United Kingdom, funding for VR agencies has often necessitated taking whatever work placements are available in order to trigger payments. There has often been insufficient attention paid to placing options and longer-term retention issues.

There are a number of reasons as to why an employer may wish to consider employing, retaining or providing a work trial for someone sustaining injury/developing a health condition. Many employees who become disabled, or develop a health condition, retain skills, knowledge and experience that can continue to be utilised. Recruiting new staff can be both time consuming and expensive, besides which the DDA requires employers to make 'reasonable adjustment' to facilitate employment. Although there is a need for vocational agencies to establish good working relationships with employers, too frequently this does not occur other than in insurance-funded cases. VR support may only be provided long after injury, or there are limited resources to visit employers, so that employers' experience of injured or ill workers returning to work is often one of them first 'getting better'.

If placement and retention rates are to be improved then, with the consent of the service user, it is considered that there is always potentially a need to offer the employer advice on the disability, intervention techniques required at the job site, medical implications that can accompany the employee's performance, social problems and possible methods to minimise stressful situations, and how to contact a support worker should problems arise.

Key points to placement (adapted from Corthell, 1993)

Effective placement is based on an analysis of work requirements. Details in respect of job requirements, characteristics of the work environment and other features that might influence job retention are considered essential for matching job requirements with client abilities. The second key point is that job placement can take place with clients who do not possess all the necessary work, cognitive or social competencies for immediate job success. However, this requires careful consideration as to the consequences of any placement failing. There are a number of pre-placement factors and placement options to consider:

1 Ideally, the job should be compatible in some way with the service user's previous work experience. Work placements might be rejected if they do not conform to the client's expectations of the work role and identity. For example, someone with a clerical background might have difficulty accepting a manual placement. Certain work placements have a neutral character, such as garden centres and charity shops. Although a work trial could lead to a job, at this stage the most important issue is a return to a 'real' working environment.

2 The service user has realistic attitudes about the purpose of work. Attitudes to work often include placing a value on one's time. An attitude may exist of 'I am not working for nothing'. The issue of payment should be addressed as part of pre-placement planning. It might be necessary to ensure the service user sees the trial as a continuation of the rehabilitation process. Service users might need to be helped to realise that work is not just about money, but also about providing a structure to their life, restoring direction, assisting with interpersonal and cognitive skills and restoring a sense of self-esteem and confidence. There is a need to check travel arrangements. In some cases there will be a need to have a 'trial run'.

3 The position matches the service user's mental and physical ability. It is important to ensure that the first placement is likely to succeed. If the job initially conforms to the client's expectations in respect of status, identity and previous experience, but the client fails to settle into the work role because it is too physically or mentally demanding, the consequences could lead to a loss of motivation and confidence.

4 The work role is compatible with the service user's interpersonal skills and emotional stability. If a work placement is to be successful, then acceptable interpersonal skills must be demonstrated. Although a brain-injured VR service user might be able to accept the principle that the customer is always right, in practice they might not always show such discretion. A gradual exposure to customers is preferable to subjects being left on their own.

5 There is appropriate and sufficient supervision available. Many VR service users are likely to take longer than other employees to learn and settle into a work routine. They will respond faster if there is some structure in the workplace. This might be in the form of supervision from another employee. Initially, the client, and job coach, will need to have regular meetings with supervisors to discuss progress, review the job description and determine if the level of supervision can be reduced.

6 There are flexible working hours and conditions. Many VR service users are likely to need a gradual reintroduction to the workplace and need to resume/start work by spending 1 or 2 hours, two or three times a week, at the workplace, gradually increasing the hours and frequency of attendance as their stamina improves. It is also necessary to show that skills relating to the work role have been consolidated before work hours are increased. This should mean that the subject becomes more independent in the workplace, so that an increase in working hours does not increase supervision time.

7 The placement needs to be accessible and safe. If the client has to spend time travelling to and from work, then performance and tolerance of work might suffer. Quality of the workplace needs to be considered in respect of such matters as health and safety requirements, reliability and good quality of supervision throughout the day, commitment to the placement(s) and the opportunity for personal development, as opposed to being perceived to be 'cheap labour'.

Placement options

The implications of both trial and permanent placements need to be considered:

1 Return to previous employer – same position: A return to the previous position might facilitate regaining previous financial and personal status, although many VR service users are incapable of this. This placement might require advocacy to enhance skill acquisition and maintain performance standards, including orientation, communication and counselling, and on-site assistance such as work restructuring. If a positive employer–employee relationship existed prior to injury, this situation may be re-established. On the other hand, the employer and work colleagues might have difficulty if the worker is 'not the same person'. A negative aspect of returning to the former job occurs when the client does not have the skills to return to the same position or there are safety reasons as to why such a return would be inappropriate. An inability to return to the same work can produce issues in respect of disability acceptance and generate frustration. Such matters are best addressed before alternative placement options are considered.

2 Return to previous employer – different position: This placement offers the potential security of familiar surroundings and experience of the work routine and co-workers. Difficulties with this placement can occur when the client is unwilling to accept a position below his/her previous status and ability.

3 Same job – different employer: The same job but different employer option provides a familiarity with the required job skills but introduces challenges from a different setting. An assessment that deals with the physical, social and organisational aspects of the work site can provide information that might have an impact on the work performance. Emphasis needs to be placed on the required level of interpersonal skills and the establishment of natural supports to reinforce and monitor social interaction. Employer and co-worker education might be necessary to prepare both parties for this work placement.

4 New job – new employer, (a) subjects with prior work experience: In some cases, physical injuries will prevent a client returning to a former occupation. Placement will require an assessment of residual skills and the exploration of options allowing for the transfer of skills. For example, a former mechanic might have all of the cognitive abilities to work in his field but not the agility or strength required to physically perform the required job tasks. On the other hand, a parts counter person might require knowledge similar to that of a mechanic but not the physical ability to competently undertake the work. During the VR assessment stage, residual skills should be noted, and vocational development should be planned around these abilities. If the individual does not wish to return to a position related to former skills, other options need to be pursued. Personal qualities (ability to work well with others, mathematical abilities, cognitive levels, previous academic records, capabilities and so on) can be assessed, and appropriate jobs can be pursued.

(b) Subjects without prior work experience: A person acquiring an injury at an early age might have limited or no previous work experience to bring to the placement process. In such a circumstance, it is often best to develop career options relying on intermediate goals to determine the appropriate way forward. In addition to open employment, some VR clients will require consideration for supported employment or permitted work. In all placement options, it is advisable to have the support of the family. The family might assist with transportation, completion of application forms and in encouraging the acceptance of suitable positions, although, on occasions, the family might have a negative impact.

Home-working and self-employment

A minority of VR service users might not be able to return to their former employer for environmental reasons but, nevertheless, be capable of undertaking most, if not all, aspects of the required work from home. Indeed, in some cases, such a measure might be regarded as a 'reasonable adjustment'. Such cases might not only require technological considerations but also practical ones, such as whether or not Council approval is required to work from home, and the social impact of working in isolation from colleagues.

Self-employment offers at least the theoretical prospect of organising one's own workload to suit circumstances. People with cystic fibrosis are particularly prone to infections and often have an above average sickness absence level. Examples of self-employed people with CF include a mobile hairdresser, solicitor and dry-stone-wall builder.

Step 11: Work-site evaluations, job design and adjustments

Prior to placement, a work-site evaluation is recommended. This can serve a number of purposes, such as allowing the opportunity to provide the client with objective data to prepare him/her for the job and 'designing' aspects of the job to accommodate the client, such as providing advice to the employer on reasonable adjustments. Essentially, the objective is to achieve a 'good fit' between the client and the job. The necessary work-site tasks to undertake to achieve this (with some overlapping between them) are:

(a) job analysis
(b) assessing workstation accessibility and usability
(c) job design
(c) compensatory strategies and making adjustments.

Job analysis

Chapter 7 observes that the characteristics of clients of private and public sector VR services vary, the former being more likely to have a job or, at least, an employer to return to. Theoretically this means that private sector VR counsellors are likely to have a greater opportunity than their public sector counterparts to undertake a job analysis as part of the job–client matching process; 'theoretically', because practical difficulties are recognised. This means that VR counsellors without the opportunity to undertake a job analysis must consider alternative means of job information gathering.

It might seem a matter of common sense that matching a disabled client against a potential job requires information about not only the client's work competencies but the demands of a particular job. The reality is that, in many VR services, job analysis is not undertaken to any great extent, if at all. It is time consuming, it can be intrusive, and there is not always funding for it. Nevertheless, job analysis is a task that *should* be undertaken. Many organisations carry out their own job analyses as part of good recruitment and selection procedure and in order to develop a job profile and personal specification. The analysis details the core and peripheral functions of the job, how it is organised, its setting/location and the qualifications required. When this task has already been done, there is little to be gained from repetition, other than gaining a familiarity with the work environment.

The first skill a VR practitioner is likely to require is one of convincing an employer of the benefits of an 'outsider' undertaking any such analysis. Occupational psychology and HR publications abound with information on job analyses, but few approach the subject from the perspective of placing a person with a disability. There is no model job analysis, and it is a matter of developing an approach and format that do the job. Whatever job analysis is used, it is important to recognise that:

- it is undertaken in a systematic fashion, to ensure that nothing is missed;
- information needs to be gathered from more than one source, for example a job description and the views of a supervisor; and
- for many clients, there might be an issue of breaking down tasks into subtasks.

What aspects of a job are analysed?

Data need to be collected in the following areas:

1 **Duties and tasks**: Information to be collected about such items might include movements carried out during the work and awkward postures associated with constrained body positions; frequency and duration of work cycles, for example highly repetitive movements; strengths needed in different tasks, complexity, equipment and standards.
2 **Environment**: This can have a significant impact on the ability to do a job. Factors to look for include access, flooring, lighting, air quality, cleanliness/hygiene, substances (toxic and non-toxic), temperature and humidity, any hazards and vibrations.
3 **Tools and equipment**: Some duties and tasks are performed using specific equipment and tools. Equipment can include protective clothing. These items need to be specified. To reduce the risk of work-related MSDs, tools should allow the work to be done with the wrist in a slightly extended functional position, avoiding excessive flexion, extension, ulnar and radial deviations; be of a balanced weight (centre of gravity should correspond to the centre of the hand grip); and be capable of being used by both hands, so they can be alternated during the task.
4 **Relationships**: This covers supervision and relationships with co-workers and external people.
5 **Requirements**: This covers the knowledge, skills and abilities required to perform the job, such as the general skills and any specific training requirements (and where it can be obtained).

Undertaking a job analysis

As indicated, practitioners can devise their own means of recording essential information. Typically, a job analysis is the process of breaking down aspects of the job into component parts. For example, there is a need to make a list of duties and tasks necessary to perform the job. Next, the following questions require answering:

1 How often does the task take place?
2 How is the task performed? What methods, techniques or tools are used?

3   How much time does the task take? Any variation?
4   Where is the task performed?
5   How is task accomplishment measured?
6   What happens if the task is done wrong?
7   What aptitudes (potential to learn and accomplish a skill) are necessary?
8   What general knowledge is necessary?
9   What skills are necessary?
10 How much physical exertion is needed (lifting, standing, sitting etc.)?

Essential functions

Once there are answers to these questions, the essential functions of the job need to be determined – what are the bottom-line skills needed to be successful at the job? What is the relationship between the tasks involved in the job? Is there a special sequence that must be followed?

Associated questions might be:

11 What physical activities are required to undertake the job?
12 How is the job organised in the overall work environment? Could some reorganisation improve the opportunity for their client with a disability?
13 Would removing some of the tasks to accommodate the client with a disability fundamentally alter the job?

Once essential functions are determined, the marginal functions, not strictly necessary for success, can begin to be eliminated. The importance of consulting co-workers and supervisors cannot be overstressed.

Work environment

Typical questions requiring an answer are:

14 Where are the essential functions of the job carried out?
15 How is the work organised for maximum safety and efficiency?
16 What are the physical conditions of the job setting (indoors, outdoors, underground, air-conditioned, dirty, greasy, noisy, sudden temperature changes etc.)?
17 What are the social conditions of the job (working alone, working around others, working with the public, working under close supervision, working under minimal supervision, working to deadlines)? This information is particularly important for people with disabilities applying for a job, so that they can decide what supports and changes to the work environment (if any) they might need to fulfil its requirements.

Such a systematic process also needs to be applied to gathering information on tools and equipment, relationships and any special job requirements. Various techniques can be used to facilitate a job analysis, including repertory-grid interview, critical-incident technique and task analysis. Case studies can be found in DiLeo *et al*. (1995).

Repertory-grid interview (Kelly, 1955)

Managers are asked to identify the attributes that make people successful in a particular role. They do this by identifying three job holders and explaining how two of them differ from the third. This is continued until an appropriate amount of attributes measuring successful job performance have been identified. Repertory grid can also be used in relation to a job performance. Respondents are provided with elements of the work in groups of three and asked how two of them differ from the third. This leads to opposites being initially identified, such as the length of a particular task. In such a fashion, data are built up regarding the requirements of a job.

Critical-incident technique (Flanagan, 1954)

This method applies more to higher-level jobs and identifies competencies and behaviour making someone successful in a particular role.

Task analysis

This method allows for a highly structured understanding of a particular task by breaking it down into its constituent parts. The main purpose is to evaluate the interactions

---

Case study: Job analysis and adjustment for short-term memory

Mick works in a nursing home as an assistant. Until some adjustments were made, his short-term memory was proving an insurmountable obstacle to successfully holding down a position.

Job analysis
During the VR process, it was identified that close relatives of Mick own a nursing home. They were willing to employ him in some capacity, provided he could work reliably without constant supervision. A job analysis identified three tasks that Mick could do and in which he expressed an interest: folding laundry, tidying a garden area and clearing the dining room after meals. A 20-hour-per-week job was created around these tasks.

Adjustment for short-term memory
At first, the duty manager tried posting a daily list of activities, but this did not work, particularly when Mick was outside and there was nobody there to prompt him. A co-worker noted that Mick regularly checked his mobile phone for text messages. His daily tasks were then posted on to his phone, appearing every time he checked it. This arrangement was successful because Mick got into such a routine that the need to prompt him declined over a period.

Co-worker support
Co-workers were encouraged to get Mick to check his phone and not to distract him from his routine.

Case study: Job analysis, job carving and equipment modification

Gabby is a clerical assistant in a government department. She is restricted by cerebral palsy. The following adjustments were made:

Job carving
Job analyses were undertaken in the department to identify tasks compatible with Gabby's capabilities. Three that did not typically get completed, and in which Gabby was interested, were identified. They performed the basis of a job description for a new post within the department.

Equipment modification
A template was purchased to put across the keyboard and reduce the prospect of hitting two keys at the same time.

Co-worker support
Female staff volunteered to accompany Gabby to the staff restaurant so that she would not feel left out.

Environmental accommodation
Gabby was located in a ground-floor office to reduce the travelling distance from the car park to the office. Grab rails were fitted in a ground-floor toilet. She continues to be brought to and from work by a taxi paid for by Access to Work.

---

between user and a work machine or system and to design jobs, taking into account the worker's limitations and capabilities. There are three main steps (Salvendy, 1987):

1 identifying and gathering information about the requirements of the task, reducing this to subtasks;
2 recording appropriate data; and
3 analysing information.

Workstation accessibility and usability

An issue with a work trial that might not occur with a permanent placement is the opportunity to make some adjustments to a workstation. A workstation is any 'area with equipment for the performance of a specialised task by a single individual' (Merriam-Webster On-Line Dictionary) and not just a computer desk. Workstations not based on the physical and mental capabilities of their users are, at best, likely to be inefficient and, at worst, harmful. For example, poor posture and movement caused, or exacerbated, by a badly designed or ill-considered workstation can lead to musculoskeletal injuries (Dul and Weerdmeester, 2001). On the other hand, appropriately considered workstations have the capacity to reduce the impact of a disability. For example, software or input devices are available for people with perceptual difficulties (Sears, 2003).

Factors to consider when analysing a workstation are: (a) a workstation may have more than one user, and (b) a user may move from one station to another. In such cases, it is necessary to consider the main usage, although health and safety legislation requires the needs of all users to be taken into account (HSE, 1998).

A starting point when assessing a workstation often involves ensuring that an employee can maintain a neutral posture, that is one in which the muscles and ligaments spanning the joints are stretched to the smallest possible extent but are also able to deliver their greatest force. Practically, this often requires the employee's elbows to be at a working height, this being achieved by adjusting the height of the seating, lowering the work surface or workpiece itself. Guidelines (Dul and Weerdmeester, ibid.) are:

Posture

In respect of posture, standing for long periods is tiring for the whole musculoskeletal system, particularly the back and legs. Similarly, sitting for long periods can be tiring, particularly if a neutral position cannot be maintained and an employee sits hunched or has to stretch excessively. Obviously, individual differences and environmental circumstances make the definition of a 'long period' unrealistic, but the HSE's (2002) upper-limb-disorder risk assessment checklist makes reference to durations of 2 hours or more.

Fit-for-purpose equipment

In considering fit-for-purpose equipment, there are a number of guidelines, including:

- BSI EN ISO 9241–5 (BSI, 1998a): Ergonomic requirements for office work with visual display terminals (VDTs): Workstation layout and postural requirements.
- BSI EN ISO 9241–5 (BSI, 1998b): Ergonomic requirements for office work with VDTs: Guidance on usability.
- BS EN ISO 14738 (BSI, 2002): Safety of machinery. Anthropometric requirements for the design of workstations at machinery.
- HS (G) 57 (HSE, 1998): *Seating at work*.
- Work with display screen equipment Health and Safety Regulations (HSE, 2003).

Generally, these guides provide dimensions, such as a suitable working height, to suit most users, but also discuss the background and criteria that enable the practitioner to apply the correct principles to individual cases.

Tools

Time and budget constraints rarely lend themselves to much consideration of tools, accessories, IT and software. When equipment is designed or bought specifically for a disabled employee, it does not have the benefit of widespread usage.

Labelling

Some years ago, Marks and Spencer (M&S) redesigned its warehouses so that each area housing a particular category of stock, for example clothing, was painted a different colour. For people with dyslexia, this reduced the amount of information they needed to know to locate specific items. If one looks at M&S clothes labels, one can see that a combination of colours is used to indicate different sizes. This reduces the informational demands upon all employees and customers.

Environment and task influences

There is more to providing an accessible and usable workstation than ensuring the employee fits and can use the equipment provided. The environment in which the work is conducted has a direct relationship with both the performance of the user and the equipment. Factors such as sunlight, temperature, ventilation, noise and vibration can all adversely affect the capacity to do the job.

HS(G)60 (rev) (HSE, 2002a) provides guidance on the prevention and management of upper-limb disorders, injuries historically associated with posture, repetition and force. It also highlights additional risk factors, including the working environment, and psychosocial factors, including the effects of work pace, piecework, supervisory support, attention and concentration, deadlines and seasonal changes.

When considering individual circumstances and job design, there is a danger of 'dumbing down' jobs: for example, making text bigger and bolder for the visually impaired, louder for the hard of hearing and simpler for those with cognitive impairments. People with disabilities need stimulation just as much as the able-bodied population, and an oversimplification of tasks can be demeaning and lead to frustration and boredom.

Job design

The process of successfully supporting an employee on the job starts with good job design. This necessitates bringing together the work-site and the client-assessment data and making an informed judgement in respect of:

*   the client's physical and intellectual ability to do the work, taking into account several aspects of the tasks that make up the job, including:
    *   equipment
    *   physical environment
    *   nature of the work
    *   work methods and times
    *   procedures used
    *   materials
    *   routines
    *   rules
*   environment; for some clients the will be a need to identify:
    *   location of furniture, pathways, tabletops, toilets, restaurant etc.
    *   co-workers movements and how they relate to the job;
    *   social culture: job design is not restricted to an understanding of how tasks are performed; an analysis of the social culture is necessary if the client is to be integrated into the workforce; this can include such factors as dress and grooming, rules about breaks and lunch, what is regarded as an acceptable pace of work, ways employees are initiated, oriented and released, power relationships, the 'pecking order', subgroups and their primary ties, humour, expectations of teasing and joking.

Compensatory strategies

'Compensatory strategies' refers to a group of techniques, procedures and devices that allow an individual to overcome a cognitive, physical or emotional impairment and successfully perform a specific task or behaviour (Parenté *et al.*, 1991).

Compensatory strategies are said to be suited to vocational applications because they can be designed and implemented at the job site and might result in an immediate improvement in production and self-esteem. To be effective, compensatory strategies must be developed on an individual basis, with a knowledge of the work environment. Typically:

1   The first step in developing compensatory strategies is reference to a vocational or psychological evaluation to determine the client's strengths and weaknesses with regard to areas having a direct implication for potential work performance.
2   The second step is a job or task analysis, that is an evaluation of the work setting and the step-by-step process necessary for work completion.
3   The next step involves the development of a series of specific instructions and/or materials to be utilised by the client.

At least four categories of compensatory strategy can be used in vocational settings (Table 14.1). 'Slotting' a strategy into a specific category is not a constructive activity. Some interventions can be listed in more than one bracket. To this list, one can add (5) cognitive remediation (Kreutzer *et al.*, 1988) as an appropriate intervention and support strategy for many brain-injured people, although many rehabilitation practitioners might perceive such intervention as a pre-placement activity.

1   Job analysis is covered above.
2   Environmental engineering refers to changes made to the job site or workstation to facilitate the worker's adaptation to the work setting and promote independent task performance. This can refer to mechanical changes, as well as human support and other arrangements, such as flexi-time.
3   Prosthetic aids involve the design and use of materials or devices to compensate for an inability to perform specific tasks. The process of using assistive devices to facilitate task completion is described by Parenté and DiCesare (1991). They recommend a number of devices, including checklists, electronic signalling devices, telememo devices, personal directories and microcassette recorders. Wright *et al.* (2001) compared two styles of pocket computer memory aids for people sustaining closed head injury. It was found that all twelve volunteers could use the memory aids, and most found them useful. The authors considered that there is a need to distinguish ability from the willingness to use such aids.
4   Cognitive orthotic devices refer to a specific type of prosthetic aid that performs a specific cognitive process or task required in a certain job (Parenté *et al.*, 1991).

Table 14.1 Categories of compensatory strategy used in vocational settings

Category
1   Job analysis
2   Environmental engineering
3   Prosthetic aids
4   Cognitive orthotic devices

Many of these devices take the form of microcomputer software, such as spell-checkers.

Cognitive remediation and accommodating neurological impairments imposes specific challenges. There are several ways in which cognitive deficits can be addressed, including role-playing, environmental engineering and the use of prosthetic aids and assistive devices, as well as cognitive orthotic devices.

Matching compensatory strategies to presenting problems

Briel (1996) describes an approach used to maximise the use of compensatory strategies for individuals with TBI participating in a SE programme. Key components included assessing residual skills, identifying potentially effective compensatory strategies through situational assessments, and incorporating compensatory strategies into training on the job.

It needs to be remembered that one support model will not be appropriate for every person's needs, and a series of different options might be required.

VR clients sometimes have difficulty accepting the use of compensatory strategies for a variety of reasons, such as embarrassment, considering they do not have a problem, or being pessimistic about their value. Suggestions for ensuring the optimal use of compensatory mechanisms include capitalising on strengths, fully involving the client in the development of strategies, helping the client to understand the potential value of the technique, and gradually introducing strategies to avoid overwhelming the client. Because needs and abilities will change over time, in an ideal situation VR practitioners should monitor the effectiveness and value of strategies.

Crossover between compensatory strategies and workplace adjustments

It is possible to view the introduction of compensatory strategies as no more than the making of workplace adjustments. Whether or not they are 'reasonable' is likely to depend upon the resources of the employer. For example, whereas a VR professional might be aware of certain psychological techniques to facilitate the employment of a brain-injured client, an employer, even one with OH support, is unlikely have any knowledge unless told. Certainly, the examples of reasonable adjustments provided in the 1995 DDA are readily identifiable (Chapter 5). Hence, taking the example of a brain-injured VR service user with commonly found behavioural and memory problems, while the rehearsal of appropriate behaviour might facilitate employment, this is unlikely to be regarded as a reasonable adjustment to be made by the employer. On the other hand, allowing the use of notebooks for recording important information; watches and electronic devices with alarms being used as reminders of important daily events; improving attention by reducing distractions in the work environment; and providing rest breaks may all be regarded as reasonable adjustments.

Making reasonable adjustments

Employers regularly make adjustments for disabled and non-disabled employees. In connection with the former, common examples are the:

- provision of adapted equipment, for example split-screen software for a clerical worker who could not read a computer screen past the left mid-line, or a ladder with locking castors and side rails to allow a worker with a balance problem to replace ceiling lights;
- modification of the workplace or premises;
- change of location of job from one place to another;
- redesign of working duties, e.g. allowing a worker reporting stress a period of time without telephone interruptions so that he can concentrate on production;
- reallocation of a worker to another job;
- provision of flexible working patterns;
- special leave or additional time off;
- provision of additional support on the job, for example using one worker as a mentor for another.

There is a need to recognise that individuals with similar characteristics and job duties can have different adjustment needs. For example, one person with cognitive problems as a result of a brain injury might have difficulty organising their daily schedule and benefit from the use of a computerised pocket organiser. On the other hand, another person with a brain injury might find such devices difficult to program or confusing to use and might benefit more from a simple paper-and-pencil organiser with a 'things to do today' section.

In order to assess for and implement adjustments, there is a need to bring employers and employees together. While aware that performance problems could be occurring, employers might not realise the extent of the individual's functional limitations as a result of injury. For example, the employer might know that an employee has suffered a brain injury, yet not identify this as the reason why reports are disorganised.

The need for adjustments can stem from the following.

Symptoms of the condition

Examples of adjustments falling within this category include work-schedule changes allowing for medical appointments and allowing telephone calls during work hours for support or counselling. The DDA says nothing about addressing specific conditions, although, given the extent to which MH problems are encountered in the workplace, there is a case for giving this subject additional consideration. In order to avoid any unfounded assumptions about the nature of conditions, what needs to be addressed is how the symptoms (B) affect job performance (C) (Figure 14.1).

Specific tasks requirements

Tasks obviously vary from job to job. Making adjustments requires an assessment of the VR service user's strengths and limitations and matching the findings against job

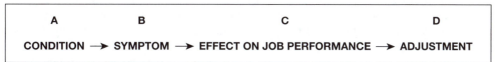

Figure 14.1 From a condition to an adjustment

and task analyses. Although tribunals are not necessarily interested in whether or not the person concerned is consulted over any adjustments (as long as they are made, the process whereby adjustments are determined is not of paramount significance), taking on board the opinion of the person concerned is not only likely to result in an identifcation of areas requiring adjustment but also to facilitate implementation. Line management and work colleagues might also have significant contributions to make. This is a matter that can be particularly important in the context of MH, where the process of adjustment is often a social process. In a study of 194 employees with psychiatric disabilities, MacDonald-Wilson *et al.* (2003) identified the most frequent functional limitations as (1) social, (2) emotional, (3) cognitive and then (4) physical.

Working circumstances

These include, for example, hours or method of training.

Environmental circumstances

Environmental circumstances include, for example, access to premises. An example of an adjustment within this category is reserving an enclosed office/cubicle for a worker who might have difficulty concentrating.

External circumstances

Examples of adjustments within this category are making travel-to-work arrangements and permitting an employee to work at home.

Identifying a need for an adjustment

Employers have a legal responsibility to provide reasonable adjustments (Chapter 5), but they cannot do so unless they know there is an issue. Finding a reasonable adjustment is not always easy. There is no 'one solution fits all' method to use. Although a VR service user might not initially appear to need adjustments in order to RTW, this can change if the job changes, tasks change, health or disability needs change, the employment moves location, or if new systems, policies or procedures are brought in. In the first instance, there is a need to identify what is causing the difficulty:

- Is it the physical environment, the chair, the lighting?
- Is it an inability to do a part of the job because of the impairment?
- Is it having to move equipment?
- Is it taking part in training/meetings, perhaps because of communication issues?
- Is having too much to do causing stress and anxiety?

On most occasions, the employees themselves will be able to identify a need for an adjustment. On other occasions, advice might be required from someone such as a medical expert or OT. The use of pro formas will help establish need covering the five areas listed above. Tables 14.2 and 14.3 illustrate.

In addition to job functions, the working environment also needs to be considered (Table 14.3).

Table 14.2 Identifying a need for an adjustment: assessing essential job functions

Tick any essential job functions or conditions that pose a problem for you. Describe the two most important job adjustments that you need, for example modifying existing equipment, adding new technology, or changing the type of work you do.

Physical abilities	Problem ✓	Cognitive abilities	Problem ✓	Social abilities	Problem ✓
Working 8 hours Standing all day Standing part of day Walking for 8 hours Some kneeling Some stooping Some climbing Much pulling Much pushing Much talking Seeing well Hearing well Handling work Raising arms above shoulders Using both hands Using both legs Using left hand Using right hand Using left leg Using right leg Lifting (specify object/weight) Prolonged sitting		Immediate memories Short-term memory Judgement/safety Judgement/ interpersonal Thought processing Problem-solving Planning Organising Short-term memory		Working alone Working around others Long-term memory Interacting with supervisors Supervising others	
		Task-related abilities		*Working conditions*	
		Repetitive work Pace sequencing Variety of duties Performing under stress/deadlines Little feedback Reading written instructions Ability to drive Attending to precise standards Following specific instructions Writing Remembering Speaking / communicating Initiating work activities		Too cold Too hot Temperature changes Too wet Too humid Slippery surfaces Obstacles in path Dust Fumes Odours Noise Outdoors Inside	

Company policies

Work schedules
Inflexible work
Lack of flexitime
Inflexible job description
Vague job description
Rigid sick-leave policy

Describe the two job adjustments that would be most helpful to you, e.g. restructuring of the job, modification of work schedules, reassignment to another position, modification of equipment or provision of readers and interpreters:

1 ....

2 ....

Table 14.3 Assessing accessibility/environmental issues

Tick any problems you have getting to, around or from your job. List any other access problems not included in the list. Describe solutions for the two most important access issues.

	Problem ✓		*Problem* ✓		*Problem* ✓

Parking
Entrance
Access to office
Stairs/steps
Floors/covering
		Temperature
		Ventilation
		Hazards
		Lighting
		Evacuation routes
				Lifts
				Toilets
				Identifying
				  signs/labels
				Access to general-
				  use areas
				Seating/tables	

List any other access/environment problems:
1 ....
....
2 ....
....

Describe solutions for the two most significant problems:
1 ....
....
2 ....
....

From this point, it is possible to draw up an adjustment plan that is likely to include arrangements falling into the following categories:

1   Procedural: in this category are likely to be arrangements such as:
    • reduction of hours in the working day
    • flexi-time arrangements
    • job restructuring
    • reassigning some tasks to co-workers
    • job-sharing
    • working from home
    • supervisory/co-worker support
    • provision of some physical assistance.
2   Equipment: this might include:
    • memory aids
    • fans (to combat heat)
    • larger computer screen.
3   Work-site modifications: for example:
    • easing access to the work site
    • easing access to the workstation
    • appropriate toilet and rest facility access.

Factors emerging from research are that the *perception* of costs in accommodating disabled employees influences decisions, and adjustments follow different patterns for retention and recruitment (Needles and Schmitz, 2006). For existing employees, employers will generally adapt the work to suit the needs of the employee, such as providing special leave, whereas, for new recruits, the work remains the same, but adjustments are used, such as special equipment, to help the recruit fit the job.

Identifying the appropriate adjustment

In the United Kingdom, Access to Work teams have developed considerable expertise in providing advice on adjustments. The Job Accommodation Network (JAN) (Morgantown, West Virginia) provides a searchable online accommodation resource (SOAR) system designed to let users explore various accommodation options for people with disabilities in work (http://askjan.org/soar/index.htm). Regrettably, there is no UK equivalent, which means that sourcing some of the recommended technical solutions might be problematic.

Technology

Some conditions require extra consideration, and it is difficult to see how employers can be aware of what is available without specialist consultation. The suitability of technological products requires expert assessment. For example, there are different types of computer screen reader available for blind and visually impaired people. Through a synthetic voice, some relay back what is being typed. Others read what is on a web page. There are also readers that have a Braille output device. Magnification software products enlarge a particular part of a computer screen. Closed-circuit-camera systems can magnify print and text and then display an enlarged version on a television or computer screen. Although this is excellent for some who are visually impaired, for others with tunnel vision such magnification would just reduce the field of vision. There are also 'standalone', portable versions, which do not require a television or computer. Stickers can be put on to standard keyboard keys that either present the letters and numbers as Braille or simply increase the size of the characters.

Examples of technological products suitable for some people with a physical disability include a larger keyboard if someone has difficulties with dexterity. Devices are available that take the place of keyboards but are smaller and need less effort to press the keys. An 'on-screen keyboard' means the user only needs a mouse to select characters on the screen. Alternatives to using a standard mouse include joysticks or trackerballs, which can be easier to control and use. Pointers and sticks are available that can be attached to the head and used to press keys on a keyboard. As with mobile phones, predictive text can help increase the rate of typing – after typing two or three letters, the user is given a selection of words to choose from.

Commonly found adjustments for employees with specific conditions

The DDA does not provide illustrations of disability-specific adjustments. The probable explanation is that not everyone with the same diagnosis requires the same adjustment. However, some adjustments are more commonly associated with certain conditions than others; for instance, people with a SCI and wheelchair users are likely to require a car parking space adjacent to the employment location, appropriate access and egress, suitable toileting facilities and so on.

Neurological conditions

Examples of modifications for people with a range of neurological conditions, such as an acquired brain injury, include:

1   **Modifying work activities**: such modifications often take the form of flexible scheduling, colour-coding materials and modifying communication formats, with supervisors and co-workers, for example, receiving/giving written as opposed to verbal instructions.
2   **Using an assistive device**: typical adjustments in this category include time-management systems (either computer- or paper-based), buying headsets to reduce extraneous sounds and purchasing modified keyboards.
3   **Workstation modifications**, such as erecting sound barriers to reduce distractions, repositioning materials for easier access, and individual task lighting.
4   **Addressing fatigue**: most adjustments involve schedule changes and allowing for breaks or flexi-time. In addition, providing products that might prevent fatigue can be useful, for example a cart to reduce the physical burden of moving heavy objects.

Multiple sclerosis

MS reinforces the need to focus on specific individual circumstances. MS is a complex disability from an employment perspective. People with the disability are often well educated and appear to encounter disability onset and its associated impairments in mid career, although this is not always the case. It needs to be recognised that MS creates particular resettlement problems because of:

*   unpredictability
*   pervasiveness
*   gravity
*   cumulative psychological effects.

Once diagnosed, the prognosis in individual cases is difficult for clinicians to determine, and this means that the employment position needs to be regularly monitored. Some people experiencing symptoms such as an episode of visual deterioration, ataxia or sensory disturbance in a limb might make a full recovery; others will go on to experience more attacks. Although there are widespread individual variations, major clinical issues include:

*   impaired mobility and motor function
*   cognitive deficits
*   fatigue
*   vision impairment
*   mood fluctuations
*   difficulties with micturition/continence
*   heat sensitivity.

Job retention is likely to be the focus of most VR intervention. This is likely to have implications for the realistic assessment of:

- performance difficulties (assessing the individual)
- worksite barriers (job and task analyses)
- compensatory and/or other adjustments strategies.

This represents a return to the points made previously in respect of what needs to be assessed, and, in a case such as MS, this can rarely be done without some structured assessment format that involves the client, even if this only involves asking them to complete a checklist. In addition to the pro forma above, there might be a need to prepare a checklist that identifies the symptoms, from which adjustments might flow, as indicated in Table 14.4 (based on a study by O'Connor *et al.*, 2005).

O'Connor's study is based on 100 patients with MS attending an MS outpatient clinic at the National Hospital for Neurology and Neurosurgery. The employment difficulties most identified were difficulties with walking and access at work. For example, a 51-year-old solicitor who had had MS for 8 years said, 'I travel by minicab because I can't use public transport, so I only go to the office twice a week'.

Learning disability

People with a learning disability often require visual cues, such as charts and checklists, using written instructions as a supplement to verbal ones. Tasks are often learned more efficiently if demonstrated rather than simply explained.

Table 14.4 Impact on work questionnaire

On the right-hand side of the list rank, from 1 to 17, in order of significance, the symptoms and factors you consider most commonly adversely impact upon your employment.

How much does the symptom impact on your work (please circle)? Rank 1–17				
Fatigue	Not at all	A little	Moderately	Quite a bit	Extremely
Balance	Not at all	A little	Moderately	Quite a bit	Extremely
Walking difficulties	Not at all	A little	Moderately	Quite a bit	Extremely
Visual problems	Not at all	A little	Moderately	Quite a bit	Extremely
Weakness	Not at all	A little	Moderately	Quite a bit	Extremely
Handwriting	Not at all	A little	Moderately	Quite a bit	Extremely
Pain	Not at all	A little	Moderately	Quite a bit	Extremely
Coordination	Not at all	A little	Moderately	Quite a bit	Extremely
Speech	Not at all	A little	Moderately	Quite a bit	Extremely
Swallowing	Not at all	A little	Moderately	Quite a bit	Extremely
Continence	Not at all	A little	Moderately	Quite a bit	Extremely
Concentration	Not at all	A little	Moderately	Quite a bit	Extremely
Memory	Not at all	A little	Moderately	Quite a bit	Extremely
Mood	Not at all	A little	Moderately	Quite a bit	Extremely
Travel to work	Not at all	A little	Moderately	Quite a bit	Extremely
Access at work	Not at all	A little	Moderately	Quite a bit	Extremely
Public attitudes	Not at all	A little	Moderately	Quite a bit	Extremely

Mental health

Examples of adjustments for people with MH problems include:

- altering the work content
- providing support
- shortening or altering work hours
- increased tolerance of absenteeism
- allowing extra holiday or unpaid leave
- permitting absence for treatment
- allowing rehabilitation following absence.

For most people with commonly found conditions, it is unlikely that much more than these adjustments will be required. However, more severe conditions are likely to require extra consideration, as illustrated in Figure 14.1. By focusing on the consequences of the symptoms, one can begin to move from a diagnostic label to appropriate adjustments, as illustrated in Figure 14.2. (Again the crossover between introducing compensatory strategies and making adjustments appears, and it becomes a matter of judgement as to how far an employer is expected to go. A tribunal will take into consideration such factors as the status of the employee, their health, length of service and the employer's resources. It will be evident that adjustments cannot be seen, nor should be viewed, in isolation from other disability management strategies.)

In case of any misperception that adjustments will always be required, Dewson *et al.* (2005) found that 41 per cent of employers made no adjustment to retain a disabled employee, and 56 per cent made no adjustment to recruit one.

Additional retention strategies

In addition to compensatory approaches and adjustments, placement and retention strategies can be enhanced by utilising:

(a) self-management
(b) natural supports in the workplace.

Self-management strategies

The term self-management is frequently used interchangeably with self-control or self-regulation. Because self-management approaches are implemented by the individual, they have a number of advantages in a work setting. The various components of self-management involve:

- self-recording and self-monitoring
- functional assessment
- self-instruction and self-reinforcement.

Self-recording refers to the use of conventional observation and data-collection strategies to measure one's behaviour. For example, someone attempting to meet a production standard of so many units per hour might simply record each unit as it is completed. Self-monitoring is similar to self-recording. Functional assessment in this

Mood disorder

Depression and the effect on work
- Low motivation.
- Poor ability to stick to a task.
- Mistakes.
- Irritability.
- Sensitivity to criticism.
- Poor stress tolerance.

Vocational strategies and adjustments
- Straightforward tasks to aid memory and concentration and help develop a sense of mastery.
- Predictability, little change in tasks from day to day.
- Clear guidelines and protocols, possibly written down.
- Flexibility with regard to the pace of work, timing of breaks and so on.
- Work as part of a team to minimise isolation.

Bipolar disorder (manic phase)
- Inflated self-concept, reduced level of interpersonal functioning.
- Excessive, inappropriate motivation.
- Distractibility.
- Distracting to others.
- Poor judgement.
- Poor stress tolerance.
- Workplace danger.

Vocational strategies and adjustments
- Role for OH in checking medication is taken to reduce severity of mood swings.
- Structured work setting with clear guidelines and expectations to help modulate mood.
- Clear and predictable time frames and deadlines.
- Clear limits with regard to behaviour and dress.
- Flexible scheduling to accommodate effects of medication and fluctuations in energy level.
- Regular feedback about job performance and social interaction, if appropriate.

Anxiety disorder

Post-traumatic stress disorder (PTSD)
- Inconsistency.
- Reduced stress tolerance.
- Low energy, poor endurance, high error rate.

Vocational strategies and adjustments
- Predictability, reducing fear of unknown.
- Option of working independently (but not in isolation) to control the working space.
- Opportunity to arrange the workspace as needed.
- Flexible scheduling to accommodate medication effects and fluctuations in symptom severity.
- Social support.

Figure 14.2 Mental health: examples of moving from the diagnostic label to adjustments (adapted from Fischler and Booth, 1999)

Personality disorder (characterised by problems 'getting along')

Schizophrenia
- Unusual interpretation of ordinary events.
- Aloof and disinterested, or oddly intense and excited.
- Ostracised by others.
- Unusual ways of processing information.

Vocational strategies and adjustments
- Work alone to accommodate poor social skills.
- Work under close supervision and consistent levels of accountability.
- Prevent inappropriate 'creativity' or unusual interpretation of reality applied to ordinary events.
- Clear expectations with regard to work performance, behaviour and appearance, in order to maximise marginal levels of motivation.
- Have mistakes pointed out in a direct manner, in order to correct them.

Figure 14.2 continued

case involves an examination of the setting events, antecedents and consequences of the target behaviour to determine the control and function of the behaviour itself. Self-instruction refers to a number of strategies in self-management programmes in which the individual delivers a visual or auditory prompt to set the occasion for the targeted behaviour to occur. When designing self-management programmes:

- the individual should be involved with setting the goal for the programme;
- the goal must be practical and attainable;
- all the principles of behaviour management should apply; hence, principles such as reinforcement schedules, fading, maintenance and generalisation must all be considered and addressed in the design and implementation of the programme.

In vocational settings, rehabilitation counsellors, employers and family members may all assist the individual with a disability to develop a plan appropriate to a particular situation.

Natural supports

Most people are accommodated in some way at work. Arrangements such as flexi-time, job-sharing, compressed working weeks and restructured job tasks are commonplace. The use of natural supports focuses on accommodating the disabled employee by relying on co-workers and other individuals to undertake training, observe and record work behaviour, provide feedback and act as an advocate on the worker's behalf (Callahan, 1992; Hagner, 1992). The use of natural supports has two main advantages:

1   co-workers and supervisors are usually always present at the work site;
2   there is no intrusion from a job coach or other support worker.

Much of what it takes to facilitate natural supports involves providing technical assistance and advice to the employer on integrating the employee into a work team, such as:

(a) intervention techniques used at the job site (and how to implement these techniques);
(b) social problems and possible methods to minimise stressful situations;
(c) the disability and medical implications that might accompany the worker's performance;
(d) instructions regarding contact of support workers should problems arise.

Building on existing practices

A vital aspect of using natural supports is to use existing resources. In this respect, an organisation's training functions are particularly important, and it is necessary to:

• analyse existing training functions;
• understand the learning style of the client;
• provide consultation to the employer on effective training approaches relevant to the client;
• help the client access all relevant training opportunities, both formal and informal;
• advise the employer on adaptations and modifications to training and tasks;
• supplement the training in non-intrusive ways, both on or off the job when necessary.

It needs to be remembered that not all employers have formal training approaches, such as a handbook for a new employee, but nearly all offer some sort of job orientation, even if it is only 'sitting with Nelly'. Job development should not entail taking over the training of the client from the employer – and the employer losing control over a critical aspect of the business – but should be a case of providing advice on 'reasonable adjustment'. In addition, promising an employer to take over training creates the wrong impression, that only a disability specialist can do this.

Providing training expertise to co-workers

Co-worker(s) responsible for training need to be aware of effective teaching strategies. They might need guidance in two broad areas:

(1) enabling the client to display appropriate social behaviour: difficulties in this area are more commonly found among some clients with an acquired brain injury, a MH problem or learning disability; and
(2) ensuring that adequate skill training is provided to enable the client to do the job.

These two requirements influence each other. How skill training occurs can affect how the client is viewed by other employees and whether he or she is accepted as part of the team. Some guidelines for teaching trainers are:

• Recognise that each person learns in different ways: some prefer to listen to instructions, others prefer to learn by following manuals or through a 'hands-on' approach.

- Be consistent when you teach.
- Provide frequent practice, but remember too much repetition can be boring.
- Keep a record of learning activity, date, supervision required, time needed, accuracy etc.; this will help when planning the next session.
- Use task analysis to break down the sequence and elements of a task.
- Use natural prompts – vocal, visual and tactile.
- Use natural reinforcers. An example of using natural supports is in the following example (adapted from DiLeo *et al.*, 1995):

Jane: Modification to equipment and co-worker training

Jane is a visually impaired 19-year-old who enjoys cooking. A trial placement was arranged for her with a fast-food chain, although the manager had concerns regarding Jane's sight. Jane's personality persuaded him to 'give her a chance' to show that she would make a good employee.

Transport: the job coach worked with Jane and her parents to get her to and from work. Trial runs were made on the bus, and Jane's mum helped out by driving Jane to work when this was necessary.

Modifications: indelible marks were made on oven dials to facilitate the right settings.

Co-worker training: during her induction, Jane was given step-by-step instructions, accompanied by a sequenced picture chart. Whenever Jane had difficulty remembering a task, co-workers referred to the chart. Staff taking written orders were given felt-tip pens and asked to record them legibly for Jane and to state the nature of the order.

Social mentoring: Jane is now employed part-time. She occasionally becomes frustrated when unable to keep up with orders, and her output declines. In such a circumstance, Jane has been encouraged to do what other staff do, complain and ask for assistance. One particular member of staff has befriended Jane and often chooses to work alongside her when the restaurant is busy.

Systematic training

In the late 1970s, researchers such as Marc Gold (1980) popularised a systematic approach to training people with learning disabilities known as systematic instruction (SI) (Callahan and Garner, 1997). The approach (Box 14.1) works with many other conditions.

Step 12: Job retention, follow-up and case closure

James *et al.*, (2003) were commissioned by the HSE to identify issues that employers and employees need to address to facilitate continuing employment through VR. They posit a conceptual framework referred to as the 'cycles of vulnerability' faced by

---

Box 14.1 Steps to systematic instruction

1 Break down complicated tasks to individual steps.
2 Cluster steps into teachable chunks, or content steps.
3 Provide the smallest number of prompts needed to remind the learner how to perform each step.
4 Provide feedback and natural reinforcement as the client learns.
5 Consider changing the content steps, prompts or reinforcers if learning is problematic.
6 Expand the chunks into bigger sets of skills.
7 Help the learner perform independently of prompts.
8 Help the learner generalise the skill.

---

ill, injured and disabled workers (Figure 14.3). The central tenet is that appropriate rehabilitation action can be utilised to address the identified problems.

Seven management processes and practices are said to contribute to the development and operation of effective workplace rehabilitation programmes and address the cycles (Table 14.5). These practices work best when embedded within a comprehensive disability management strategy.

Organisational disability management practice

As indicated in Chapter 1, VR is just one element of comprehensive DM. This aspect requires addressing organisational issues emphasising the benefits of VR, namely quicker RTW, reduced sickness-absence costs, the retention of skilled staff, improved morale and improved productivity. There is a need to dispel a number of myths that have built up around the employment of people with health conditions, including the need for the employee to be 100 per cent fit before RTW; a notion that the health of employees is not the employer's problem; the employer should not contact workers off sick; and a GP sick note (now fit note) means the worker cannot work. It is also necessary to address issues such as concern over any risk of re-injury through work activities and what is meant by 'light duties'. A major problem is that many companies have policies (of variable quality), but managers and supervisors are either unaware of them, do not understand them or do not implement them. An organisation's DM policy serves little purpose without all line managers and supervisors understanding the aims and objectives of such a policy, such as complying with anti-discrimination legislation; ensuring 'the best' candidates are not rejected because of unfounded assumptions; ensuring the workforce remains integrated and motivated; identifying and promoting talent; providing a safe working environment; managing absence and RTW; facilitating the retention of employees who become disabled or develop a health condition; and developing an awareness of internal and external supports.

Policies require implementation. In turn, this involves consultation (including union and/or staff representatives), maintaining a dialogue with employees and monitoring. There are implications for the required information and skill needs of managers and

Cycles of vulnerability

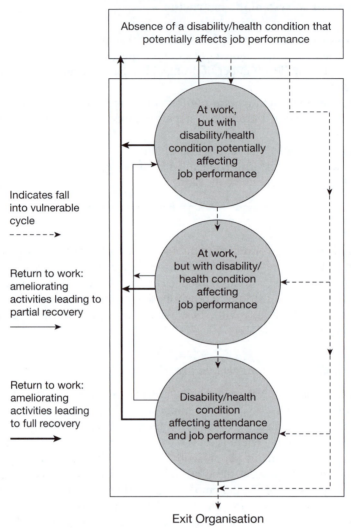

Figure 14.3 The cycles of vulnerability

Source: James *et al.* (2003).

Table 14.5 Management processes to facilitate job retention

1   Provision of rehabilitation support, for example treatment, adjustment, functional evaluations
2   The co-ordination of the rehabilitation process (joined-up services)
3   Access to worker representation to encourage openness and trust
4   The establishment of a policy framework, that is who is responsible for what
5   Systematic action
6   Mechanisms that allow any framework weaknesses to be addressed
7   'The early and timely identification of vulnerable workers through health checks,
    maintenance and regular contact with absent workers, return to work interview, etc.'

supervisors responsible for implementing any company disability policy, in particular what the policy is and the practical aspects of meeting its objectives, their own role and that of others in delivering the policy, who in the organisation can provide information and guidance on action to be taken, and what advice and information staff should receive on the policy in order to maximise its effectiveness. When making decisions on the employment of disabled people, managers and supervisors need guidance in the areas identified in Table 14.6.

Developing point 3 in Table 14.6, Induction, managers and supervisors are likely to need the knowledge, information and skills identified in Table 14.7 if a new employee, or one transferring from another work area because of a health condition, is to be successfully integrated into the workforce (adapted from Smith *et al.*, 1991).

It is possible to develop all of the points in Table 14.6 in a similar fashion. For instance, with regard to point 9, fluctuating and poor performance, see Table 14.8.

Sickness absence management

A fundamental aspect of managing job retention relates to point 7 in Table 14.5 and the early identification of a potential problem. Too often, when VR is provided in insurance claims, it is only when the problem has become protracted and entrenched. Even when companies have sickness absence procedures including VR, it is often not even considered as an intervention and support strategy until the employee has been off work for 6 months.

Absence management systems vary, but generally include:

- reporting of absence by employees;
- communicating absence to line managers and/or HR;
- recording absence dates, reasons, etc.;
- RTW interviews;
- involvement of OH services;
- triggers to deal with persistent absence; and
- using absence rates as performance indicators, consideration of absence in promotion decisions, bonus or incentive schemes.

Table 14.6 Improving job retention prospects: organisational disability management training

---

1 Recruitment and selection
2 Allocating people to jobs and jobs to people
3 Induction
4 Training
5 Building and maintaining a team
6 Working relationships
7 Health and safety
8 Motivating staff
9 Fluctuating or poor performance
10 Career development
11 Promotion and transfer
12 Dealing with organisational and work changes
13 Relations with customers (not considered entirely relevant to VR)
14 Implementing the organisation's disability policy

Table 14.7 Induction knowledge and skills required of managers and supervisors

Key issues	Knowledge and information	Skills
Taking time to prepare the work group and new employee with a disability to ease induction and reduce the prospect of later difficulties	What to raise when discussing job requirements, and the needs of the person and how they can both be met	How to obtain relevant information from a new employee without causing offence or embarrassment
Standard induction procedure might need modifying	What to say to co-workers	How to provide information when a disability might make it difficult to follow standard format
A talk to the new employee before starting work about any assistance they might require and who is responsible for providing it will clarify needs and responsibilities	What to say to a person joining a group including a disabled person	How to make co-workers aware of a person's needs in order to encourage integration
A new employee joining a work group including a person with a disability might need advice to minimise any discomfort or apprehension	How to address staff fears and concerns	
Once inducted, person with a disability needs to be treated as 'normally' as possible		

It is unlikely that there are many employers not operating some kind of absence management system. Although most organisations report that they undertake a variety of absence management practices, many are using only the most straightforward methods (CBI/Axa, 2007). Furthermore, it is impossible to know if these practices are being performed well. The UK record, especially on short-term absence, suggests that more effective methods need to be introduced, particularly to prevent short-term absences developing into long-term ones.

The CBI report (op. cit.) highlights the potential effectiveness of different absence-management policies, showing that OH provision can have the most positive effective in reducing levels of absence among small businesses. Indeed, among the smallest organisations, the biggest gains are to be made. OH provision ought to have a critical role in the identification of employees requiring VR services, but this is not always the case.

The importance of occupational health

Although there are limitations on the availability of company OH services, there is always NHS Plus, a network of more than 100 OH departments providing, on a commercial basis, support to non-NHS employers, particularly SMEs. In addition, NHS Plus provides

Table 14.8 Fluctuating and poor performance: knowledge and skills required of managers and supervisors

Key issues	Knowledge and information	Skills
Inadequate or fluctuating performance may be related to inappropriate management of a disability, e.g. inadequate aids	What the organisation's policy is if the performance is due to a health problem	How to elicit sensitive information from an employee
Boredom, resulting in mistakes, as a consequence of a narrow range of tasks	When and how to intervene	How to set and agree realistic goals and timetables and provide training for an individual to improve their performance
A person with a deteriorating or fluctuating condition might need help to retain maximum independence and dignity within the constraints imposed by the work environment	What to do if symptoms of illness or stress are detected or reported	How to generate supportive mechanisms
A person with a deteriorating or fluctuating condition might be unaware of aspects of their work causing problems for others because of a lack of willingness to criticise	What training is available within and outside the organisation to help the individual improve their performance or train them for alternative work	How to minimise problems for others
The self-esteem of some people with particular problems might be very low	Where help and advice is available within and outside the organisation	How to recognise when it is appropriate to seek external support
A manager might have to explain the acceptance of a reduced performance or unusual behaviour to colleagues of the person	What alternative working arrangements are available	How to counsel an individual unable to carry out a job satisfactorily
Unpredictable or inappropriate behaviour might be linked to a change in medication or a fluctuating medical condition	Where an individual who has to be redeployed can be assessed and receive guidance	How to relate medical information to the workplace
Where to go for help should a person be unable to continue in their work	The organisation's policy on early retirement and available alternatives	How to assess the capability of an individual who has to be redeployed

website guidance to employers and employees about how to deal with common OH problems. In the private sector, service delivery models include 'in-house' and external private providers. They are often nurse-led, with sessional OH physician support. The level of expertise available to provide advice on adjustments and other aspects of RTW procedures varies considerably. Two major limitations are the lack of any requirement for OH practitioners to hold OH qualifications, and their knowledge of workplace practice and the requirements of a specific job. This is particularly the case when services are provided by external providers. It will have been noted in Chapter 6 that the EAT determined that, in respect of adjustments, it is not sufficient for a tribunal to accept OH recommendations. They must also explore *how* any recommendations would prevent substantial disadvantage. Despite such limitations, the role of OH can be critical to successful job retention (and recruitment). OH specialists are typically asked questions in respect of:

- likely duration of any absence;
- likely residual disability on RTW and ability to do the job;
- likely duration of any limitations and future attendance;
- adjustments to overcome the limitations;
- impact of disability on health and safety.

VR professionals working with the employee of a company have a crucial role to play in keeping the OH professional informed of RTW developments. In turn, these will inform the OH of advice given to the company. The case study (Chapter 7) provided by the independent VR practitioner draws attention to the need to keep informed all the parties with an interest in the employee. In general, successful VR intervention is likely to focus on managing workplace performance, rather than reducing the impairment arising from a condition.

A problem is that short-term sickness absence is broadly defined as frequent, recurring periods of sickness absence that do not relate to an underlying health issue. Frequent short-term absences, often self-certified, are more likely to trigger capability issues rather than the recognition of a more deep-seated problem.

A question arises, however, if employers do become aware of a deep-seated problem, such as depression or alcoholism, triggering periodic short-term absences: would they perceive it to be their problem or would capability dismissal follow? (Employees with such problems might not reveal them, and, hence, they would not be covered by the DDA; in any event, although a tribunal might conclude that the employer has a duty to allow above-average sickness absence for an employee covered by the DDA, they are unlikely to find an employer at fault for following agreed dismissal procedure on the grounds of capability.) Roles and responsibilities in monitoring sickness absence need to be clearly defined in relationship to identifying and addressing problems (Table 14.9).

All employees need to be aware of whom they should contact if they are absent sick, and they must understand the notification procedure. When staff initially phone in sick, there is a need to obtain certain information:

- What are the reasons for the sickness?
- Have they been to the doctor? If so, what was their advice?
- When do they expect to return-to-work?
- Agreement on how contact will be maintained should they be unable to return on the expected date.
- Confirmation, if needed, of any current telephone numbers and/ or contact address. Some conditions, such as work-related stress, are likely to require immediate consideration of the RTW process, workload or environment and its effect upon health or ability to cope with the demands of their job.

Table 14.9 Roles and responsibilities in identifying potential problems arising from sickness absence

Managers	Responsible for ensuring there are systems to record and monitor absence.
	Provide a safe working environment for staff.
Managers and supervisors	Have awareness of an employee's circumstances and, where possible, identify (potential) problems at an early stage.
Managers and HR	Establish a point of contact when employees are off sick and ensure employees are aware of the correct notification procedures.
	Make employees aware of any support mechanisms available, such as a counselling service (EAP) and OH.
	Provide information to the employee regarding their sickness-absence record.
	Consider and implement reasonable adjustments where appropriate, e.g. a phased return from long-term sickness absence.
HR	Provide managers and supervisors with guidance and support.
	Provide employees with advice on the policy and their entitlements.
	Advise the manager on the most appropriate course of action for the employee.
	Advise on what further information should be sought, e.g. from OH.
Trade union/staff association	Be consulted on the policy.
	Advise members at any stage of the process, in particular, accompanying them at any formal meetings.
OH	Provide specialist medical advice to managers and employees.
	Identify where an underlying medical condition exists and provide advice in relation to the condition and the employee's work.
	Provide advice on reasonable adjustments where appropriate.
	Support the employee's RTW and their continued attendance at work.

Maintaining contact

It is important to keep in contact with an employee while they are absent owing to sickness. Maintaining contact allows the employer to be aware of changes in an employee's circumstances, offer appropriate support and keep the employee informed of developments within the workplace, thereby facilitating an eventual return. This is particularly important where the employee is absent for an extended period of time. The frequency and tone of contact needs to reasonable and necessary, to avoid any perceived harassment/bullying, particularly in MH cases. Agreed contact procedure needs to be established.

Notice of a meeting

Employees should be given no less than three working days' notice of a formal meeting. However, should the employee be unable to attend or cannot be accompanied by a work colleague or a trade union representative on this date, the meeting should be arranged for an alternative date.

Home visits

As a rule, home visits should not be undertaken unaccompanied (VR counsellors may have no option) and can only be undertaken with the express permission and agreement of the individual and by prior arrangement.

Return-to-work interview

When an employee returns from sickness absence, a discussion should be held in order to:

*   discuss the reasons for the absence and if they are likely to recur;
*   update the employee on any developments that have occurred;
*   let the employee know if their absence has triggered any requirement for an informal or formal meeting under the sickness-absence policy;
*   consider whether any adjustments should be made;
*   consider whether a risk assessment is required of the area and procedures, in the light of information, e.g. relating to an accident at work.

This discussion should be informal and should be held as soon as practicably possible on an employee's RTW. It allows the employer to discover any underlying problems, with a view to resolving them at an early stage, before the absence reaches problematic levels. A record needs to be taken and kept of the meeting and the employee informed of this, with an explanation that the notes might be referred to in the future if necessary. Notes might include requests for adjustments; informal arrangements in relation to agreed adjustments; reasons why adjustments could not be made; concerns raised by the employee; or any actions that should be followed up after the discussion. Figure 14.4 is a a typical RTW template form.

When to consider vocational rehabilitation

There is no one point when VR should be considered. Although, generally, employees on long-term sickness absence are more likely to need such intervention, some aspects of the VR process, for example the consideration of reasonable adjustments, might be appropriate for some employees after only one period of short-term absence.

Issues to consider are when:

*   specialist advice is required on managing a particular disability in the workplace;
*   an employee sustains a permanent injury or develops a long-term health condition;
*   an employee is having frequent, health-related, short-term absences;
*   advice is required on making reasonable adjustments;
*   an employee with a disability/health condition is no longer able to undertake all the required aspects of their usual work; and
*   an employee and employer are likely to require advice and support on the RTW process.

Name:	Work location:		
Length of absence:			
Number of absences in the last 12 months and durations:			
Any capability triggers?			
Reason/s for absence:			
How is your current health? Are you fully recovered?			
Did you seek medical attention?		Yes	No
Do you have any follow up appointments?		Yes	No
Is there anything we can do to help?		Yes	No
If yes, note:			
Brief the employee on how work covered whilst absent:			
Note any other operational issues for the employee to be aware of:			
Signed by interviewer		Date:	
Signed by employee		Date:	

Figure 14.4 Return to work template form

Case closures and follow-up

VR counsellors have a responsibility not to leave their clients 'in the lurch', but there is rarely funding for long-term support. On occasions, counsellors might have to transfer a client to another counsellor or service. When this occurs, the same standards of practice can be followed as when closing a case, such as ensuring that all file notes are up to date, and the client and employer are kept fully informed. In addition, there is a need to ensure that the new provider receives the documentation in adequate time to review before meeting the referred person. In an ideal world, closure should occur only when the client is successfully resettled and able to self-manage. In the real world, VR plans can fail for reasons outside the control of the service provider, and funding can run out. Closure must be included as part of the VR plan and include liaison with the family, employer, funding agency and any other relevant party.

These circumstances focus attention on the need to be able, at any time, to determine the client's progress against predetermined milestones, record the amount of support needed to achieve the milestones, identify possible amendments or options for continuing support that might enable the client to achieve the specified aim, and identify and suggest any follow-up or other activity, such as adjustments, that might help improve the client's situation.

It is important to keep communication lines open following a placement. This can serve as a channel for future concerns and support needs. Even after a case closure, there are a number of reasons for maintaining a follow-up procedure with the employer, such as giving reassurance to both the client and employer that, should there be any future problem, then the support service is potentially available, for data-collection purposes and for keeping doors open for other placements.

Summary

Too often in the past, public sector VR agencies in the United Kingdom have focused on placing service users in any available job in order to trigger funding. There has been little incentive to investigate all available options and concentrate on longer-term job retention, involving, as it can, the development of compensatory strategies, the identification of workplace adjustments and the use of natural supports. Even in the private sector, when there is an inability to return to an employer, there is a temptation to encourage the client to take the first job that comes along, in order to reduce or stop insurance payments.

As job retention can be an even more significant problem for some disabled people than job acquisition (Langman, 2007), ensuring that the VR service user is placed in the 'right job' in the first place, with all available support mechanisms in place, can be the most critical aspect of the VR process.

Some employees are always going to remain more vulnerable than others to losing their jobs because of their health and issues surrounding capability. In such circumstances, comprehensive DM policies and practices are required to support such workers (while minimising disruption and maximising productivity). An obvious problem relates to the resources of employers, particularly SMEs, although both the Scottish NHS VR model and the Fit for Work pilots (Chapter 9) might be considered to offer ways forward, while another one is the growing relationship between ELCI and access to VR services (Chapter 4).

Student exercises

14.1 Case study: JP

JP is a 44-year-old word processor operator who has periodically suffered from bouts of severe depression. She was dismissed from her last job on the grounds of capability. This exacerbated her condition, and she has not worked for nearly a year. She now feels that she needs to get back to work for financial reasons, but she has lost a great deal of confidence. You have found a trial placement for her, working part-time in a PCT HR office.

Devise a feedback form for completion by JP's supervisor.

14.2 Case study: RS

RS was in her mid 30s when she sustained a SCI as a consequence of a RTA. Prior to injury, she had worked in middle management in banking. She has a degree in economics. She has significant physical limitations, including being confined to a wheelchair, occasional spasms and fatigue.

(a) What should RS say about herself when asked for a medical history on an application form?
(b) What arrangements should she request for an interview?
(c) What should she ask for by way of 'reasonable adjustments'?

14.3 Case study: MW

MW, an experienced word processor, sustained a serious injury to her non-dominant hand in a freak gardening accident. She is now self-conscious about the hand and frustrated by her limitations, including being only able to use her little finger for typing. She does not want to go back into the typing pool and has suggested 'an office job'. There is a vacancy for a receptionist.

How do you consider her return to work should be managed?

14.4 Case study: BC

BC, a middle manager in his late 50s, is employed in the planning department of a local authority. He has developed Parkinson's Disease. His work output has slowed to the point that two members of the office in which he works have voiced an opinion to HR that they are 'carrying him'. BC is a proud man and he has given long service after an earlier career as a professional footballer. In his last annual report, before his condition was known, he indicated that, as a late entrant, he wanted to carry on working as long as possible to maximise his pension. You suspect that you have been brought in to ease his departure from the employer.

What measures do you consider should be taken?

15 Considering the future

Key issues

- Vocational rehabilitation skills for the twenty-first century.
- Addressing quality and increasing accountability.
- VR education, training and research needs.
- Incentivising the RTW process and integrating VR into absence-management practice.
- The failure of the compensation system to address employment.

Learning objectives

- Understanding significant issues affecting the continuing development of VR in the United Kingdom.
- Understanding the need to develop 'joined-up' services.

Where are we?

For many post-war years, no private sector VR services existed in the United Kingdom. Employers did not consider such services were needed, and only the advocacy and support of the insurance sector has contributed to a growing awareness of the benefits. However, even now, employers addressing sickness absence are more likely to have stand alone absence-management systems than comprehensive DM policies and practices incorporating VR. In the circumstances, it is not surprising to find that the promotional literature of a number of rehabilitation companies entering the UK market from the 1990s onwards very much emphasises their role in absence management and employee well-being, while offering case-managed graduated RTW programmes (see, for example, Rehab Works: www.rehabworks.co.uk, and hcml Employment Services: www.hcml. co.uk). Understandably, a common feature of such companies is to stress their professional expertise, so that, for example, Rehab Works draws attention to a national network of occupational physiotherapists and their role in supporting employees with MSDs; Rehab Options (www.rehaboptions.co.uk) stresses the role of occupational therapy in providing functional assessments; and Ways to Work (www.waystowork. co.uk) highlights psychological expertise in assessing and supporting people with neurological and other conditions. Yet all such organisations are essentially doing the same job (returning employees to work), and, although a particular disciplinary background provides an advantage with regard to working with certain conditions (particularly with regard to the use of some assessment tools), there is no evidence for any particular discipline being the critical factor in the RTW process or having a monopoly of VR skills and knowledge. Other common factors are invariably more important than discipline, such as early intervention, establishing a rapport with the service user, counselling skills, an accommodating employer, workplace adjustments and income considerations. Regrettably, if understandably, within the United Kingdom, disciplines and their professional bodies are more likely to promote their own interests, rather than recognise, develop and promote mutidisciplinary practice cutting across established boundaries. Hence, VR has been slow to develop as a professional discipline. Practitioners are far more likely to describe themselves in terms of their first qualification than as a VR professional. To what extent this situation is desirable is a matter of conjecture. There are many experienced personnel who would maintain that the lack of a requirement for a common professional post-graduate qualification impedes a market reliant on generic skills and knowledge in order to be effective. What is clear is that the lack of any such qualification requirement has contributed to a lack of awareness of VR among employers, although government must take prime responsibility for this situation.

New Labour considered the need to require employers to provide VR, but, on rejecting this, supported research into the identification of evidence-based practice and the development of organisational and individual standards. However, as the cost of long-term absence swiftly passes to the state, there remains a need to incentivise employers.

In the public sector, New Labour recognised the limitations on the availability of VR services and the cost to the public purse and sought to address the problems arising through:

- creating Jobcentre Plus;
- delivering new public sector employment programmes, either containing aspects of, or directly delivering, VR;
- reforming the specialist disability services within Jobcentre Plus, particularly the SE programme;
- developing NSFs for the NHS, containing specific VR requirements;
- addressing the most prevalent health conditions found on the IB registers, particularly MH, with joined-up NHS/Jobcentre Plus CMPs; and
- promoting other NHS-led VR primary care initiatives.

Along the way, many other central government-funded bodies, such as the Social Exclusion Unit, private sector and voluntary organisations such as the Association of British Insurers, British Society of Rehabilitation Medicine, Royal College of Psychiatrists, Scottish Centre for Healthy Working Lives, United Kingdom Rehabilitation Council and the Vocational Rehabilitation Association have all played significant roles.

Hard evidence suggests that, although the measure taken by New Labour did not turn back the tide of IB claimants, at least the surging waves were being checked. It was always recognised that it would take time for policies to produce a substantial downturn in the claimant count, because of the difficulties in moving long-term claimants off benefits. Hence, much of the thrust of intervention has been based on preventing short-term claims developing into long-term ones.

For a while, it began to look as though the United Kingdom would develop VR services comparable with those found elsewhere in the Western world, such as in North America and Australasia, but without the same legislative underpinning, ensuring that injured and sick employees would receive support as a matter of course. In the meantime, the expansion of public sector funded services, paid for by benefits savings, would ensure that the VR needs of unemployed sick/disabled people would not be overlooked.

The reality is that, if not exactly in a random or ad hoc fashion, VR services have developed in both the public and private sectors in the absence of any overarching strategy, legislation, mandatory services or practitioner standards, driven by the insurance sector and New Labour's love affair with the Third Sector. Given the reluctance of the Conservative/Liberal Democrat coalition to intervene in the market, it is highly probable that, at least in the private sector, this situation will continue for the foreseeable future, although it is to be hoped that the case for kite-marking agencies able to meet PAS 150 standards and the case for individual VR accreditation can be progressed.

The public sector is a source of concern. Although the DWP has supported and endorsed the development of standards, it has not asked for the standards to be observed in its contractual arrangements with agencies, although a number of voluntary and not-for-profit organisations have adopted the VRA standards on a voluntary basis. There are a number of possible explanations for the DWP's position. One is the absence of any bureaucracy to police the standards. Another is that the DWP probably perceives the standards as being more applicable to the private sector than publicly funded services (analogous to the Framework document, DWP, 2004).

Of even greater concern is the development of the Work Programme and its funding mechanism. Although New Labour can be accused of producing a market of Byzantine complexity, at least, in theory, services reflected the diverse nature of the unemployed/sick population and their resettlement needs. To what extent the Work Programme providers will subcontract their work to specialist providers or, indeed, the level of outcome-related funding will support the needs of people with severe conditions remains to be seen. What is clear is what is already being lost. CMPs have reflected a ground-breaking liaison between Jobcentre Plus and the NHS serving a neglected population. Although resettlement figures (and the way they were compiled) often left much to be desired, the failure to renew contracts in the absence of any cost–benefit analyses reflects policy driven by ideology and not need.

The troubling concern is that, while the private sector continues to make some progress, not withstanding economic blips, in the public sector the United Kingdom may be re-entering the dark ages of neglect and indifference – an economic view of disability, no matter how IB history and associated costs to the NHS reflect the short-sightedness of such a strategy. In the meantime, VR professionals need to continue to make the economic case for their services.

Vocational rehabilitation skills for the twenty-first century

VR in the United Kingdom is at a crossroads. Historically, public sector VR services in the United Kingdom have routinely faced the vicissitudes of political indifference and financial restrictions. Although the contracting out and devolution of services have contributed to the lack of a national VR strategy (to the extent that the availability of an appropriate service remains a postcode lottery), the period from 1997 to 2010 may be regarded as a golden age, as the underlying political philosophy, aided by a decade of economic growth, recognised both the financial and social costs of excluding large numbers of people with a health problem from the labour market. Times have changed. The sector now faces the twin challenges of financial constraints and increased accountability (Figure 15.1).

Services relying on public sector funding face major challenges as financing is restricted. Similarly, in the private sector, pressures on costs during a period of low economic growth will result in demands for higher accountability and value for money. The futures of both the public and private sectors will rest on being able to produce results. There is a risk that one of the main driving forces for VR over the last decade, a reduction in social exclusion, will no longer remain a priority.

The political demand will be to achieve more with less, and this will require public services to improve the quality of existing and developing services. In turn, this should result in:

- increased professionalism reflected in an increasing emphasis on organisational standards, individual accreditation and continuing professional development;
- increased specialisation, for example case management, working with a specific condition, job coaching, focus on assessment practices, use of technology etc.;
- increased awareness and expectations from the public with regard to VR services;
- an increased recognition of the importance of managing disability as sound business practice (with consequential demands on public and private sector services, particularly relating to the implementation of the DDA and Equality Act); and
- a need for increased business awareness.

Education and training

Education and training are critical to the success of achieving more for less. The application of standards requires the recognition of professional standards. In this respect, the UK's VR sector faces unique problems. VR has either never appeared, or it has disappeared off, undergraduate syllabi during the years of post-war indifference. Although there are belated attempts to introduce the subject on a number of clinical courses, the reality is that most core and non-core VR practitioners in the United

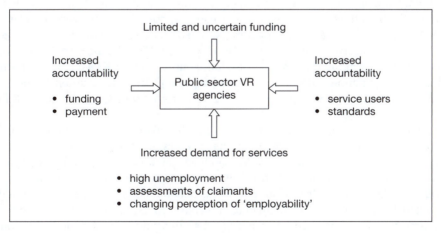

Figure 15.1 Multiple demands on public sector VR agencies

Kingdom have undertaken little or no VR training leading to a professionally recognisable qualification in VR practice.

In the circumstance, one would have thought that, during the growth period in the first part of the twenty-first century, there would be a significant demand for education and training. During the latter part of the twentieth century, only City University, London, offered an MSc in Disability Management in Work and Rehabilitation. Despite over 180 graduates, this course declined as staff retired, not to be replaced. Sheffield Hallam University saw a gap in the market and began a successful MSc in Vocational Rehabilitation, with teaching taking place at weekends, recognising the participants' full-time occupations. It is understood that about half the students are OTs, building on the department's undergraduate training in this discipline. The other students have a range of backgrounds, being well represented by the voluntary and non-profit sectors. In the latter respect, employers have been prepared to support the students financially, but, as organisational finances have become tighter, so support has become more difficult to obtain.

Bearing in mind that most prospective students are not in particularly well-paid jobs; are working full-time, at an age when they are likely to have family and other domestic commitments; already have a related undergraduate qualification; and are are not professionally required to have a recognised VR qualification, it becomes understandable as to why a perceived bandwagon in demand for VR courses has not taken off.

While finances are tight in the public sector, the position of some employers towards education and training is disconcerting, with frequent failure even to support short-course attendance from the NHS in England and Wales. The cost of courses is likely to increase, and the support and funding that clinicians have traditionally accessed from their Strategic Health Authorities may go as these organisations dissolve. A question remains as to whether or not GP commissioners will recognise this.

The situation in Scotland is different. NHS Education Scotland recognised both the need for, and absence of, professional VR training and, in 2008, organised a conference of interested parties to address the situation. Measures taken include support for course development and funding staff attendance.

Chapter 4 records how the sale of GIP policies has had an impact on the development of private sector VR in the United Kingdom. UNUM has recognised the shortage of VR education and training in the United Kingdom and has established its own training arm, Workmatters. It has also vigorously supported the delivery of Canadian NIDMAR courses in the United Kingdom (National Institute of Disability and Research, www.nidmar.ca/certification/CertificationProcess.pdf). The licence for delivering NIDMAR courses in the the United Kingdom is now held by KPMG Health Partners, working in conjunction with partners to deliver the CDMP designation (Table 15.1), and there are plans to develop the Certified Return-to Work Co-ordinator (CRTWC) course.

A number of the modules have been specifically adapted for the United Kingdom. They are thorough, and course members have reported enjoying and benefiting from them. At the present time, the NIDMAR modules cannot be compared to studying for a Masters-level qualification, and, in any event, many prospective VR students are likely to require a foundation qualification. The assessment methodology does not sit alongside the United Kingdom's highly regulated university course accreditation system, and, at the time of writing, Salford University is examining the means of accreditation and adapting the assessments to different levels of academic study. In the absence of further

Table 15.1 NIDMAR modules (available in the UK)

Unit	Title
A	Effective disability management programmes
B	Introduction to return-to-work co-ordination
C	Physical impairments, rehabilitation services and return to work
D	Mental health issues, rehabilitation services and return to work
E	Job analysis
F	The role of assessment
G	Communication and interviewing skills
H	Interviewing and helping skills
I	Legislation and disability management
K	Insurance and other benefits
L	Problem-solving with groups
M	Disability management in unionised organisations
N	Disability and diversity in the workplace
O	Disability management from a human-resource perspective
P	Management and organisational skills for return-to-work co-ordinators
Q	Assistive technology and accommodation
R	Managing change
S	Evaluating the return-to-work process and disability management programmes
T	Marketing and education in disability management and return-to-work
U	Information management
V	Injury prevention and health promotion
W	Professional conduct
X	Managing the return-to-work process

development, any consideration of the NIDMAR courses as a United Kingdom-recognised, post-qualifying VR accreditation (on top of basic undergraduate study), by bodies such as the Qualifications and Curriculums Development Agency or the Health Professionals Council, is likely to run into difficulty (the recognition of qualifications is devolved to the Scottish government and Welsh Assembly), although there is evidence of private, public and Third Sector organisations in the United Kingdom embracing NIDMAR as one of the few accessible education and training programmes.

An interesting development is Travors2 (www.travors-2), funded by the European Commission to develop a European Disability Employment Practitioner Certificate for staff involved in employment rehabilitation. This has the support of the DWP, and it is said that the certificate content will be based on learning-needs analyses of staff working across nine European countries. DWP Training Design: Research Principles and Implementation Guidance and work-based assessment techniques will be integral to the course. A development partner within the United Kingdom is Rehabilitation Network (travors@rehabilitationnetwork.com).

There remains a need for:

- short courses for both non-core and core VR practitioners addressing specific subjects;
- the inclusion of VR on a number of undergraduate courses (a matter that is already taking place for some disciplines, but is by no means universal, even for potential core practitioners);

- foundation education for non-core and many core practitioners, enabling them to take their VR studies to a higher level if required;
- post-graduate education and training for core practitioners (building on graduate-level qualifications). In the United States, Frain *et al*. (2006) undertook a meta-analysis of VR studies, examining the benefits of rehabilitation counsellors having a rehabilitation-counselling MSc. They compared the employment outcomes of those holding MScs in rehabilitation counselling with a combined group of all other degrees, which included Bachelor degrees and Masters degrees in related and unrelated fields. The analysis revealed a statistically significant relationship. Translated into practice, the researchers concluded that approximately 20,000 more people with disabilities would have positive employment outcomes every year if all rehabilitation counsellors held an MSc in rehabilitation.

Although credit needs to be given to organisations such as the Royal College of Nursing for showing one way forward and providing an online learning opportunity, 'Vocational rehabilitation – the health worker's role', such provision is no substitute for accredited learning for a recognised professional qualification against which standards can be measured. One interesting development has been made by a private sector company, Harrison Training (www.harrisontraining.co.uk), in having a number of its courses accredited by the University of the West of England (Bristol), so that collected points can contribute towards a recognised academic qualification.

The situation in the United Kingdom with regard to education, training and accreditation in VR should be a national embarrassment. From 2002, when HOST Policy Research undertook its ground-breaking survey into the employment and disability sector, every organisation and numerous commentators reporting on VR services in the United Kingdom have recognised a skills and training gap. Although the sector deals with some of the most vulnerable people in the United Kingdom's 'big society', anybody, and any organisation, can designate themselves as VR practitioners. Although it might be maintained that individuals have a responsibility to themselves and their clients (and a disciplinary professional body if they belong to one) to ensure an appropriate level of skills and knowledge, evidence from course take-ups suggests that, in the absence of a mandatory required VR qualification and employer support, the costs and time required to study are prohibitive, even for core practitioners. In additon, access to local education and training is also an issue.

Such matters can only be addressed on a national basis. Yet what we have is the perverse situation of the DWP supporting and endorsing the development of standards, contingent on professional expertise, which it then fails to demand and monitor among its own contractors and their subcontracors. To its credit, the ABI has supported the development of standards to enable its members to instruct quality services, but, in the absence of any mandatory required standards, and any organisation responsible for policing such matters, implementation of such matters as PAS 150 is likely to remain an uphill struggle. There is a strong case for raising the status and authority of the UKRC beyond its current advisory role, but, in a larger labour market in which deregulation is likely to be the norm, it is diffcult to envisage any substantial changes in the immediately foreseeable future. Inevitably, this will continue to result in the disparate provison and quality of services. For example, after much delay, the guidance to the NHS on delivering VR for LT(N)Cs has recently been published (BSRM, 2010), but there are no mechanisms for validating any observance of recognised qualitative standards.

VR research

Related to education is the need to improve research into VR and the development of a uniform language. DWP reports emanate from annual ministerial priorities being contracted to preferred organisations. Although this generally results in high-quality research reports, the DWP is not averse to representation on steering groups influencing the way the research is undertaken and burying bad news (as invaluable as this may be). The HOST Policy Research report (2002) identified the need for an independent national education and training centre, which could also serve as a source of research expertise. In contrast to approximately thirty-eight Vocational Rehabilitation and Education Centers in the United States, the United Kingdom has none. An independent centre would, no doubt, have had something to say about the DWP's preferred VR research methodology (notwithstanding Treasury influence). Randomised controlled trials were the preferred methodology of Jobcentre Plus during 2002–2005 in the pilot musculoskeletal condition management programme (Back to Work) and the Job Retention and Rehabilitation Pilot. The methodology failed. It is highly questionable as to whether or not the circumstances of a clinical trial can be applied to large samples of benefits claimants based in different locations. Realistic evaluation (Pawson and Tilley, 1997) is the preferred methodology of those undertaking research into the provision of VR for long-term neurological conditions, and this approach has much more to offer the sector. This approach acknowledges the importance of context to the understanding of why 'interventions' work, for whom, how and in what circumstances.

Although it is some time since the DWP funded any large-scale VR research, a number of smaller programmes are currently running or have recently been concluded, using a variety of quantitative and qualititative methodologies. They include *Return-to-work after traumatic brain injury: a cohort comparison study and evaluation* (the final report is yet to be published; a related paper is Phillips, 2010), a project funded by the College of Occupational Therapists; *Changing perceptions of work ability in people with low back pain: a feasibility and economic evaluation*, a project funded by Arthritis UK (papers relating to earlier stages of the study are Coole *et al.* 2010a–e); an evaluation of the cost–benefits of VR and 'best practice' at trial sites identified by Macmillan Cancer Support, a project led by Dr Diane Playford of the University College Hospitals Trust (UCHT); and a 5-year programme exploring VR for people with MS, funded by the College of Occupational Therapists in conjunction with the Multiple Sclerosis Society and, again, led by a team from UCHT. Although such programmes are to be welcomed, it will be noted that they are being driven by particular interests, such as a large professional body or a particular disability interest group. This follows the lack of a national co-ordinated research programme to prioritise and address the knowledge and skills gaps in the UK VR market. What is at least an equally significant issue is the lack of any mechanisms for ensuring the roll-out of lessons learned to the diverse market of service providers.

The difficulties arising from any consistently used research criteria are nowhere more evident than when interpreting RTW studies and the means used to describe functioning and work problems.

Understanding RTW studies

There are considerable difficulties in comparing and contrasting studies that have taken place; a lack of homogeneity often contributes to problems in understanding the impact of intervention. Although identifying RTW statistics at a particular period post-VR and contrasting with pre-VR employment rates, or a matched sample, might seem simple, the sector is beset with the lack of a common language. Measuring any social phenomenon requires an understanding of the meaning of key concepts. What does 'return-to-work' mean? Work varies by:

*   level (status): there is clearly a big difference in outcome if a former teacher returns to work in their normal role, or a classroom assistant, yet both placements are likely to be counted as positive outcomes;
*   regularity (hours worked);
*   level of productivity;
*   amount of structure needed to maintain it; and
*   tenure.

There is also an argument that social productivity should be taken into account. In the circumstances, studies that fail to clarify what is covered by a reported RTW rate are not necessarily adding much to the sum of VR knowledge. In addition, it is generally difficult to compare studies, because programmes are different, as are the evaluation methods.

In the United Kingdom, it is not so much a question of research 'failing', but one of good quantitative VR research being undertaken at all. The United Kingdom needs more intervention-related studies (quasi-experimental and experimental) and fewer ad hoc studies regarding employment outcomes. Research effort needs to be theoretically based, with clear definitions of variables, populations and interventions. Data, such as effect size, need to be routinely included in research reports to maximise the ability to use meta-analysis and other statistical procedures when this is required. In order to meaningfully address knowledge translation, and the development of evidence-based practice, there is a need for the replication of previous research in order to establish coherent findings serving to inform future policy and practice.

Regrettably, what the United Kingdom experienced with New Labour was public-policy announcements and commitments being made before the research evidence became available, and, even worse, at the present time, with the Conservative/Liberal Democrat coalition, plans to introduce fundamental influences to the funding of the Work Programme – differential payments, likely to have a significant impact on the prospects of unemployed people with health conditions, without any evidence as to the impact this will have on the hard-to-place. No one knows the level of funding required to ensure appropriate support.

Describing functioning

There remains a matter of developing joined-up, holistic services and, underlying this, a uniform understanding of the VR process reflected in a common language, together contributing towards practical measures enhancing the RTW process. Describing functioning is an example of the way a common language and understanding can enhance the VR process.

VR programmes aim to facilitate the RTW process, but there is no universal description of functioning for those who participate. Chapter 11 records a recommendation that a medical evaluation for VR purposes should use the ICF to describe human functioning

(Chamberlain *et al.*, 2009). It is recognised that RTW depends on numerous factors, and the ICF classification is subdivided into:

- body functions
- body structures
- activities and participation
- environmental factors
- personal factors.

Such factors are systematically addressed in an ICF framework for job placement (Homa, 2007).

However, there is an issue as to the extent that assessment tools can be mapped on to the ICF. Two approaches to doing this have been identified, one based on the aim of an assessment tool ('goal-oriented') and another consisting of allocating several items ('assessment domains') to ICF categories by means of linking (Cieza *et al.*, 2002, 2005). Although some tests, such as ERGOS and Blankenship (detecting sub-maximal effort) are said to map well, there remains a substantial task in selecting measurements and instruments to assess functioning and work capacity in clinical situations.

In recognising this problem, the WHO has developed a Core Set for VR, based on the ICF, to serve as a reference framework and practical tool to classify and describe an individual functioning more efficiently. An ICF Core Set is a short list of ICF categories, with alphanumeric codes relevant to a health condition or a health-related event. These ICF classifications complement WHO's International Classification of Diseases (ICD-10) describing people by their medical diagnoses, but not how they function. A significant advancement is the integration of medical and social aspects of an individual's health condition in the ICF classifications. There is now:

- an ICF Comprehensive Core Set for VR to guide multidisciplinary interventions and assessments; and
- an ICF Brief Core Set for VR for use with all service users.

The Core Sets can serve as a guide in the evaluation of patients and in planning appropriate intervention within VR programmes. These Core Sets could also provide a standard and common language among clinicians, researchers, insurers and policymakers in the implementation of successful VR. The Core Sets are so new that they have yet to be adopted in the United Kingdom, but, given the extent to which other WHO classifications have been adopted, will undoubtedly begin to gain ground, even though there remains a huge amount of work to identify and adapt.

Providing services that work

The incentivising effects of the costs of absence

Research from the International Monetary Fund (2007) found that where the balance of cost falls has an effect on levels of absence. When employers share a greater part of the costs of absence, they are more likely to make changes that impact upon absence from work. The OECD (2007) found that, 'The longer employers have the financial responsibility for sick workers, the larger their interest should be in keeping workplaces and working conditions healthy and safe.'

As UK employers are responsible for the first 28 weeks of sickness absence, the IMF and OECD argument looks misplaced. In contrast, in Sweden and Norway, the state begins paying benefits after 15 and 16 days, respectively. In Germany, it is 6 weeks; in Austria, employers pay for a maximum of 16 weeks; in Denmark, 2 weeks.

There appears to be little appetite for major reform to SSP in the United Kingdom. The burden of short-term absence costs on employers has not succeeded in keeping down levels of absence. The problem is that the longer absences drag on, the less incentive there is for employers to take action to return a person to work.

It appears that, in the United Kingdom, among the major causes of high short-term absence are high levels of labour market participation and relatively long working hours. Among the causes of long-term absence resulting in high levels of benefit claims are the adverse incentive for low-paid workers represented by high levels of benefit replacement and the disincentive for employers to invest in measures to help the long-term sick back to work. (Although the IMF found that high levels of public sickness benefits act as an incentive for employees to take more long-term absence, given that sickness benefits in the United Kingdom are among the lowest in Western Europe, on its own this is not a convincing explanation for the UK level of sickness absence. However there is evidence that those who are long-term sick come from among the lowest paid, and, not withstanding any chicken and egg argument, benefits represent a high proportion of any net-earned-income capacity.)

A solution to encouraging employers to take action, such as recognising the potential value of VR in some cases of short-term absence, could be found in changing the incentives, so that it is cost-effective for them to invest in early measures to help absent employees back into the workplace. The problems in the United Kingdom are that, in the absence of robust evidence as to the benefits of large-scale absence-management and VR programmes, the CBI and other employer organisations are likely to resist what they perceive to be any additional burdens on employers. On the other hand, the TUC and claimant organisations are unlikely to accept that benefits act as a disincentive to work, especially given the generally low levels of benefits within the United Kingdom. Hence, the 2004 vocational rehabilitation framework document showed no political will from New Labour to make any radical changes, and the Conservative/Liberal Democrat coalition is even less likely to be seen to impose any additional requirements on employers.

Costs of public health issues and 'presenteeism'

It needs to be recognised that, beyond absence, four major public health issues also impose a significant burden on employers: first, 'presenteeism', that is the cost of working while not fully fit; second, healthcare costs to the state; third, social costs, in the form of the pressures on families, children and individuals; and, fourth, longer-term health and personal consequences. This is particularly prevalent in the case of mental health.

Costs and benefits of absence-management systems

An efficient absence-management system can be provided quite cheaply, although the potential range of services is broad and can make the system more expensive. A high-quality, effective absence-management system can be put in place for less than £20 per employee per year. This provides the key tools for a company that needs to improve its handling of absence, including notification, reporting, monitoring and managing information about absences. Such services are key to linking together other responses, such as the involvement of OH and VR when needed. Smaller employers need to be encouraged to equip themselves with absence-management systems. This can be done in two ways: by removing VAT on such products, and by providing an incentive for smaller firms to purchase such a product.

Case for a VR code of practice

Good-quality absence management can contain and potentially reduce absence and its effects, highlight ongoing problems, provide employees with guidance, give employers more and better information, ensure that underlying issues can be dealt with, and improve efficiency. Employers have to observe the Advisory Conciliation and Arbitration Service (ACAS) Codes of Practice when considering dismissing an employee, so why not a Code of Practice for addressing sickness absence, including reference to VR intervention and/or OH when:

- an underlying and persistent health problem is identified;
- adjustment(s) and advice are required;
- redeployment is being considered;
- absence becomes protracted (with a fixed time span); and
- capability dismissal is being considered?

Although a prescriptive approach may fail to win acceptance among employers, and could create unnecessary fixed costs, regulation that follows the style of other UK health and safety regulations might achieve the objective of increased uptake of RTW/ rehabilitation without imposing fixed costs. Such an approach might include employers having a written rehabilitation policy; making arrangements to ensure they have access to OH rehabilitation providers should the need arise; securing competent assessments; making a rehabilitation and RTW plan for an employee injured or made ill by their work; making arrangements to ensure RTW interviews are carried out by managers or other service providers, within one month of absence; making suitable workplace modifications; and co-operating with recognised RTW and rehabilitation practices.

The employer perspective

The role of employers is obviously critical to the management of sickness absence and the VR process. Policies, laws and regulations attuned to employers' goals will have a greater chance of success. VR interventions need to support existing employer–employee relations, particularly with regard to retention. There is much that remains to be done to enhance the prospects of sick and disabled workers that VR practitioners can facilitate, including:

- raising awareness of the benefits of rehabilitation with unions, employees and employers;
- encouraging early intervention;
- aligning health-care support with the RTW process, e.g. treating clinicians being made aware of work circumstances.

The need for joined-up services

In an ideal world, anyone with employment and health difficulties would receive appropriate support. Figure 15.2 illustrates the sorts of pathway that need to be developed. In the absence of services and mandatory requirements, the United Kingdom is a long way from having such comprehensive support. Nevertheless, there remains the need for VR practioners to develop their own networks to ensure the best possible client support to obtain and retain employment.

What's wrong with the litigation system?

The United Kingdom's compensation system badly fails those claimants who can and want to return-to-work. Despite the protocols that exist, it remains the case that litigation:

*   undervalues the importance of getting people back to good health and back to work as quickly as possible;
*   lacks incentives for claimants to return-to-work as soon as reasonably possible;
*   provides little or no incentive to employers to take RTW action for an employee on long-term sickness; and
*   provides little incentive to employers' liability insurers.

On the contrary, besides being complex and adversarial, the compensation system:

*   diverts money that could be used for rehabilitation to 'claims handlers' (£2 billion every year: nearly 40p for every £1 paid in PI compensation, with more money going to claims handlers than claimants in many small claims);

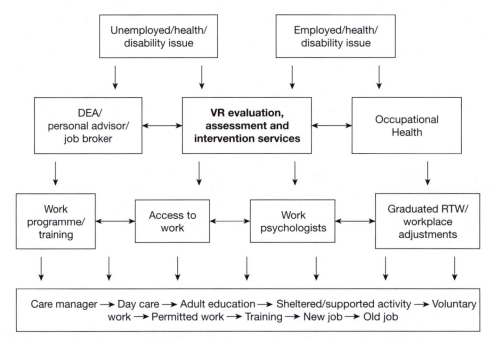

Figure 15.2 The need for joined-up services

- takes too long for liability issues to be addressed and to get compensation to claimants (for ELCI claims, an average of 1,000 days);
- rewards poor and sometimes misleading advice for claimants.

No-fault compensation

The 2004 Framework for Vocational Rehabilitation (DWP) states that in the longer-term, insurers should consider the benefits of VR as not just limited to an environment framed by liability or third-party insurance. Society still benefits if an individual injured outside the workplace gets back to work quickly, but, in such cases, there is no insurance policy to be triggered. Therefore, insurers considering the long-term vision should be focused on assembling the body of evidence and stakeholder education to promote 'no-fault' rehabilitation, uncoupling it from fault-based PI compensation. Alongside this, other insurance products, such as income protection and private medical insurance, could provide rehabilitation outside the liability arena, without the complications of proving negligence. As the framework document acknowledges, savings are an issue: 'insurers would add that cost effectiveness is a critical element of rehabilitation and that it may not always be desirable to achieve an individual's return-to-work regardless of cost', but 'insurers may also offer rehabilitation not to achieve a return-to-work, but to maximise quality of life, reduce the need for ongoing care and so reduce the cost of claims.'

A missed population

Of particular concern are PI claimants sustaining injury serious enough to have an adverse impact on their employment, but not so severe as to require case management services. Although GIP and a growing number of ELCI claimants are being identified and provided with RTW support, there is little evidence of PI solicitors efficiently identifying such cases, or of the courts approving the instruction of VR agencies. It remains the case, particularly among members of the Bar, that 'success' is measured in terms of the size of the claim, and not the quality of life of the injured person and their ability to provide for themselves once the compensation has run out.

Summary

Although both public and private sector VR services have made substantial progress over the last decade, externally imposed and internal limitations could still derail the process and leave the United Kingdom lagging many years behind its main Western competitors.

Individual and organisational standards have been developed in the absence of any statutory requirments to provide VR services, meaning that, for the main part, standards remain voluntary and implicit. The absence of legislation means that there is no executive body to ensure compliance with the standards at the service provider level, and, at the practitioner level, professional organisations to which practitioners may belong have no brief (or competence) to validate the member's VR practice against the standards that have been developed.

The absence of organisational standards is of particular concern to the insurance sector, the ABI wishing to promote VR by being able to point its membership towards qualitative services. (Despite a general consensus of support among the membership, there are still some grumblings in some cases over costs and outcomes.) In the public sector, the DWP does little more than pay lip service (the 'little more' being some funding to help develop standards). It is doubtful that NHS commissioners in England and Wales have any notion of PAS 150 or VRA standards.

In the circumstances, it is not surprising that VR continues to struggle to become a recognised profession within the United Kingdom. In the absence of legally prescribed boundaries, it is improbable that this will ever occur. However, this does not prevent the recognition of organisational and individual expertise. PAS 150 offers a means to kite-mark practices, but, if the development of these standards is to be anything more than another paper exercise, then at least the UKRC, if not the BSI, needs to be given the means to advance these standards.

At an individual level, practitioners need to clearly establish their expertise. Ordinarily, the main means is the possession of a recognised UK qualification (or an overseas one with 'equivalency'). Although there is much to be said for NIDMAR, this offers overseas qualifications without equivalency. In particular, there remains a need to validate core practioners. This is also one means by which organisations can meet some of the PAS 150 standards. No undergraduate course in the United Kingdom suffiently equips any discipline to consider itself a source of VR expertise and able to meet the developed standards. As such, one might be excused for thinking that there would be a rush for generic, post-graduate training. Evidence suggests that the lack of any mandatory requirement to hold a specific VR-related qualification, limitations on employer support, access to such courses, costs and the personal circumstances of practitioners all conspire against this. The situation is different in Scotland, where the Scottish government has grasped the nettle, particularly with regard to rolling out VR services from NHS Scotland.

In all the circumstances, including a government loath to intervene in the labour market, progress in the VR sector is likely to slow down in the coming years, particularly in the public sector. Indeed, it is to be hoped that the availability of intervention and support services does not go backwards for some vulnerable groups. The detail is always what counts, and it remains to be seen what the final version of the Work Programme looks like; likewise, the progress made in delivering the VR components of the NSFs within the NHS will ultimately need to be examined once the final delivery date in 2015 is reached. The private sector is likely to continue to advance, with a watchful eye on value for money. Education, training and research will also suffer from tight financial constraints.

Lessons from the past in respect of the financial and social costs of long-term unemployment and sickness/disability have not been fully learned. Much can be done without imposing any significant burden on employers, but short-term policies driven by ideology and a need to reduce public expenditure are likely to prevail for the immediately foreseeable future.

Notes

Introduction

1 Strictly speaking, there are a number of *incapacity benefits*, although the acronym IB is commonly used.

1 Recognising vocational rehabilitation

1 In the mid 1970s, the ERRC was established and produced papers identifying such factors as the characteristics of the clients and service efficacy. These papers are kept in the DWP library at the Adelphi, London, and are accessible by prior appointment.
2 Insurance companies, supported by the courts, strongly resisted claims to pay for such support. The argument was that such services were either not necessary or provided by the state. The rising cost of compensation heralded a sea change in attitude, and so, by the late 1990s, the ABI was vigorously promoting rehabilitation among its membership.
3 Discussions with the author in 2009.

2 The nature of the problem: sickness, disability, absenteeism, worklessness and a developing compensation culture

1 Occupational Sick Pay is the level of income that an employer agrees to pay an absent, sick employee, for example half pay for a defined period. This usually includes the mandatory minimum Statutory Sick Pay.

4 The private sector response: the legal profession and insurance industry

1 The International Underwriters Association tends to concentrate on the more technical aspects of writing policies covering the insured, whereas the Association of British Insurers is concerned more with broader aspects of policy and market strategy.
2 Unpublished ABI survey, 2008.
3 Data supplied to the author and collected for the 2008 survey by the ABI.
4 Discussions with the author in January and February 2010.
5 Data provided to the author by the ABI, January 2010.
6 Data provided to the author by the ABI, January 2010.

5 The legal context

1 Readers are more likely to require practice guidance than an ability to cite case law. Case details can be obtained by googling the case and consulting the Additonal Reading for the chapter.
2 Observation made by the OT to the author, on a visit to the Scottish NHS pilot VR programme in Dundee during November 2008.

References

Advisory Committee for Disabled People in Employment and Training (2001) In the mainstream: Recommendations on removing barriers to disabled people's inclusion in mainstream labour market interventions, DWP, London.

Ahrens, C. S., Lane Frey, J. and Senn Burke, S. C. (1999) 'An individualized job engagement approach for persons with severe mental illness', *Journal of Rehabilitation*, Oct/Nov/Dec: 17–24.

Alcock, P. (2009) 'Devolution or divergence? Third Sector policy across the UK since 2000', Briefing Paper 2, Third Sector Research Centre.

Allen, S., Rainwater, A., Newbold, N., Deacon, N., Slatter, K. *et al.* (2004) 'Functional capacity evaluation reports for clients with personal injury claims: A content analysis', *Occupational Therapy International*, 11(2): 82–95.

American Physical Therapy Association (1992) 'Guidelines for programs in industrial rehabilitation', *Magazine of Physical Therapy*, 1: 69–72.

Anyadike-Danes, M. and McVicar, D. (2008) 'Has the boom in Incapacity Benefit claimant numbers passed its peak?', *Fiscal Studies*, 29(4): 415–34.

Association of British Insurers (2006) *Improving health at work: employers' attitudes to occupational health*, ABI, London.

Arksey, H., Thornton, P. and Williams, J. (2002) 'Mapping employment focussed services for disabled people' DWP In-house Report 93.

Armstrong, T. J. (2000) 'Analysis and design of jobs for control of work related musculoskeletal disorders', in Violante, F., Armstrong, T. and Kilbom, A. (eds), *Occupational ergonomics: work related musculoskeletal disorders of the upper limb and back*, Taylor and Francis, London, pp. 51–81.

Association of Chief Executives of Voluntary Organisations (2009) 'Making it personal: a social market revolution. Interim report of the Commission on Personalisation, ACEVO, London.

Aylward, M. (2004) 'Needless unemployment: the public health crisis', in Holland-Elliot, K. (ed.), *What about the workers?*, Royal Society of Medicine Press, London.

Bambra, C., Whitehead, M. and Hamilton, V. (2005) 'Does "welfare- to-work" work? A systematic review of the effectiveness of the UK's welfare-to-work programmes for people with a disability or chronic illness', *Social Sciences and Medicine*, 60.

Bandura, A. (1995) *Self-efficacy: the exercise of control*, Freeman, New York.

Banks, P., Riddell, S. and Thornton, P. (2002) *Good practice in work preparation: Lessons from research*, WAE Research Series 135, DWP, London.

Barham, C . and Begum, N. (2005) 'Sickness absence from work in the UK', *Labour Market Trends*, 150–8.

Barham, C. and Leonard, J. (2002) 'Trends and sources of data on sickness absence', *Labour Market Trends*, 110(4): 177–85.

Bartlett, P. and Sandland, R. (2007) *Mental health law: policy and practice*, Oxford University Press.

Beard, J. (2007), *VocRe 5*, NVRA, Glasgow.

Beaumont, D. G. (2003) 'The interaction between general practitioners and occupational health professionals in relation to rehabilitation for work: a Delphi study', *Occupational Medicine*, 53(4): 249–3.

Becker, D., Whitley, R., Bailey, E. L., Drake, R. E. (2007) 'Long-term employment trajectories among participants with severe mental illness in supported employment', *Psychiatric Services*, 58(7): 922–8.

Becker, D. R. and Drake, R. E. (2003) *A working life for people with severe mental illness*, OUP.

Becker, D. R., Xie, H., McHugo, G. J., Halliday, J. and Martinez, R. A. (2006) 'What predicts supported employment program outcomes?', *Community Mental Health Journal*, 42(3): 303–13.

Ben-Yishay, T., Silver, S. M., Piasetsky, E. and Rattok, J. (1987) 'Relationship between employability and vocational outcome after intensive holistic cognitive rehabilitation', *Journal of Head Trauma Rehabilitation*, 2(1): 35–48.

Bertram, M. and Howard, L. (2006) 'Employment planning and occupational care planning for people using mental health services', *Psychiatric Bulletin*, 30: 48–51.

Boardman, J., Grove, B., Perkins, R. and Shepherd, G. (2003) 'Work and employment for people with psychiatric disabilities', *The British Journal of Psychiatry*, 182(6): 467–8.

Bolderson, H. (1991) *Social security, disability and rehabilitation*, Jessica Kingsley Publishers, London.

Bolton, B. and Roessler, R. (1986a) *Manual for the work personality profile*, Arkansas Research and Training Center in Vocational Rehabilitation, University of Arkansas, Fayetville.

Bolton, B. and Roessler, R. (1986b) 'The work personality profile: factor scales, reliability, validity and norms', *Vocational Evaluation and Adjustment Bulletin*.

Bond, G. R., Drake, R. E. and Becker, D. R. (2008) 'An update on randomized controlled trials of evidence-based supported employment', *Psychiatric Rehabilitation Journal*, 31(4): 280–90.

Bond, G. R., Picone, J. , Mauer, B., Fishbein, S. and Stout, R. (2000) 'The quality of supported employment implementation scale', *Journal of Vocational Rehabilitation*, 14(3): 201–12.

Bond, G. R., Salyers, M. P., Dincin, J., Drake, R., Becker, D. R., Fraser, V. W. and Haines, M. (2007) 'A randomized controlled trial comparing two vocational models for persons with severe mental illness', *Journal of Consulting and Clinical Psychology*, 75(6): 968–82.

Booth, D., Francis, S. and James, R. (2007) 'Finding and keeping work: issues, activities and support for those with mental health needs', *Journal of Occupational Psychology, Employment and Disability*, 9(2): 65–97.

Bradshaw, L. M., Curran, A. D., Eskin, F. and Fishwick, D. (2001) 'Provision and perception of occupational health in small and medium-sized enterprises in Sheffield', *UK Occupational Medicine*, 51(1): 39–44.

Brantner, G. L. (1992) 'Job coaching for persons with traumatic brain injuries employed in professional and technical occupations', *Journal of Applied Rehabilitation Counselling*, 23(3): 3–14.

Braveman, B., Robson, C., Veloso, C., Kielhofner, G., Fisher, G., Forsyth, K. and Kerschbaum, J. (2005) 'The worker role interview', Version 10.0, Chicago MOHO Clearing House (available at: www.moho.uic.edu/assess/weis.html).

Briel, L. W. (1996) 'Promoting the effective use of compensatory strategies on the job for individuals with traumatic brain injury', *Journal of Vocational Rehabilitation*, 7: 151–8.

British Society of Rehabilitation Medicine (2000) *Vocational rehabilitation: the way forward – Report of a Working Party*, BSRM, London.

British Society of Rehabilitation Medicine (2003) *Vocational rehabilitation: the way forward – Report of a Working Party* (2nd edn), BSRM, London (available at: http://bsrm.co.uk/Publications/VocRehabUpdate2ndEd.pdf).

British Society of Rehabilitation Medicine (2010) *Vocational assessment and rehabilitation for people with long-term neurological conditions: recommendations for best practice*, BSRM, London.

British Society of Rehabilitation Medicine, Royal College of Physicians, Jobcentre Plus (2004) *Vocational rehabilitation and assessment after acquired brain injury, Inter-agency guidelines*, RCP, London.

Bubb, S. (2006) 'In the right hands', *Public Finance*, 3.

Burchardt, T. (2000) *Enduring economic exclusion: Disabled people, income and work*, York Publishing and Joseph Rowntree Foundation, York.

Burns, T., Catty, J., Becker, T., Drake, R. E., Fioritti, A., Knapp, M., Lauber, C., Rössler, W., Tomov, T., Van Busschbach, J., White, S. and Wiersma, D. (2007) 'The effectiveness of supported employment for people with severe mental illness: A randomised controlled trial', *The Lancet*, 370: 1146–52.

Bustillo, J. R., Lauriello, J., Horan, W. P. and Keith, S. J. (2001) 'The psychosocial treatment of schizophrenia: An update', *American Journal of Psychiatry*, 158(2): 163–75.

Callahan, M. J. (1992) 'Job site training and natural support', in Nisbet, J. (ed.), *Natural supports in school, at work, and in the community for people with severe disabilities*, Paul H. Brookes, Baltimore, pp. 257–76.

Callahan, M. J. and Bradley Garner, J. (1997) *Keys to the workplace: skills and supports for people with disabilities*, Paul H. Brookes Publishing, Baltimore.

Care Programme Approach Department of Health (2001) *The journey to recovery – the government's vision for mental health care*, Department of Health, London.

Casillas, J. M., Smolick, H. J. and Didier, J. P. (2006) 'Cardiac rehabilitation and vocational rehabilitation', in Gobelet, C. and Franchigoni, F., *Vocational rehabilitation*, Springer-Verlag, Paris.

Chamberlain, M. A., Moser, V. F., Ekholm, K. S., O'Connor, R. J., Herceg, M. and Ekholm, J. (2009) 'Vocational rehabilitation: an educational review', *Journal of Rehabilitation Medicine*, 41: 856–69.

Chandler, D., Levin, S. and Barry, P. (1999) 'The menu approach to employment services: philosophy and five year outcomes', *Psychiatric Rehabilitation Journal*, 23(1): 24–33.

Cieza, A., Brockow, T., Ewert, T., Amman, E., Kollerits, B., Chatterji, S., Ustün, T. B. and Stucki, G. (2002) 'Linking health-status measurements to the international classifications of functioning, disability and health', *Journal of Rehabilitation Medicine*, 34: 205–10.

Cieza, A., Geyh, S., Chatterji, S., Kostanjsek, N., Ustün, T. B. and Stucki, G. (2005) 'ICF, linking rules, an update based on lessons learned', *Journal of Rehabilitation Medicine*, 37: 215–18.

Cochrane Review (2004) 'Functional restoration for workers with back and neck pain', 1, The Cochrane Library.

Commission for the Accreditation of Rehabilitation Facilities (1988) *Work hardening guidelines*, Tucson.

Cook, J. A. and Razzano, L. (2000) 'Vocational rehabilitation for persons with schizophrenia: Recent research and implications for practice', *Schizophrenia Bulletin*, 26(1): 87–102.

Coole, C., Drummond A., Watson, P. J. and Radford, K. (2010a) 'What concerns workers with low back pain? Findings of a qualitative study of patients referred for rehabilitation', *Journal of Occupational Rehabilitation*, 20(4): 472–80.

Coole, C., Watson, P. J. and Drummond, A. (2010b) 'Work problems due to low back pain: what do GPs do? A questionnaire survey', *Family Practice*, 21(1): 31–7.

Coole, C., Watson, P. J. and Drummond, A. (2010c) 'Staying at work with back pain: patients' experiences of work-related help received from GPs and other clinicians. A qualitative study', *BMC Musculoskeletal Disorders*, 11: 90.

Coole, C., Watson, P. J. and Drummond, A. (2010d) 'Low back pain patients' experiences of work modification; a qualitative study', *BMC Musculoskeletal Disorders*, 11: 277.

Coole, C., Drummond, A., Sach, Th. and Watson, P. J. (2010e) 'Assessing the feasibility of collecting health care resource use data from general practices for use in an economic evaluation of vocational rehabilitation for back pain', *Journal of Evaluation in Clinical Practice*.

Corthell, D. (ed.) (1993) *Employment outcomes for persons with acquired brain injury*, Research and Training Center, Stout Vocational Rehabilitation Institute, University of Wisconsin-Stout.

Crewe, N. M. and Athelstan, G. T. (1984) *Functional assessment inventory: manual*, Materials Development Center, Stout Vocational Rehabilitation Institute, University of Wisconsin-Stout.

Crowther, R. E., Marshall, M., Bond, G. R. and Huxley, P. (2001) 'Helping people with severe mental illness to obtain work; a systematic review', *British Medical Journal*, 322: 204–8.

Crowther, R., Marshall, M., Bond, G. and Huxley, P. (2004) 'Vocational rehabilitation for people with severe mental illness (Cochrane Review)', in The Cochrane Library, Issue 3, Chichester, John Wiley & Sons.

Coleman, N., Rousseau, N. and Carpenter, H. (2004) 'Jobcentre Plus service delivery survey (Wave 1)', DWP RR 223, CDS, Leeds.

Caulkin, S. (2006) 'How the not-for profit sector became big business', *The Observer*, 12 February.

Chamberlain, M. A. (2007) Work, disability and rehabilitation: making the best job of it', *Clinical Medicine*, 7(6): 603–6.

Chartered Institute of Personnel and Development (2008) *Absence management: annual survey report 2008* (available at: www.cipd.co.uk).

Chartered Institute of Personnel and Development (2009) *Absence management annual survey report 2009* (available at: www.cipd.co.uk).

Collings, J. A. and Chappell, B. (1994) 'Correlates of employment history and employability in a British epilepsy sample', *Seizure*, 3: 255–62.

Corden, A., Harries, T., Hill, K., Kellard, K., Sainsbury, R. and Thornton, P. (2003) 'NDDP National Extension: findings from the first wave of qualitative research with clients, job brokers and Jobcentre Plus staff', Social Policy Research Unit Report 169 for DWP, Leeds.

Confederation of British Industry (2007) *Attending to absence: absence and labour turnover survey 2007*, CBI/AXA, London.

Confederation of British Industry (2008) *CBI survey of sickness absence*, CBI/Axa, London.

Cornes, P. (1982) *Employment rehabilitation: the aims and achievements of a service for disabled people*, HMSO, London.

Cornes, P. (1990) 'The vocational rehabilitation index: a guide to accident victims' requirements for return-to-work assistance', *Disability and Rehabilitation*, 12(1): 32–6 (available at: www.informaworld.com/smpp/title~db=all~content=t713723807~tab=issueslist~branches=12 – v12).

Crepeau, F. and Scherzer, P. (1993) 'Predictors and indicators of work status after traumatic brain injury: a meta-analysis', *Neuropsychological Rehabilitation*, 3(1): 5–35.

Cutler, R. B., Fishbain, D. A., Stelle-Rosconoff, R. *et al*. (2003) 'Relationship between functional capacity measures and baseline psychological measures in chronic pain patients', *Journal of Occupational Rehabilitation*, 13: 249–58.

Danieli, A. and Woodhams, C. (2005) 'Disability frameworks and monitoring disability', in Roulstone, A. (ed.), *Local authorities in working futures: disabled people, policy and social inclusion*, The Policy Press, Bristol, pp. 91–105.

Davies, R. and Jones, P. (2005) 'Trends and contexts to rates of workplace injury', HSE RR 386 (available at: www.hse.gov.uk./research/rrpdf/rr386.pdf).

Deal, J. and James-Brown, S. (1997) *Job coaching: integrating people with disabilities into open employment: a trainer's training manual*, The Enham Trust, Andover.

Department of Health (1999) *National Service Framework for mental health*, TSO, London.

Department of Health (2000) *Improving working lives standards*, DH, London.

Department of Health (2001) *National Service Framework for older people*, DH, London.

Department of Health (2004a) *Choosing health: making healthy choices easier*, HMSO, London, and (2008) *Next stage review*, (available at: www.dh.gov.uk/en/Publications).

Department of Health (2004b) *10 high impact changes for service improvement and delivery: a guide for NHS leaders*, Leicester DH, London.

Department of Health (2005) *National Service Framework for long-term conditions*, TSO, London.

Department of Health (2008) *National Service Framework for chronic pulmonary disease*, DH, London.

Department of Health (2009) 'New horizons: towards a shared vision for mental health', Consultation, London.

Department for Works and Pensions (2001) 'Strategy for increasing the employment rates of disabled people', DWP Research Paper, DWP, London.

Department for Works and Pensions (2002) *Pathways to work: helping people into employment*, Cm 5690, HMSO, Norwich.

Department for Works and Pensions (2003) *Helping people into employment. The government's response and action plan*, HMSO, Norwich.

Department for Works and Pensions (2004) *Building capacity for work: a UK framework for vocational rehabilitation*, HMSO, Norwich (available at: www.dwp.gov.uk/asd/asd5/report_abstracts/rr_abstracts/rra_224.asp).

Department for Works and Pensions (2006) *A new deal for welfare: empowering people to work*, Green Paper Cm 6730, TSO, Norwich.

Department for Works and Pensions (2007) *Ready for work: full employment in our generation*, Cm7290, HMSO, London.

Department for Work and Pensions Public Consultation (2007) 'Helping people achieve their full potential: improving specialist disability employment services' (available at: www.dwp.gov.uk).

Department for Work and Pensions Summary of Responses (2008) 'Helping people achieve their full potential: improving specialist disability employment services' (available at: www.dwp.gov.uk).

Department for Work and Pensions (2009) *Working our way to better mental health: a framework for action*, Cm. 7756, TSO, London.

Department for Works and Pensions, Department of Health, Department for Education and Skills (2005) *Health, work and well-being – caring for our future*, HMSO, London.

Department for Work and Pensions, Department of Health (2008a) *Working for a healthier tomorrow*, TSO, London.

Department for Works and Pensions, Department of Health (2008b) *Dame Carol: a healthier tomorrow*, TSO, London.

Department for Works and Pensions, Department of Health (2008c) *Improving health and work: changing lives, the government's response to Dame Carol Black's review of the health of Britain's working age population*, TSO, London (available at: www.workingforhealth.gov.uk).

Department for Social Security (1990) *A new contract for welfare support for disabled people*, CM 4103, DSS, London.

Department for Social Security (1998) *Ambitions for our country: A new contract for welfare*, DSS, London (available at: www.dwp.gov.uk/asd/asd5/report_abstracts/rr_abstracts/rra_224.asp).

Disability Discrimination Act (1995) (available at: www.legislation.gov.uk/ukpga/1995/50/contents).

Disability Discrimination Act (2005) (available at: www.equalityhumanrights.com/uploaded_files/disability_discrimination_act_2005.pdf).

Demers, L. M. (1992) *Work hardening. A practical guide*, Andover Medical Publishers, Boston.

Dewson, S., Ritchie, H. and Meager, N. (2005) 'New deal for disabled people: survey of employers', DWP RR 301, CDS, Norwich.

DiLeo, D., Luecking, R. and Hathaway, S. (1995) *Natural Supports in action training resources*, Network, St. Augustine.

Dixon, L., Hoch, J. S., Clark, R., Bebout, R., Drake, R., McHugo, G. and Becker, D. (2002) *Cost effectiveness of two vocational rehabilitation programs for persons with severe mental illness psychiatric services*, 53, 1118–1124.

Drake, R. E., Becker, D. R. and Bond, G. R. (2003) 'Recent research on vocational rehabilitation for persons with severe mental illness', *Current Opinions in Psychiatry*, 16(4): 451–5.

Dul, J. and Weerdmeester, B. (2001) *Ergonomics for beginners, a quick reference guide*, Taylor and Francis, London.

Employment Act (Dispute Regulations) (2002) 'Adopting statutory minimum dismissal, disciplinary and grievance procedures' (available at: www.opsi.gov.uk/Acts/acts2002/ukpga_20020022_en_1).

Employment-Related Services Association/Association of Chief Executives of Voluntary Organisations (2006) *A new deal for welfare. Empowering people to work*, Welfare Reform Green Paper, ERSA/ACEVO joint submission April 2006 (available at: wwloiw.ersa.org.uk/files/welfare-reform-green-paper-submission.pdf).

Escorpizo, R., Ekholm, J., Gmünder, H.-P. , Cieza, A., Kostanjsek, N. and Stucki, G. (2010) 'Developing a core set to describe functioning in vocational rehabilitation using the International Classification of Functioning, Disability, and Health (ICF)', *Journal of Occupational Rehabilitation*, Springer Netherlands.

Equality Act (2010) (available at: www.equalities.gov.uk/equality_act_2010.aspx).

European Union (2000) *Charter of the fundamental rights of the European Union* (2000/C364/01), Articles 21 and 26 (available at: www.europarl.europa.eu/charter/pdf/text_en.pdf).

Evans, A. and Walter, M. (2003) *From absence to attendance*, 2nd edition, CIPD, London.

Evans, J. and Repper, J. (2000) 'Employment, social inclusion and mental health', *Journal of Psychiatric and Mental Health Nursing*, 7: 15–24.

Fabian, E. S. and Luecking, R. G. (1991) 'Doing it the company way', *Journal of Applied Rehabilitation Counselling*, 22(2).

Fairbank, J. C., Couper, J., Davies, J. B. and O'Brien, J. P. (1980) 'The Oswestry Low Back Pain Disability Questionnaire', *Physiotherapy*, 66(8): 271–3.

Farrell, C., Nice, K., Lewis, J. and Sainsbury, R. (2006) 'Experience of the job rehabilitation and retention pilot', DWP RR 339, CDS, Leeds.

Fischler, G. and Booth, N. (1999) *Vocational impact of psychiatric disorders: a guide for rehabilitation professionals*, Aspen Publishers.

Fisher, G. S. (1999) 'Administration and application of the worker role interview: looking beyond functional capacity', *Work*, 12(1): 13–24.

Flanagan, J. C. (1954) 'The critical incident technique', *Psychological Bulletin*, 51(4).

Floyd, M. (ed.) (1997) *Vocational rehabilitation and Europe*, Jessica Kingsley Publishers, London.

Floyd, M., Pilling, D., Garner, K. and Barrett, P. (2004) 'Vocational rehabilitation; what works for whom and in what circumstances', *International Journal of Rehabilitation Research*, 27(2): 99–103.

Ford, J., Parker, G., Ford, F., Kloss, D., Pickvance, S. and Sawney, P. (2008) *Rehabilitation for work matters*, Radcliffe Publishing, Oxon.

Frain, M. P., Ferrin, J. M., Rosenthal, D. A. and Wampold, B. E. (2006) 'A meta-analysis of rehabilitation outcomes based on education level of the counselor', *Journal of Rehabilitation*, 72(1): 10–18.

Frank, A. O. and Sawney, P. (2003) 'Vocational rehabilitation', *Journal of the Royal Society of Medicine*, 96(11): 522–4.

Frank, A. O. and Thurgood, J. (2006) 'Vocational rehabilitation in the UK: opportunities for health-care professionals', *International Journal of Therapy and Rehabilitation*, 13(3): 126–34.

Frank, J. W., Sinclair, S., Hogg-Johnson, H., Shannon, C., Bombardier, C., Beaton, D. and Cole, D. (1998) 'Preventing disability from work-related low back pain. New evidence gives new hope – if we could just get all the players onside', *Journal of the Canadian Medical Association*, 158: 1625–31.

Freud, D. A. (2007) 'Reducing dependency: increased opportunity: options for the future of Welfare to Work', An Independent Review to the Department for Works and Pensions Services, CDS, Leeds.

Genskow, J. K. (1973) 'Evaluation, the multi-purpose proposition', *Journal of Rehabilitation*, 39(3): 22–5.

Gibson, L. and Strong, J. (2003) 'An occupational therapy framework of functional capacity evaluation in work rehabilitation', *Australian Journal of Occupational Therapy*, 50: 64–71.

Gilworth, G., Bhakta, B., Eyres, S., Carey, A., Chamberlain, M. A. and Tennant, A. (2007) 'Keeping nurses working: development and psychometric testing of the Nurse-Work Instability Scale (Nurse-WIS)', *Journal of Advanced Nursing*, 57(5): 543–51.

Gilworth, G., Chamberlain, M. A., Harvey, A., Woodhouse, A., Smith, J., Smyth, M. G. and Tennant, A. (2003) 'Development of a work instability scale for rheumatoid arthritis', *Arthritis and Rheumatology*, 49(3): 349–54.

Gilworth, G., Carey, A., Eyres, S., Sloan, J., Rainford, B., Bodenham, D., Neumann, V. and Tennant, A. (2006) 'Screening for job loss: development of a work instability scale for traumatic brain injury', *Brain Injury*, 20(8): 835–43.

Gilworth, G., Emery, P., Barkham, N., Smyth, M. G., Helliwell, P. and Tennant, A. (2009) 'Reducing work disability in ankylosing spondylitis – development of a Work Instability Scale for AS', *BMC Musculoskeletal Disorders*, 10: 68.

Gilworth, G., Haigh, R., Tennant, A., Chamberlain, M. and Harvey, A. (2001) 'Do rheumatologists recognize their patients' work related problems?', *Rheumatology*, 40(11): 1206–10.

Gilworth, G., Smyth, G., Smith, J, and Tennant, A. (March 2008) 'The development and validation of the Office Work Screen', *Occupational Medicine*, 58(4): 289–94.

Gobelet, C., Luthi, F., Al-Khodairy, A. T. and Chamberlain, M. A. (2007) 'Vocational rehabilitation: a multi-disciplinary intervention', *Disability and Rehabilitation*, 29(17): 1405–10.

Gold, M. (1980) *Try another way: training manual*, Research Press, Champaign, IL.

Gold, P. B., Meisler, N., Santos, A. B., Carnemolla, M. A., Williams, O. H. and Keleher, J. (2006) 'Randomized trial of supported employment integrated with assertive community treatment for rural adults with severe mental illness', *Schizophrenia Bulletin*, 32: 378–95.

Goldstone, C. and Douglas, L. (2003) *Pathways to Work from incapacity benefits: A pre-pilot exploration of staff and customer attitudes*, DWP, Sheffield.

Gowdy, E. L., Carlson, L. S. and Rapp, C. A. (2003) 'Practices differentiating high-performing from low-performing supported employment programs', *Psychiatric Rehabilitation Journal*, 26: 232–8.

Greenstreet Berman (2003) *Costing of a UK no fault compensation scheme*, Greenstreet Berman, Reading.

Greenstreet Berman, in association with Callund Consulting for the ABI(2004) *Cost and benefits of return-to-work and vocational rehabilitation in the UK*, Greenstreet Berman, Reading (available at: www.abi.org.uk/Publications/Cost_and_Benefits_of_Return_to_Work_ and_Vocational_Rehabilitation_in_the_UK1).

Grewal, I., McManus, S., Arthur. S. and Reith, L. (2004) 'Making the transition: addressing barriers in services for disabled people', DWP RR204, DWP, Sheffield.

Gross, D. P., Battie, M. C. and Asante, A. (2006) 'Development and validation of a short-term functional capacity evaluation for use in claimants with low back disorders', *Journal of Occupational Rehabilitation*, 16: 53–62.

Gross, D. P., Battie, M. C. and Asante, A. K. (2007) 'Evaluation of a short-form functional capacity evaluation: less may be best', *Journal of Occupational Rehabilitation*, 17: 422–35.

Gross, D. P., Battie, M. C. and Cassidy, J. D. (2004) 'The prognostic value of functional capacity evaluation in patients with chronic low back pain, part 1: timely return-to-work', *Spine*, 29: 914–19.

Groswasser, Z., Melamed, S., Agranov, E. and Keren, O. (1999) 'Return-to-work as an integrative measure following traumatic brain injury', *Neuropsychological Rehabilitation*, 9: 493–504.

Grover, C. (2007) 'The Freud Report on the future of Welfare to Work: some critical reflections', *Critical Social Policy*, 27(4): 534–45.

Grover, C. (2009) 'Privatising employment services in Britain', *Critical Social Policy*, 29(3): 487–508.

Grubbs, L. A., Cassell, J. L. and Mulkey, S. W. (2006) *Rehabilitation case-load management: concepts and practice*, 2nd edition, Springer Publishing, New York.

Gunnari, H., Evjenth, O. and Brady, M. (1984) *Sequence exercise. The sensible approach to all-round-fitness*, Dreyers-Forlag, Oslo.

Habeck, R. V., Hunt, H. A. and Van Tol, B. (1998) 'Workplace factors associated with preventing and managing work disability', *Rehabilitation Counselling Bulletin*, 42: 98–143.

Hagner, D. (1992) 'The social interactions and job supports of supported employees', in Nisbet, J. (ed.), *Natural supports in school, at work, and in the community for people with severe disabilities*, Paul H. Brookes, Baltimore, pp. 217–39.

Halstead, W. C. (1947) *Brain and intelligence: a quantitative study of the frontal lobe*, University of Chicago Press, Chicago.

Hanson, M. A., Burton, A. K., Kendall, N. A. S., Lancaster, R. J. and Pilkington, A. (2006) *The costs and benefits of active case management and rehabilitation for musculoskeletal disorders*, Hu-Tech Associates for HSE (available at: www.hse.gov.uk/research/rrpdf/rr493.pdf).

Harder, H. G. and Scott, L. R. (2005) *Comprehensive disability management*, Elsevier Churchill Livingstone, London.

Harding, V. R., Simmonds, M. J. and Watson, P. J. (1998) 'Physical therapy for chronic pain', *Pain Clinical Updates*, VI.

Harrington, M. (2010) *An independent review of the Work Capability Assessment*, TSO, London (available at: www.dwp,gov.uk/docs/wca-review-2010.pdf).

Hasluck, C. and Green, A. (2007) *What works for whom? A review of evidence and meta-analysis for the Department for Works and Pensions*, DWP RR407, CDS, Norwich.

Hathaway, S. R. and McKinley, J. C. (1967) *Minnesota multiphasic personality inventory manual*, The Psychological Corporation, New York.

Health and Safety at Work Act (1974) (Available at: www.hse.gov.uk/pubns/law.pdf).

Health and Safety Executive (1998) *Seating at work*, HS(G) 57, HSE Books, Sudbury.

Health and Safety Executive (2002a) *Upper limb disorder in the workplace*, HS(G)60 (rev) HSE Books, Sudbury.

Health and Safety Executive (2002b) 'Survey of use of occupational health support', Contract Research Report 445/2002.

Health and Safety Executive (2003) *Work with display screen equipment: Health and Safety (Display Screen Equipment) Regulations 1992*, as amended by the Health and Safety (Miscellaneous Amendments) Regulations 2002 – guidance on regulations, HSE Books, Sudbury.

Health and Safety Executive (2004) *Managing sickness absence and return-to-work: an employer's and manager's guide*, HSE Books, Norwich.

Health England (2007) 'Measures of preventative health spending', Report No 1 (available at: www.healthengland.org/publications/HealthEnglandReportNo1.pdf).

Heller, A. (1997) 'Developing an ergonomics task force', in *Strategies for success: disability management in the workplace*, National Institute of Disability Management and Research, Port Alberni, BC.

Henderson, M., Glazier, N. and Elliot, K. H. (2005) 'Long-term sickness absence', *British Medical Journal*, 330: 802–5.

Hershenson, D. (1990) 'A theoretical model for rehabilitation counseling', *Rehabilitation Counselling Bulletin*, 33.

Hoff, D., Gandolfo, C., Gold, M. and Jordan, M. (2000) *Demystifying job development. Field-based approaches to job development for people with disabilities*, Training Resources Network, St Augustine.

Holosko, M. J. and Feit, M. D. (eds) *Evaluation of employee assistance programs*, The Haworth Press, New York

Holmes, J. (2007) *Vocational rehabilitation*, Blackwell, Oxford.

Homa, D. B. (2007) 'Using the International Classification of Functioning, Disability and Health (ICF) in job placement', *Work*, 29: 277–86.

Home Office (1998) 'The compact on relations between the government and the voluntary and community sector', Cm 4100, Home Office, London.

Honey, S. and Williams, M. (1998) 'Supply and demand for supported employment', DfEE RR70, HMSO.

Hooper, R. (2003) 'Work personality profile – reviewed', *Journal of Occupational Psychology, Employment and Disability*, 5(2), DWP, Sheffield.

House of Commons Committee of Public Accounts (2006) 'Gaining and retaining a job. The DWP's support for disabled people', Sixth Report of Session 2006–7, HC112.

House of Commons Works and Pensions Committee (2006) 'The Efficiency Savings Programme in Jobcentre Plus', Second Report of the Session 2005/06, oral and written evidence, 8 March.

House of Commons Work and Pensions Committee (2007) 'The government's employment strategy', Third Report HC 63.11, oral and written evidence, 21 February.

HOST Policy Research (2002) 'A report for the Employment National Training Organisation on functional mapping in the employment and disability sector' HOST Policy Research, Horsham.

Howard, M. and Thornton, P. (2000) 'Job retention in the context of long-term illness', A paper prepared for the Joseph Rowntree Foundation Seminar 1 March 2000. Unpublished. SPRU, University of York.

HM Treasury (2002) *The role of the voluntary and community sector in service delivery; a cross cutting review*, HM Treasury, London.

HM Treasury (2004) *Releasing resources for the frontline: independent review of public sector efficiency*, HM Treasury, London.

Hudson, B. (2005) '"Sea change or quick fix?" Policy on long-term conditions in England', *Health and Social Care in the Community*, 13(4).

Income Data Services (July 2010a) 'Swapping roles was reasonable adjustment', Employment Law Brief 909.

Income Data Services (Nov 2010b) 'Reasonable adjustments –tribunals must give adequate reasons', Employment Law Brief 913. National Institute for Mental Health (England) (available at: www.equalityhumanrights.com/en/Pages/default.aspx).

ICAS Absence Survey (2006) (available at: www.axa-icas.absencemanagement.php).

International Monetary Fund (2007) 'Work absence in Europe', *IMF Staff Papers*, 54(3).

IRS Employment Review (2001) 'Return-to-work', *Policies and practices*, 741: 40–7.

Isernhagen, D. D. (2000) 'A model system: integrated work injury prevention and disability management', *Work*, 15(2): 87–94.

Isernhagen, S. J., Hart, D. L. and Matheson, L. N. (1999) 'Reliability of independent observer judgements of level of lift effort in a kinesiophysical Functional Capacity Evaluation', *Work*, 12: 45–50.

Jackson, T., Everatt, G. and Beyer, S. (undated) 'Reforming the supported placement scheme to promote career development and access for people with greater support needs' (available at: www.afse.org:uk/pages 8.htm).

James, P., Cunningham, I. and Dibben, P. (2003) *Job retention and vocational rehabilitation: the development and evaluation of a conceptual framework*, Research Report 106, Middlesex Business School and the University of Strathclyde for the Health and Safety Executive, HSE Books, Sudbury.

James, P., Cunningham, I. and Dibben, P. (2006) 'Job retention and return-to-work of ill and injured workers', *Employee Relations*, 28(3).

Japp, J. (2005) *Brain injury and returning to employment: a guide for practitioners*, Jessica Kingsley, London.

Jastak, J. F. and Jastak, S. R. (1965) *The wide range achievement test. Manual of instructions*, Guidance Associates, Wilmington.

Johnson, K. L., Yorkston, K. M., Klasner, E. R., Kuehn, C. M., Johnson, E. and Amtmann, D. (2004) 'The cost and benefits of employment: a qualitative study of experiences of persons with multiple sclerosis', *Archives of Physical Medicine and Rehabilitation*, 85: 201–9.

Kaiser, H. and Kersting, M. (2000) 'Der Stellenwert des Arbeitssimulation-serates', *ERGOS als Bestandteil der leistungsdiagnostichen Begutacktung Rehabilitation*, 39: 175–84.

Kielhofner, G. (2002) *Model of human occupation, 3rd edition: theory and application*, Lippincott, Williams and Wilkins, Philadelphia.

Kelly, G. (1955) *The psychology of personal constructs*, Norton, New York.

Kemp, P. A. and Davidson, J. (2008a) 'Routes into Incapacity Benefit: findings from a survey of recent claimants', DWP RR 469, CDS, Leeds.

Kemp, P. A. and Davidson, J. (2008b) 'Routes onto Incapacity Benefit: findings from a follow-up survey of recent claimants', DWP RR 516, CDS, Leeds.

Kendall, N. A., Burton, A. K., Main, C. J. and Watson, P. J. (2009) *Tackling musculoskeletal problems, a guide for the clinic and workplace – identifying obstacles using the psychosocial flags framework*, TSO, London.

Klonoff, P. S., Lamb, D. G. and Henderson, S. W. (2001) 'Outcomes from milieu-based neurorehabilitation at up to 11 years post-discharge', *Brain Injury*, 15(4).

Krause, N., Dasinger, L. K. and Neuhauser, F. (1998) 'Modified work and return-to-work: a review of the literature', *Journal of Occupational Rehabilitation*, 8: 113–19.

Krause, N. and Ragland, D. R. (1994) 'Occupational disability due to low back pain: a new interdisciplinary classification based on a phased model of disability', *Spine*, 19: 1011–120.

Kreider, J. (1983) 'Rehabilitation in the private sector', Paper reported in Grubbs *et al.* (2006).

Kreutzer, J. S., Wehman, P., Morton, M. V. and Stonnington, H. (1988) 'Supported employment and compensatory strategies for enhancing vocational outcome following traumatic brain injury', *Brain Injury*, 2(3): 205–24.

Labour Party (2005) *Britain forward not back*, Labour Party Manifesto.

Lakey, J. and Simpkins, R. (1994) *Employment rehabilitation for disabled people*, Policy Studies Institute, London.

Langman, C. (2007) 'Accounting for vocational outcomes following traumatic brain injury', unpublished PhD thesis, City University, London.

Latimer, E. A., Lecomte, T., Becker, D. R., Drake, R. E., Duclos, I., Lahaie, N., St-Pierre, M., Therrein, C. and Xie, H. (2006) 'Generalizability of the individual placement and support model of supported employment. Results of a Canadian randomized controlled trial', *British Journal of Psychiatry*, 189: 65–73.

Lawlis, G. F., Cuencas, R., Selby, D. and McCoy, C. E. (1989) 'The development of the Dallas pain questionnaire for illness behaviour', *Spine*, 14: 511.

Layard, R. (2005) 'Therapy for all on the NHS'. Speech. Sainsbury Centre for Mental Health, London, 6 September 2007 (cited in Booth *et al.*, 2007).

Lehman, A. F., Goldberg, R., Dixon, L. B., McNary, S., Postrado, L., Hackman, A. and McDonnel, K. (2002) 'Improving employment outcomes for persons with severe mental illness', *Archives of General Psychiatry*, 59: 165–72.

Lelliott, P., Tulloch, S., Boardman, J., Harvey, S., Henderson, M. and Knapp, M. (2008) 'Mental health and work', *Health, Work, Wellbeing* (available at: www.workingforhealth.gov.uk/documents/mental-health-and-work.pdf).

Lewis, F. D. and Bitter, C. F. (1991) 'Applied behavioural analysis and work adjustment training in work worth doing', in MacMahon, B. T. and Shaw, M. (eds), *Advances in brain injury rehabilitation*, Deutsch Press, Orlando.

Lewis, J., Corden, A., Dillon, L. and Thornton, P. (2005) 'An in-depth study of job broker service delivery', DWP RR246, CDS, Leeds.

Lissenburgh, S. and Marsh, A. (2003) 'Experiencing Jobcentre Plus Pathfinders; overview of earlier evaluation evidence', A study carried out on behalf of the DWP. In-house Report 111, DWP, London.

Loisel, P., Abenhain, L., Durand, P., Esdaille, J. M., Suissa, L., Gosselin, L., Simard, R., Turcotte, J. and Lemaire, J. (1997) 'A population based randomized clinical trial on back pain management', *Spine*, 22: 2911–18.

Loisel, P., Durand, M., Berthelette, D., Vezina, M., Baril, R., Gagnon, D., Larivière, C. and Tremblay, C. (2001) 'Disability prevention, new paradigm for the management of occupational back pain', *Disease Management and Health Outcomes*, 9(7): 351–60.

Loveland, D., Driscoll, H. and Boyle, M. (2007) 'Enhancing supported employment services for individuals with serious mental illness: A review of the literature', *Journal of Vocational Rehabilitation*, 27: 177–89.

Lucy, D., Tyers, C. and Savage, J. (2009) 'Healthy workplaces, Milton Keynes Pilot: evaluation findings', Prepared for Institute for Employment Studies, HSE RR809, Norwich.

MacDonald-Wilson, K. L., Rogers, E. S. and Massaro, J. (2003) 'Identifying relationships between functional limitations, job accommodations and demographic characteristics of persons with psychiatric disabilities', *Journal of Vocational Rehabilitation*, 18: 15–24.

MacErlean, N. (2005) 'Social enterprise: the issues', *The Observer*, 20 November.

Macias, C., Rodican, C. F., Hargreaves, W. A., Jones, D. R., Barreira, P. J. and Wang, Q. (2006) 'Supported employment outcomes of a randomized controlled trial of ACT and clubhouse models', *Psychiatric Services*, 57: 1406–15.

Main, C. J. and Spanswick, C. C. (2000) *Pain management. An interdisciplinary approach*, Churchill Livingstone.

Malec, J. F., Smigielski, J. S., DePompolo, W. and Thompson, J. M. (1993) 'Outcome evaluation in a comprehensive integrated post-acute brain injury rehabilitation program', *Brain Injury*, 7(1): 15–29.

Mansour, J. and Johnson, R. (2006) *Buying quality performance: procuring effective employment services*, Work Directions UK, London.

Marchington, M. and Wilkinson, A. (2003) *People management and development: human resource management at work*, CIPD, London.

Matheson, L. N. (1995) 'Getting a handle on motivation: self-efficacy in rehabilitation', in Isernhagen, S. J. (ed.), *The comprehensive guide to work injury management*, Aspen Publishers, Gaithersburg, Maryland, pp. 514–42.

Matheson, L. N. (2003) 'Functional capacity evaluation', in Demester, S. L., Anderson, G. B. J. and Smith, G. M. (eds), *Disability evaluation*, 2nd edition, Mosby Yearbook, Chicago, IL.

Matheson, L. N., Isernhagen, S. J. and Hart, D. L. (2002) 'Relationships amongst lifting ability, grip force, and return-to-work', *Physical Therapy*, 82: 249–56.

Matheson, L. N. and Matheson, M. L. (1996) 'Spinal function sort', Swiss Association for Rehabilitation, Working Group Ergonomics (available at: www.sar-rehab.ch).

Mathiason, N. (2005) 'Social enterprise: business phenomenon of the century', *The Observer*, 20 November.

Mayer, T. G., Barnes, D., Kishino, N. D., Nichols, G., Gatchel, R. J., Mayer, H. and Mooney, V. (1988) 'Progressive isoinertial lifting evaluation 1. A standardized protocol and normative database', *Spine*, 13: 993–7.

McHugo, D. J., Drake, R. E. and Becker, D. R. (1998) 'The durability of supported employment effects', *Psychiatric Rehabilitation Journal*, 22: 55–61.

Mclean, C., Carmona, C., Francis, S., Wohlgemuth, C. and Mulvilhill, C. (2005) *Worklessness and health – what do we know about the causal relationship?*, Evidence Review Health Development Agency, London.

Melzack, R. (1975) 'The McGill Pain Questionnaire: major properties and scoring methods', *Pain*, 1: 277–99.

Menchetti, B. (1991) 'Should vocational assessment and supported employment be partners or competitors? A research perspective', in *Vocational Evaluation and Work Adjustment Association Fifth National Forum on Issues in Vocational Assessment*, Menomonie, Materials Development Center, Stout Vocational Rehabilitation Institute, University of Wisconsin-Stout, pp. 49–5.

Mitchell, T. (2008) 'Utilization of the functional capacity evaluation in vocational rehabilitation', *Journal of Vocational Rehabilitation*, 28: 21–8.

Moore-Comer, R. A., Kielhofner, G. and Olsen, L. (1998) 'The work-environment impact scale, 2.0', MOHO Clearing House, Illinois (available at: www.moho.uic.edu/assess/weis.html).

Morritt, P. and Clark, F. (1997) *The Papworth experience*, Papworth Trust, Papworth Everard, Cambridgeshire.

Mosey, A. C. (1974) 'An alternative: the biopsychosocial model', *The American Journal of Occupational Therapy*, 38(3): 137–40.

Moss, N. and Arrowsmith, J. (2003) 'A review of "what works" for clients over 50', DWP W174, Sheffield.

Mowlam, A. and Lewis, J. (2005) 'Exploring how general practitioners work with patients on sick leave', DWP RR 257 CDS, London.

Mueser, K. T., Clark, R. E., Haines, M., Drake, R. E., McHugo, G. J., Bond, G. R., Essock, G. R., Becker, D. R., Wolfe, R. and Swain, K. (2004) 'The Hartford Study of supported employment for people with severe mental illness', *Journal of Consulting and Clinical Psychology*, 72: 479–90.

Nachemson, A. L. and Jonsson, E. (2000) *Neck and back pain*, Lippincott, Williams and Wilkins, Philadelphia.

National Audit Office (1987) *Employment assistance to disabled adults*, HMSO, London.

National Audit Office (2005) 'Gaining and retaining a job; the Department for Works and Pensions support for disabled people', Report by the Comptroller and Auditor General, HC 455 Session 2005–6.

National Audit Office (2006) 'Jobcentre Plus: delivering effective services through personal advisors', HC24 Session 2006–2007.

NHS Tayside (2009) Report No 04/09, Dundee CHP Committee, 19 February, Working Health Services Dundee, Vocational Rehabilitation Pilot Project Update.

Needles, K. and Schmitz, R. (eds) (2006) 'Economic and social costs and benefits to employers of retaining, recruiting and employing disabled people and/or people with health conditions or an injury: A review of evidence', DWP RR 400, CDS, Leeds.

Nice, K. and Thornton, P. (2004) 'Job retention and rehabilitation pilot: employers' management of long-term sickness absence', DWP RR 227 CDS, Norwich.

Nisbet, J. and Hagner, D. (1988) 'Natural supports in the workplace: a re-examination of supported employment', *Journal of the Association of Persons with Severe Handicaps*, 13: 260–7.

O'Connor, R. J., Cano, S. J., Ramio, I., Torrenta, L., Thompson, A. J. and Playford, E. D. (2005) 'Factors influencing work retention for people with multiple sclerosis: cross sectional studies using quantitative and qualitative methods', *Journal of Neurology*, 252.

Office for National Statistics (2002a) *Social trends*, TSO, London.

Office for National Statistics (2002b) *Labour force survey: Annual local area statistics digest*, TSO, London.

O'Flynn, D. (2001) 'Approaching employment: mental health, work projects and the care programme approach', *Psychiatric Bulletin*, 25: 169–71.

Olivieri, M. (2006) 'Functional capacity evaluation', in Gobelet, C. and Franchigoni, F. (eds) *Vocational rehabilitation*, Springer-Verlag, Paris.

Olsheski, J. A., Rosenthal, D. A. and Hamilton, M. (2002) 'Disability management and psychosocial rehabilitation: considerations for integration', *Work*, 19: 63–70.

Organisation for Economic Co-operation and Development (2006) *Sickness, disability and work: breaking the barriers, Vol.1: Norway, Poland and Switzerland.*

Organisation for Economic Co-operation and Development (2007) *Sickness, disability and work: breaking the barriers, Vol.2: Australia, Luxembourg, Spain and United Kingdom.*

Paetzold, R. L., Fernanda Garcia, M. and Colella, A. (2008) 'Peer perceptions of accommodation unfairness', *Journal of Occupational Psychology, Employment and Disability*, 10(1): 13–26.

Parenté, R. and DiCesare, A. (1991) 'Retraining memory: theory, evaluation and applications', in Kreutzer, J. and Wehman, P. (eds), *Cognitive rehabilitation for persons with traumatic brain injury*, Paul H. Brookes, Baltimore.

Parenté, R., Stapleton, M. C. and Wheatley, C. J. (1991) 'Practical strategies for vocational reentry after traumatic brain injury', *Journal of Head Trauma Rehabilitation*, 6(3): 35–45.

Parker, R. M. and Bolton, B. (2005) 'Research in rehabilitation counseling', in Parker, R. M. and Patterson, J. B. (eds), *Rehabilitation counselling: basic and beyond*, 4th edition, Pro-Ed, Austin, TX, pp. 335–62.

Pawson, R. and Tilley, N. (1997) *Realistic evaluation*, SAGE, London,

Perkins, R., Farmer, P. and Litchfield, P. (2009) *Realising ambitions: better employment support for people with a mental health condition*, TSO, Norwich.

Phillips, J. (2010) 'Return-to-work after traumatic brain injury: recording, measuring and describing occupational therapy intervention', *British Journal of Occupational Therapy*, 73(9): 422–30.

Prigatano, G. P., Fordyce, D. J., Zeiner, H. K., Roueche, J. R., Pepping, M. and Wood, B. (1984) 'Neuropsychological rehabilitation after closed head injury in young adults', *Journal of Neurology, Neurosurgery and Psychiatry*, 47: 505–13.

Purdon, S., Stratford, N., Taylor, R., Natarajan, L., Bell, S. and Wittenburg, D. (2006) 'Impacts of the job retention and rehabilitation pilot', DWP RR 342, CDS, Leeds.

Prime Minister's Strategy Unit (2004) 'Improving the life chances of disabled people', Interim report, PMSU, London.

Prime Minister's Strategy Unit, DWP, DH, Department for Education and Skills, Office of the Deputy Prime Minister (2005) 'Improving the life chances of disabled people' (available at: www.cabinetoffice.gov.uk/strategy/work_areas/disability.aspx).

Raptosh, D. (2005) 'Functional capacity evaluation: The Bureaus of Workers' Compensation', 4th Annual Workers' Compensation Conference handout (available at: www.dli.state.pa.us/landi/cwp/view.asp?A=138&Q=22715&tx=1).

Reiman, M. P. and Manske, R. C. (2009) *Functional testing in human performance*, Human Kinetics, Champaign, IL.

Riddell, S. (2002) *Work preparation and vocational rehabilitation: a literature review*, WAE Research Series, DWP, Sheffield.

Riddell, S. and Banks, P. (2005) Disabled people, employment and the Work Preparation programme in Working Futures? Disabled people, policy and social exclusion, Roulstone, A. and Barnes, C. T. (eds), The Policy Press, Bristol, pp. 59–74.

Rinaldi, M. and Perkins, R. (2007a) 'Vocational rehabilitation for people with mental health problems', *Psychiatry*, 6(9): 373–6.

Rinaldi, M. and Perkins, R. (2007b) 'Implementing evidence-based supported employment', *Psychiatric Bulletin*, 31: 244–9.

Rinaldi, M., Perkins, R., Glynn, E., Montibeller, T., Clenaghan, M. and Rutherford, J. (2008) 'Individual placement and support: from research to practice', *Advances in Psychiatric Treatment*, 13: 50–60.

Roessler, R. and Bolton, B. (1983) *Assessment and enhancement of functional vocational capabilities. A five-year research strategy*, Richard J Baker Memorial Monograph Series, Vocational Evaluation and Work Adjustment Association.

Roessler, R. and Bolton, B. (1985) 'The work personality profile: an experimental rating instrument for assessing job maintenance skills', *Vocational Evaluation and Work Adjustment Bulletin*.

Roessler, R. , Kirk, M. H. and Brown, P. L. (1997) 'Chronic illness and return-to-work: a social cognitive perspective', *Work*, 8: 189–96.

Rogan, P.and Hagner, D. (1990) 'Vocational evaluation in supported employment', *Journal of Rehabilitation*, 56(1): 45–51.

Ross, J. (2007) *Occupational therapy and vocational rehabilitation*, John Wiley and Sons, Chichester.

Royal College of Psychiatrists (2002) *Employment opportunities and psychiatric disability*, RCP, London.

Rubin, S. and Roessler, R. (2001) *Foundations of the vocational rehabilitation process*, 5th edition, Pro-Ed, Austin, TX.

Rumrill, P. D., Steffen, J. M., Kaleta, D. A. and Holman, C. A. (1996) 'Job placement interventions for people with multiple sclerosis', *Work*, 6: 167–75.

Saal, J. A. and Saal, J. S. (1991) 'Postoperative rehabilitation and training', in Mayer, T. G., Mooney, V. and Gatchell, R. J. (eds), *Contemporary conservative care for painful spinal disorders*, Lea and Febiger, Philadelphia, pp. 318–27.

Sainsbury Centre for Mental Health (2008) *Mental health at work: developing the business case*, Sainsbury Centre for Mental Health.

Sainsbury Centre for Mental Health (2009) 'Doing what works', Briefing 37, SCMH, London.

Sainsbury, R. and Davidson, J. (2006) 'Routes into Incapacity Benefit: findings from qualitative research', DWP RR 350, CDS, Leeds.

Sainsbury, R., Nevill, C., Wood, M., Dixon, J. and Mitchell, M. (2008) 'The Pathways Advisory Service: placing employment advisers in GP surgeries', DWP RR494, DWP, Sheffield.

Salvendy, G. (1987) *Handbook of human factors*, John Wiley, New York.

Salyers, M. P., Becker, D. R., Drake, R. E., Torrey, W. C. and ,Wyzik, P. F. (2004) 'A ten year follow-up of a supported employment program', *Psychiatric Services*, 55(3): 302–8.

Sandqvist, J. L. and Henrikson, C. M. (2004) 'Work functioning: a conceptual framework', *Work*, 23(2): 147–57.

Saunders, J. L., Leahy, M. J., McGlynn, C. and Estrada-Hernandez, N. (2006) 'Predictors of employment outcomes for persons with disabilities: an integrative review of potential evidence-based factors', *Journal of Applied Rehabilitation Counselling*, 37(2): 3–20.

Sawney, P. and Challoner, J. (2003) 'Poor communication between health professionals is a barrier to rehabilitation', *Occupational Medicine*, 53(4): 246–8.

Schaafsma, F., Schonstein, E., Whelan, K. M., Ulvestad, E., Kenny, D. T. and Verbeek, J. H. (2010) Schonstein, E., Kenny, D. T., Keating, J. and Koes, B. W. (2002) 'Work conditioning, work hardening and functional restoration for workers with neck and back pain (Cochrane Review)', Cochrane Library Issue 1, John Wiley and Sons, Chichester (available at: www.cochrane.org).

Schneider, J. (2005) 'Getting back to work: what do we know about what works?', in Grove, B., Secker, J. and Seebohm, P., *New thinking about mental health and employment*, Radcliffe Publishing, Oxford.

Scottish Executive (2007) *Co-ordinated, integrated and fit for purpose: a delivery framework for adult rehabilitation in Scotland*, Scottish Executive, Edinburgh.

Sears, A. (2003) 'Universal usability and the WWW', in Forsyth, C., Grose, E. and Ratner, J. (eds), *Human factors and web development*, Lawrence Erlbaum Associates, Mahweh.

Selander, J., Marnetoft, S.-U., Bergroth, A. and Ekhom, J. (2002) 'Return-to-work following vocational rehabilitation for neck, back and shoulder problems: risk factors reviewed', *Disability and Rehabilitation*, 24(14): 704–12.

Silcox, S. (2006) 'Enabling rehabilitation: beyond the medical model', *Occupational Health Review*, 119: 21–4.

Smith, B., Povall, M. and Floyd, M. (1991) *Managing disability at work: improving practice in organisations*, Jessica Kingsley, London.

Social Exclusion Unit (2004) 'Mental health and social exclusion', Office of the Deputy Prime Minister, London.

Stafford, B. (2003) 'In search of a welfare to work solution: the New Deal for Disabled People', *Benefits*, 11(3): 181–86.

Stein, F. and Cutler, S. K. (2002) *Psychosocial occupational therapy, a holistic approach*, Delmar, Albany, NY.

Stratford, N., Farrell, C., Natarajan, L. and Lewis, J. (2005a) 'Taking part in a randomised controlled trial: a participant's view of the Job Retention and Rehabilitation Pilot', DWP RR 273, CDS, London.

Taylor, J. and Hartfree, Y. (2003) 'Deferrals in Jobcentre Plus: research into staff understanding and application of deferral guidance for non-Jobseekers Allowance customers', In-house report 126, DWP, London.

Teasdale, T. W., Christensen, A. L. and Pinner, E. M. (1993) 'Psychosocial rehabilitation of cranial and stroke patients', *Brain Injury*, 7L 535–42.

Third Sector (2006) 'Major review of the sector's role' (available at: www.thirdsector.co.uk/ Channels/Fundraising/login/613964).

Thompson, N. (March 2009) 'How vocational rehabilitation fits into HCML's model of case management', VocRe Forum 4, Vocational Rehabilitation Association, Glasgow.

Thornton, P. (2005) 'Jobcentre Plus: can specialised personal advisors be justified?', in Roulstone, A. and Barnes, C. (eds), *Working futures? Disabled people, policy and social exclusion*, The Policy Press, Bristol.

Thurgood, J. (1997) 'The Wexham Park experience: the work rehabilitation programme in one occupational therapy department following injury or physical illness', *British Journal of Occupational Therapy*, 60: 245–7.

Tomassen, P. C., Post, M. W. and van Asbeck, F. W. (2000) 'Return-to-work after spinal cord injury', *Spinal Cord*, 38(1): 51–5.

Tomlinson Report (1943) *Report of the Inter-Departmental Committee on the Rehabilitation and Resettlement of Disabled Persons*, Cmnd 9883, HMSO, London Standards of Practice.

Townsend, E. (2002) *Enabling occupation: an occupationl therapy perspective*, Canadian Association of Occupational Therapists, Ottawa.

Tyerman, A. (1999) 'Working out: a joint DoH/ES traumatic brain injury vocational rehabilitation project', Project report, Community Head Injury Service, Vale of Aylesbury NHS Trust.

Unger, K. V., Pardee, R. and Shafer, M. S. (2000) 'Outcomes of post-secondary education programmes for people with psychiatric disabilities', *Journal of Vocational Rehabilitation*, 14: 195–9.

United Nations (2008) *UN Enable – Rights and dignity of persons with disabilities* (available at: www.un.org/disabilities).

UKRC Rehabilitation Standards (2010) (Available at: www.rehabcouncil.org.uk/standards. php).

United Kingdom Rehabilitation Council (2009a) *Rehabilitation Standard: hallmarks of a good provider*, UKRC, London (available at: www.rehabcouncil.org.uk).

United Kingdom Rehabilitation Council (2009b) *Selecting rehabilitation services: a purchaser's guide to the standards expected of a rehabilitation provider*, UKRC, London (available at: www.rehabcouncil.org.uk).

United Kingdom Rehabilitation Council (2009c) *Selecting rehabilitation services: a consumer's guide to the standards expected of a rehabilitation provider*, UKRC, London (available at: www.rehabcouncil.org.uk).

United Kingdom Rehabilitation Council, Department for Business, Innovation and Skills, BSI (2010) PAS 150: 2010, *Providing rehabilitation services Code of Practice*, London (available at: www.bsigroup.com).

Van der Weide, W. E., Verbeek, J. H. and van Tulder, M. V. (1997) 'Vocational outcome of intervention for low back pain', *Scandinavian Journal of Work, Environment and Health*, 23(3): 165–78.

Vlaeyen, J. W., De Jong, J., Geilen, M., Heuts, P. H. T. and van Breukelen, G. (2001) 'Fear avoidance and its consequences in chronic musculoskeletal pain: a replicated single case experimental design', *Behaviour Research and Therapy*, 39: 151–66.

Vlaeyen, J. W., De Jong, J., Geilen, M., Heuts, P. H. T. and van Breukelen, G. (2002) 'The treatment of fear of movement/(re)injury in chronic low back pain: further evidence on the effectiveness of exposure *in vivo*', *Clinical Journal of Pain*, 18: 251–61.

Vlaeyen, J. W. and Linton, S. J. (2000) 'Fear avoidance and its consequences in chronic musculoskeletal pain: a state of the art', *Pain*, 85: 317–32.

Vocational Rehabilitation Association (2007) *Standards of practice*, VRA, Glasgow (available at: www.vocationalrehabilitation.org).

Waddell, G. (1998) *The back pain revolution*, Churchill Livingstone, pp. 223–4.

Waddell, G. and Burton, A. K. (2001) 'Occupational health guidelines for the management of low back pain at work: evidence review', *Occupational Medicine (Lond)*, 51: 124–35 (available at: www.facoccmed.ac.uk->Publications).

Waddell, G. and Burton, K. (2004) *Concepts of rehabilitation for the management of common health problems*, TSO, London (available at: www.tso.co.uk/bookshop).

Waddell, G. and Burton, K. (2006) *Is work good for your health and well-being?*, TSO, Norwich (available at: www.tsoshop.co.uk).

Waddell, G., Burton, K. and Kendall, N. A. S. (2008) *Vocational rehabilitation: what works, for whom, and when?*, TSO, London.

Wansbrough, N. and Cooper, P. (1980) *Open employment after mental illness*, Tavistock Publications, London.

Watson, P., Booker, K., Moores, L. and Main, C. (2004) 'Returning the chronically unemployed with low back pain to employment', *European Journal of Pain*, 8(4): 359–69 (available at: www.sciencedirect.com).

Wechsler, D. (1981) *Manual for the Wechsler Adult Intelligence Scale –Revised*, The Psychological Corporation, New York (Version IV (2008) available at: www.pearsonassessments.com).

Wheatley, C. and Rein, J. (1990) 'Intervention in traumatic head injury. Learning style assessment', in Hertfelder, S. and Gwin, C. (eds), *Occupational therapy in work programs*, AOTA Press, Rockville.

Wheeler, L. and Reitan, R. M. (1962) 'The presence and laterality of brain damage predicted from responses to a short aphasia screening test', *Perceptual and Motor Skills*, 15: 783–99.

Whysall, Z. and Ellwood, P. (2006) 'HSE Horizon Scanning Intelligence Group Demographic study – Report', (available at: www.hse.gov.uk/horizons/demographics.pdf).

Williams, R. M. and Westmoreland, M. (2002) 'Perspectives on workplace disability management: a review of the literature', *Work*, 1: 87–93.

Wilson, B. A., Alderman, N., Burgess, P. W., Emslie, H. and Evans, J. J. (2003) 'Behavioural assessment of the dysexecutive syndrome', *Journal of Occupational Psychology, Employment and Disability*, 5(2): 33–7.

Woolf, H., Lord, (1996) *Access to justice*, Department for Constitutional Affairs, London.

World Health Organisation (2001) *International classification of functioning, disability and health*, 1st edition, Geneva.

Wright, P., Rogers, N., Hall, C. Wilson, B., Evans, J., Emslie, H. and Bartram, C. (2001) 'Comparison of pocket computer memory aids for people with brain injury', *Brain Injury*, 19(9), 787–800.

Additional reading and sources of information

Chapter 1

International comparisons

Bruyere, S. (2000) 'Managing disability in the workplace', *Equal Opportunities Review*, 92: 26–33.

Gobelet, C. and Franchignoni, F. (2007) *Vocational rehabilitation*, Springer-Verlag, France.

O'Halloran, D. (2002*)* 'An historical overview of Australia's largest and oldest provider of vocational rehabilitation – CRS Australia', *Work*, 19: 211–18.

Rubin, S. E. and Roessler, R. (2001) *Foundations of the vocational rehabilitation process*, Pro-Ed, Austin, TX.

Shrey, D. E. and Hursh, N. C. (1999) 'Workplace disability management: international trends and perspectives', *Journal of Occupational Rehabilitation*, 9(1): 45–59.

Westmorland, R. M. and Buys, N. (2004) 'A comparison of disability management practices in Australian and Canadian workplaces', *Work: Journal of Prevention, Assessment and Rehabilitation*, 23(1): 31–41.

Defining VR

Chamberlain, M. A., Moser, V. F., Ekholm, K. S., O'Connor, R. J., Herceg, M. and Ekholm, J. (2009) 'Vocational rehabilitation: an educational review', *Journal of Rehabilitation Medicine*, 41: 856–69.

College of Occupational Therapists/Sainsbury Centre for Mental Health (2008) *Vocational rehabilitation: what is it, who can deliver it and who pays?*, COTs/Sainsbury Centre for Mental Health, London.

Disciplines in VR

Frank, A. O. and Thurgood, J. (March 2006) 'Vocational rehabilitation in the UK: Opportunities for health-care professionals', *International Journal of Therapy and Rehabilitation*, 13(3): 126–34.

Gilworth, G., Haigh, R., Tennant, A., Chamberlain, M. A. and Harvey, A. R. (2001) 'Do rheumatologists recognize their patients' work-related problems?', *Rheumatology*, 40: 1206–10.

Griffiths, J. (2005) 'The perceptions of occupational therapists regarding the use of vocational rehabilitation', *Mental health Occupational Therapy*, 10(2): 56–61.

Joss, M. (2002) 'Occupational therapy and rehabilitation for work', *British Journal of Occupational Therapy*, 65(3): 141–8.

Disability management

International Labour Organisation (2001) *Code of practice for managing disability in the workplace* (available at: http://ilo.org/public/standards/rel. . .).

Isernhagen, D. D. (2000) 'A model system: Integrated work injury prevention and disability management', *Work*, 15: 87–94.

James, P., Cunningham, I. and Dibben, P. (2006) 'Job retention and return-to-work of ill and injured workers', *Employee Relations*, 28(3).

National Institute for Disability Management and Research (2000) *Code of practice for disability management*, NIDMAR, Port Alberni, BC.

Shrey, D. E. and Hursh, N. C. (1999) 'Workplace disability management: International trends and perspectives', *Journal of Occupational Rehabilitation*, 9(1): 45–60.

Westmoreland, M. (Jan/Feb 2007) 'Disability management – a rose by any other name', *OT Now*: 10–13.

Managing sickness absence

Carroll, C., Rick, J., Pilgrim, H., Cameron, J. and Hillage, J. (2010) 'Workplace involvement improves return-to-work rates among employees with back pain on long-term sick leave: a systematic review of the effectiveness and cost-effectiveness of interventions', *Disability and Rehabilitation*, 32(8): 607–21.

Hurstfield, J., Allen, B., Ballard, J., Davies, J., McGeer, P. and Miller, L. (2003) *The extent of use of health and safety requirements as a false excuse for not employing sick or disabled persons*, HSE Research Report 167 (available at: www.hse.gov.uk/research/rrpdf/rr167.pdf).

Hayday, S., Rick, J., Carroll, C. and Jagger, N. (2007) *Guidance for primary care services and employers on the management of long-term sickness and incapacity:mappping review*, Institute for Employment Studies, University of Brighton.

Available via HSE Books (tel. 00 44 1787 881165; http://books.hse.gov.uk):
Managing sickness absence and return-to-work (HSG 249).
Off sick and worried about your job? (INDG 397).
Managing sickness absence and return-to-work in small businesses (INDG 399).

Advice is also available at www.hse.gov.uk/sicknessabsence.

National Institute for Clinical Excellence (NICE) Public Health Guideline 19, *Management of long-term sickness and incapacity for work* (available at: www.nice.org.uk/PH19).

Hayday, S., Rick, J., Carroll, C. and Jagger, N. (2007) *Guidance for primary care services and employers on the management of long-term sickness and incapacity: mapping review*, Institute of employment Studies, Brighton ((available at http://employment-studies.co.uk).

Chapter 2

Meager, N. and Hill, D. (August 2006) 'UK national public policy initiatives and regulations affecting disabled people's labour market participation', Working Paper WP2, Institute for Employment Studies (available at: www.employment-studies.co.uk/pubs/index.php).

Chapter 3

Policy development

Roulstone, A. and Barnes, C. (eds) *Working futures? Disabled people, policy and social inclusion*, The Policy Press, Bristol.

UK regional VR strategies

Scottish Executive (2007) *Co-ordinating, integrated and fit for purpose – A Delivery Framework for Adult Rehabilitation in Scotland* (available at: www.scotland.gov.uk/Publications/2007/02/20154247/0).

Related documents are *Healthy working lives, Workforce Plus: an employment framework for Scotland* and *Healthy working lives: a plan for action* (available at: www.healthyworkinglives. com/advice/vocational rehabilitation/index.aspx).

Northern Ireland's Department for Employment and Learning (2008) *Corporate plan 2008–2011* (available at: www.delni.gov.uk/corporate-plan-2008–2011).

Welsh Assembly Government (2005) *The Welsh Strategic Framework for Economic Development: Wales: a vibrant economy*, consultation document (available at: www.wales.gov.uk); also see *Workboost Wales* (available at: www.workboostwales.com).

Trade Union Congress

The TUC website details papers on rehabilitation and health and safety at work. It includes:

TUC (2008) 'Representing and supporting members with mental health problems at work: Guidance for trade union representatives' (available at: www.tuc.org.uk/extras/mental health.pdf).

TUC (2006) 'Disability and work: a trade union guide to the law and good practice' (available at: www.tuc.org.uk/extras/disabilityandwork.pdf).

TUC (2006) 'Jobs for disabled people and a three-point plan' (available at: www.tuc.org.uk/extras/ disabledjobs.doc).

Chapter 4

Association of Personal injury Lawyers (APIL) *Think rehab: best practice guide on rehabilitation* (available at: www.apil.org.uk/campaigns.aspx).

British Society of Rehabilitation Medicine, Association of Personal injury Lawyers, Royal College of Physicians (2006) *Guide to best practice at the interface between rehabilitation and the medico-legal process*, BSRM, London (available at: www.bsrm.co.uk/Publications).

Hughes, V. (ed.) (2004) *Tolley's guide to employee rehabilitation*, Lexis Nexis Tolley, London.

Rehabilitation Working Party, *The rehabilitation code* (available at: www.iua.co.uk/rehabilitation).

Bodily Injuries Claims Management Association, *Rehabilitation: a practitioners guide* (available at: www.bicma.org.uk).

Chapter 5

Disability legislation

Doyle, B. (2005) *Disability discrimination: law and practice*, 5th edition, Jordans, Bristol.

Keen, S. and Oulton, R. (2009) *Disability discrimination in employment*, OUP.

Lawson, A. (2008) *Disability and equality law in Britain: the role of reasonable adjustment*, Hart Publishing, Oxford.

Meager, N. and Hurstfield, J. (2005) 'Legislating for equality: evaluating the Disability Discrimination Act 1995', in Roulstone, A. and Barnes, C. (eds), *Working futures? Disabled people, policy and social inclusion*, The Policy Press, Bristol.

Simm, C., Aston, J., Williams, C., Hill, D., Bellis, A. and Meager, N. (March 2007) *Organisations' responses to the Disability Discrimination Act*, Research Report DWPRR 410 (available at: http://research.dwp.gov.uk/asd/asd5/rrs-index.asp).

Woodhams, C. and Corby, S. (2003) 'Defining disability in theory and practice: a critique of the British Disability Discrimination Act 1995', *Journal of Social Policy*, 32(2): 1–20.

Woodhams, C. and Corby, S. (2007) 'Then and now: disability legislation and employers' practices in the UK', *British Journal of Industrial Relations*, 45(3): 556–80.

DDA

Various codes of practice issued under the DDA are available on the Equality and Human Rights Commission's website (www. equalityhumanrights.com). They include:
Code of practice: employment and occupation.
Guidance on matters to be taken into account in determining questions relating to the definition of disability.

Equality Act

The EHRC produces codes of practice offering statutory guidance on the Equality Act's employment implications (available at: www.equalityhumanrights.com/legislative-framework/ equality-bill/equality-bill-codes-of-practice-consultation/).

Medical questionnaires

Income Data Services (Aug 2009) *Medical questionnaire: if you don't ask, you don't get*, IDS Employment Law Brief 882.
Income Data Services (Aug 2009) *No misrepresentation in employee's answers to medical questionnaire*, IDS Employment Law Brief 882.

Chapter 6

VR prediction

Kendall, E., Muenchburger, H. and Gee, T. (2006) 'Vocational rehabilitation following traumatic brain injury: a quantitative synthesis of outcome studies', *Journal of Vocational Rehabilitation*, 25: 149–60.
Nightingale, E. J., Soo, C. A. and Tate, R. L. (2007) 'A systematic review of early prognostic factors for return-to-work after traumatic brain injury', *Brain Impairment*, 8(2): 101–42.
Roessler, R. T., Rumrill, P. D. and Fitzgerald, S. M. (2004) 'Predictors of employment status for people with Multiple Sclerosis', *Rehabilitation Counselling Bulletin*, 47(2): 96–103.

Benefits

Corden, A. (2005) 'Benefits and tax credits: enabling systems or constraints', in Roulstone, A. and Barnes, C. (eds), *Working futures? Disabled people, policy and social inclusion*, The Policy Press, Bristol.
Disability Alliance (annual) *Disability rights handbook* (available at: www.disabilityalliance.org).
Doran, I. (2011) *Employment and support allowance: work capability assessment by health condition and functional impairment*, Official Statistics 1, DWP, London.

Employment barriers

Goldstone, C. (March 2002) 'Barriers to employment for disabled people', In-House Report 95, DWP, London
Harris, J. and Thornton, P. (2005) 'Barriers to labour market participation: the experience of deaf and hard of hearing people', in Roulstone, A. and Barnes, C. (eds), *Working futures: disabled people, policy and social exclusion*, The Policy Press, Bristol.
Simkiss, P. (2005) 'Work matters: visual impairment, disabling barriers and employment options', in Roulstone, A. and Barnes, C. (eds), op. cit.

Chapter 8

Condition management programmes

Barnes, H. and Hudson, M. (2006) 'Pathways to Work: qualitative research on the condition management programme', DWP RR346, CDS, Leeds.

Disability employment advisors

Goldstone, G. (2008) 'Disability employment advisor (DEA) organisation in Jobcentre Plus', RR 539 DWP, HMSO, Norwich.

Distance travelled

Dewson, S., Eccles, J., Tackey, N. D. and Jackson, A. (2000) *Guide to measuring soft outcomes and distance travelled*, Institute for Employment Studies, Brighton, for DfEE, Sheffield.
Lloyd, R. and O'Sullivan, F. (2004) *Measuring soft outcomes and distance travelled: a methodology for developing a guidance document*, HMSO, London.
Purvis, A., Lowrey, J. and Law, R. (2009) 'Exploring a distance travelled approach to Workstep development planning', DWP RR566, HMSO, Norwich.

New Deal for Disabled People

There are a number of research reports covering aspects of NDDP, available at: http://php.york.ac.uk/inst/spru/research/sums/nddp_natext.php.

Residential training

Maton, K., Smyth, K., Broome, S. and Field, P. (2000) 'Evaluation of the effectiveness of residential training for disabled people', RR243, Department for Education and Skills, Sheffield.

Supported employment

Ridley, J. and Hunter, S. (2006) 'The development of supported employment in Scotland', *Journal of Vocational Rehabilitation*, 25: 57–68.

Chapter 9

Brain injury

Japp, J. (2005) *Brain injury and returning to employment: a guide for practitioners*, Jessica Kingsley, London.
Mysiw, W. J., Corrigan, J. D., Hunt, M., Cavin, D. and Fish, T. (1989) 'Vocational evaluation of traumatic brain injury patients using the functional assessment inventory', *Brain Injury*, 3: 27–34.
Rose, F. D., Johnson, D. A. (eds) (1996) *Brain injury and after: towards improved outcome*, John Wiley and Sons, Chichester.
Tyerman, A. and Tyerman, R. (2009) 'The functional assessment inventory', *Occupational Medicine*, 59(4): 285.
Tyerman, A. and Young, K. (1999) 'Vocational rehabilitation after severe traumatic brain injury: evaluation of a specialist assessment programme', *Journal of Applied Occupational Psychology, Employment and Disability*, 2: 31–41.
Tyerman, A. and Young, K. (2000) 'Vocational rehabilitation after severe traumatic brain injury: II Specialist interventions and outcomes', *Journal of Applied Occupational Psychology, Employment and Disability*, 2: 13–20.

Tyerman, A., Tyerman, R. and Viney, P. (2008) 'Vocational rehabilitation programmes', in Tyerman, A. and King, N. S. (eds), *Approaches to rehabilitation after traumatic brain injury*, Blackwell Publishing, Oxford.

Clinical management of RTW

Beaumont, D. G. (2003) 'The interaction between general practitioners and occupational health professional in relation to rehabilitation for work: a Delphi study', *Occupational Medicine*, 53: 249–53.
Chamberlain, M. A. and Frank, A. O. (2004) 'Congratulations but no congratulations: should physicians do more to support their patients at work?', *Clinical Medicine*, 4(2): 102–4.
Pransky, G., Katz, J., Benjamin, K. and Himmelstein, J. (2002) 'Improving the physician role in evaluating work ability and managing disability: a survey of primary care practitioners', *Disability and Rehabilitation*, 24(16): 867–74.

Implementing IPS

A dedicated area of the Sainsbury's Mental Health Centre website provides up-to-date information on the international research evidence and examples of implementation in the UK (www.centreformentalhealth.org.uk/).
Drake, R. E., Becker, D. R. and Bond, G. R. (July 2003) 'Recent research on vocational rehabilitation for persons with severe mental illness', *Current Opinion in Psychiatry*, 16(4): 451–5.

Mental health

DWP, HSE, Health Work Well-being, CIPD, DH (2009) *Line managers resource: a practical guide to managing and supporting people with health conditions in the workplace*, SHIFT, National Mental Health Development Unit (available at: www.shift.org.uk).
Boardman, J. (2003) 'Work, employment and psychiatric disability', *Advances in Psychiatric Treatment*, 9: 327–34.
Groves, B. (2001) 'Making work schemes work', *Psychiatric Bulletin*, 25: 446–8.
Harvey, S. B., Henderson, M., Lelliot, P. and Hotopf, M. (2001) 'Approaching employment: mental health, work projects and the care programme approach', *Psychiatric Bulletin*, 25: 169–71.
Irvine, A. (2008) 'Managing mental health and employment', DWP RR 537, Norwich.
Ley, P., Birkin, R. and Meehan, M. (2001) 'Enabling an individual with manic depression to obtain employment – the role of personal advisors and employability', *The Application of Occupational Psychology to Employment and Disability*, 4(1): 17–26.
Lloyd, C. and Waghorn, G. (2007) 'The importance of vocation in recovery for young people with psychiatric disabilities', *British Journal of Occupational Therapy*, 70(20): 50–9.
Michon, H. W. C., van Weeghel, J., Kroon, H., Smit, F. and Schene, A. H. (2006) 'Predictors of successful job finding in psychiatric vocational rehabilitation: an expert panel study', *Journal of Vocational Rehabilitation*, 25: 161–71.
Patmore, S. (2004) 'Factors affecting the employment of individuals who report mental health difficulties: an exploratory study', *Journal of Occupational Psychology, Employment and Disability*, 6(1): 15–20.
Sainsbury, R., Irvine, A., Aston, J., Wilson, S., Williams, C. and Sinclair, A. (2008) 'Mental health and employment', DWP RR 513, DWP, Sheffield (available at: http://research. dwp.gov.uk/asd/asd5/report_abstracts/rr_abstracts/rra-513.asp). (This report addresses circumstances that lead people to claim IB because of a MH condition and what factors contribute towards RTW after a period on IB. The study also explores employers' experience of dealing with MH conditions in the workplace.)

Sainsbury Centre for Mental Health (2009) *Evening the odds: employment support, mental health and black and ethnic minority communities*, Briefing 35, London (available at: www. scmh.org.uk).

Sainsbury Centre for Mental Health (2009) *Removing barriers: the facts about mental health and employment*, Briefing 40, London (available at: www.scmh.org.uk).

Underwood, L., Thomas, J., Williams, T. and Thieba, A. (2007) 'The effectiveness of interventions for people with common mental health problems on employment outcomes: a systematic rapid evidence assessment', in Research Evidence in Education Library, London: EPPI-Centre, Social Science Research Unit, Institute of Education, University of London.

Service user perspective

Johnson, R. L., Floyd, F., Pilling, D., Boyce, M. J., Grove, B., Secker, J., Schneider, J. and Slade, J. (April 2009) 'Service users perceptions of the effective ingredients in supported employment', *Journal of Mental Health*, 18(2): 121–8.

Chapter 10

VR case management

Chan, F. and Leahy, M. J. (eds) (1999) *Healthcare and disability case management*, Vocational Consultants Press, Lake Zurich, IL.

Chan, F., Leahy, M. J. and Saunders, J. L. (eds) (2005) *Case management for rehabilitation health professionals (2nd edition), Volume I: Foundational aspects*, Aspen Professional Services.

Chan, F., Leahy, M. J. and Saunders, J. L. (eds) (2005) *Case management for rehabilitation health professionals (2nd edition). Volume II: Advanced practice: Applications with special populations*, Aspen Professional Services.

Chapman, C., Chantler, C., Harrison, J. and Saltrese, A. (2006) *Best practice guidelines for case managers*, Case Management Society UK, Sutton (available at: www.cmsuk.org. documents/tmp70.pdf).

Garcis-Iriarte, E., Balcazar, F. and Taylor-Ritzler, T. (2007) 'An analysis of case managers support of youth with disabilities transitioning from school to work', *Journal of Vocational Rehabilitation*, 129–40.

Lee, D. N. (2005) 'Musculoskeletal disorders: case management and rehabilitation; a review', *Journal of Occupational Psychology, Employment and Disability*, 7(1): 59–72.

O'Reilly, S. (2007) *Helping hands*, Occupational Health.

Roessler, R. T. and Rubin, S. E. (1998) *Case management and rehabilitation counselling*, Pro-Ed, Austin, TX.

Russo, D. and Innes, E. (2002) 'An organizational case study of the case manager's role in a client's return-to-work programme in Australia', *Occupational Therapy International*, 9(1): 57–75.

Summers, N. (2006) *Fundamentals of case management practice: Skills for the human services*, 2nd edition, Wadsworth/Thomson Learning, Belmont, CA.

VR counselling

McMahon, B. T., Shaw, L. R., Chan, F. and Danczyk-Hawley, C. (2004) '"Common factors" in rehabilitation counselling and the working alliance', *Journal of Vocational Rehabilitation*, 20(2): 101–6.

Parker, R. M., Szymanski, E. M. and Patterson, J. B. (2005) *Rehabilitation counseling: basics and beyond*, Pro-Ed, Austin, TX.

Riggar, T. F. and Maki, D. R. (eds) (2004) *Handbook of rehabilitation counseling*, Springer Publishing.

Roessler, R. T. and Rubin, S. E. (2006) *Case management and rehabilitation counseling*, 4th edition, Pro-Ed, Austin, TX.

Chapter 11

Interviewing/motivating

Graham, V., Jutla, S., Higginson, D. and Wells, A. (2008) 'The added value of motivational interviewing within employment assessments', *Journal of Occupational and Organisational Psychology*, 10(1): 43–52.

MOHO

Brenneman Baron, K. and Littleton, M. J. (1999) 'The model of human occupation: a return-to-work case study', *Work*, 12: 37–46.

Self-efficacy

Booth, D. and James, R. (2008) 'A literature review of self-efficacy and effective jobsearch', *Journal of Occupational Psychology, Employment and Disability*, 10(1): 27–42.

James, R. (2007) 'Job-capability match, adviser skills and the five self-efficacy barriers to employment', *Journal of Occupational Psychology, Employment and Disability*, 9(10).

Chapter 12

Condition-based assessments

Breeding, R. R. (2005) 'Vocational rehabilitation and sudden onset disability: Advancing proprietary consumer involvement through improved vocational assessment', *Journal of Vocational Rehabilitation*, 22(3): 131–42.

Cancer

Grunfeld, E. A., Low, E. and Cooper, A. F. (2010) 'Cancer survivors' and employers' perceptions of work following cancer treatment', *Occupational Medicine*, 60(8): 611–17.

Epilepsy

Bishop, M. (2002) 'Barriers to employment among people with epilepsy: Report of a focus group', *Journal of Vocational Rehabilitation*, 17: 281–6.

HIV/Aids

Razzano, L .A. and Hamilton, M. M. (2005) 'Health-related barriers to employment among people with HIV/Aids', *Journal of Vocational Rehabilitation*, 22(3): 179–88.

Mental health

Rogers, E. S., Sciarappa, K. and Anthony, W. A. (1991) 'Development and evaluation of situational assessment instruments and procedures for persons with psychiatric disabilities', *Vocational Evaluation and Work Adjustment Bulletin*, 61–7.

Schultheis, A. M. M. and Bond, G. R. (1993) 'Situational assessment ratings of work behaviors: changes across time and between settings', *Psychosocial Rehabilitation Journal*, 17(2): 108–19.

Spinal cord injury

Targett, P., Wehman, P., McKinley, W. O. and Young, C. (2005) 'Functional vocational assessment for individuals with spinal cord injury', *Journal of Vocational Rehabilitation*, 22(3): 149–62.

Traumatic brain injury

Thomas, D. F. and Menz, F. E. (1996) 'Functional assessment of vocational skills and behaviors of persons with brain trauma injuries', *Journal of Vocational Rehabilitation*, 7: 243–56.

Computer-based assessment

Webb, J. (2005) 'Comment on the use of AbilityMatch in employment assessments', *Journal of Occupational Psychology, Employment and Disability*, 7(1): 3–5.

Functional capacity evaluations

Buys, T. and van Biljon, H. (2007) 'Functional capacity evaluation: An essential component of South African occupational therapy work practice', *Work*, 29: 31–6.

Hart, D. L., Isernhagen, S. J. and Matheson, L. N. (1993) 'Guidelines for functional capacity evaluation of people with medical conditions', *Journal of Occupational and Sports Therapy*, 18(6): 682–6.

Innes, E. and Straker, L. (1999) 'Reliability of work-related assessments', *Work*, 13: 107–24.

Innes, E. and Straker, L. (1999) 'Validity of work-related assessments', *Work*, 13: 125–52.

King, P. M., Tuckwell, N. and Barrett, T. E. (1998) 'A critical review of functional capacity evaluations', *Physical Therapy*, 78(8): 852–66.

Mitchell, T. (2008) 'Utilization of the functional capacity evaluation in vocational rehabilitation', *Journal of Vocational Rehabilitation*, 28: 21–8.

Strong, S. (2002) 'Functional capacity evaluations – the good, the bad and the ugly', *OT Now*: 5–9.

MOHO

Kielhofner, G., Braveman, B., Baron, K., Fisher, G., Hammel, J. and Littleton, M. (1999) 'The model of human occupation: understanding the worker who is ill and disabled', *Work*, 12: 3–11.

Psychological testing

Bryson, G. J., Bell, M. D., Lysaker, H. and Zito, W. (1997) 'The work behavior inventory: A scale for the assessment of work behaviors for clients with severe mental illness', *Psychiatric Rehabilitation*, 20: 47–55.

Garland, T. (2005) 'The Wechsler Abbreviated Scale of Intelligence (WASI): an overiew and case studies in occupational assessment', *Journal of Occupational Psychology, Employment and Disability*, 7(2): 125–30.

Greig, T. C., Nichols, S. S., Bryson, G. J. and Bell, M. D. (2004) 'The Vocational Cognitive Rating Scale: a scale for the assessment of cognitive functioning at work for clients with severe mental illness', *Journal of Vocational Rehabilitation*, 21: 71–81.

Gregory, R. G. (2004) 'Neuropsychological assessment and screening', in Gregory, R. G., *Psychological testing: history, principles, and applications*, 4th edition, Boston, pp. 440–94.

Meehan, M., Birkin, R. and Snodgrass, R. (1998) 'Employment assessment (EA), Issues surrounding the use of psychological assessment material with disabled people', *Selection and Development Review*, 14: 3–9.

Wells, A. S., Parker, G. and Snodgrass, R. (2002) 'Occupationally focussed intrepetations of the WAIS-R in employment assessments', *Journal of Occupational Psychology, Employment and Disability*, 5(1): 23–41.

Chapter 13

Condition specific support

Asperger Syndrome and Autism

Muller, E., Schuler, A., Burton, B. A. Yates, G. B. (2003) 'Meeting the vocational support needs of individuals with Asperger Syndrome and other Autism spectrum disabilities', *Journal of Vocational Rehabilitation*, 18: 163–75.
Grandin, T. and Duffy, K. (2008) *Developing talents: careers for individuals with Asperger* Temple Grandin (Author) › *Visit Amazon's Temple Grandin PageFind all the books, read about the author, and more.*
See search results for this author
Are you an Author? Learn about Author Central
Syndrome and high-functioning Autism, Autism Asperger Publishing Company, Kansas (available at: http://www.amazon.co.uk/Developing-Talents-Individuals-Asperger-High-functioning/dp/1934575283/ref=pd_sim_b_3 – #).

HIV/Aids

Breuer, N. L. (2005) 'Teaching the HIV-positive client how to manage the workplace', *Journal of Vocational Rehabilitation*, 22(3): 163–70.
Conyers, L. and Boomer, K. B. (2005) 'Factors associated with disclosure of HIV/Aids to employers among individuals who use job accommodations and those who do not', *Journal of Vocational Rehabilitation*, 22(3): 189–98.

Mental health

SHIFT (DH), NMHDU, DWP, HSE, HWWB, CIPD (2009) *A practical guide to managing and supporting people with mental health problems in the workplace* (available at: www.shift.org.uk/employers).

Musculoskeletal conditions

Verbeek, J. H. (2001) 'Vocational rehabilitation of workers with back pain', *Scandinavian Journal of Work, Environment and Health*, 27(5): 346–52.

Rheumatic diseases

De Buck, P. D .M., Schoones, J. W., Allaire, S. H. and Vliet Vlieland, T. P. M. (2002) 'Vocational rehabilitation in patients with chronic rheumatic diseases: a systematic literature review', *Seminars in Arthritis and Rheumatism*, 32(3): 196–203.
Mahalik, J., Shigaki, C. L., Baldwin, D. and Johnstone, B. (2006) 'A review of employability and worksite interventions for persons with rheumatoid arthritis and osteoarthritis', *Work*, 26: 303–11.

Spinal cord injury

Marini, I., Lee, G. K., Chan, F., Chapin, M. H. and Romero, M. G. (2006) 'Vocational rehabilitation service patterns related to successful competitive employment outcomes of persons with spinal cord injury', *Journal of Vocational Rehabilitation*, 25: 1–13.

Meade, M. A., Armstrong, A. J., Barrett, K., Ellenbogen, P. S. and Jackson, M. N. (2006) 'Vocational rehabilitation services for individuals with Spinal Cord injury', *Journal of Vocational Rehabilitation*, 25: 3–11.

Use of cognitive behavioural therapy

Winspear, D. (2007) 'Using CBT to improve employment outcomes for Incapacity Benefit customers: interim report', *Journal of Occupational Psychology, Employment and Disability*, 9(1): 41–9.

Working with employers

Balser, R. M., Hagner, D. and Hornby, H. (2000) 'Partnership with the business community: the Mental Health Employer Consortium', *Journal of Applied Rehabilitation Counselling*, 31(4): 47–53.
Fraser, R. T. (2008) 'Successfully engaging with the business community in the vocational rehabilitation placement process', *Journal of Vocational Rehabilitation*, 28: 115–20.

Interview skills

Tse, T. (1996) 'Interview skills training for people with psychiatric disabilities: a review of the literature', *Work*, 7: 203–12.

Relative value of rehabilitation support services

Meager, N., Wilson, S. and Hill, D. (2007) 'ICT strategy, disabled people and employment in the UK', Working Paper WP14, Institute for Employment Studies (available at: www.employment-studies.co.uk/pubs/report).
Schonbrun, S. L., Sales, A. P. and Kampfe, C. M. (2007) 'RSA (Rehabilitation Services Administration) services and employment outcomes in consumers with traumatic brain injury', *Journal of Rehabilitation*, 73(2): 26–31.

Work hardening and work conditioning

Cooper, J. E., Tate, R. and Yassi, A. (1997) 'Work hardening in an early return-to-work program for nurses with back injury', *Work*, 8: 149–56.
Darphin, L. E. (1995) 'Work hardening and work conditioning perspectives', in Isernhagen, S. J. (ed.), *The comprehensive guide to work injury management*, Aspen Publishers, Gaithersburg, MD.
Nicholas, K. (2002) Work hardening/conditioning: Functional restoration and pain management programs for injured workers with no 'Red Flag' conditions, WorkCover, New South Wales.
Weir, R. and Nielson, W. R. (2001) 'Interventions for disability management', *The Clinical Journal of Pain*, 17(4): S128–32.

Chapter 14

Adjustments

Blitz, C. L. and Mechanic, D. (2006) 'Facilitators and barriers to employment among individuals with psychiatric disabilities', *Work*, 26: 407–19.
DiLeo, D., Luecking, R. and Hathaway, S. (1995) *Natural supports in action training resources*, Network, Florida.
Gates, L. B. (2000) 'Workplace accommodation as a social process', *Journal of Occupational Rehabilitation*, 10(1): 85–98.

Gates, L. B., Akabas, S, H, and Oran-Sabia, V. (1998) 'Relationship accommodations involving the work group: improving work prognosis for persons with mental health conditions', *Psychiatric Rehabilitation Journal*, 21(3).

Hirsh, A., Duckworth, K., Hendricks, D. and Dowler, D. (1996) 'Accommodating workers with traumatic brain injury: issues relating to TBI and ADA', *Journal of Vocational Rehabilitation*, 7: 217–36.

Mancuso, L. L. (1990) 'Reasonable accommodation for workers with psychiatric disabilities', *Psychosocial Rehabilitation Journal*, 14(2): 3–19.

Meager, N., Dewson, S., Evans, C., Harper, H., McGeer, P., O'Regan, S. and Tackey, N. D. (2002) 'Costs and benefits to service providers of making reasonable adjustments, under Part III of the Disability Discrimination Act', RR 169, DWP, CDS, Leeds (available at: www.dwp.gov.uk/asd/asd5/rrs-index.asp).

Munir, F., Jones, D., Leka, S. and Griffiths, A. (2005) 'Work limitations and employer adjustments for employees with chronic illness', *International Journal of Rehabilitation Research*, 28(2): 111–17.

Pryce, J., Munir, F. and Haslam, C. (2007) 'Cancer survivorship and work: Symptoms, supervisor response, co-worker disclosure and work adjustment', *Journal of Occupational Rehabilitation*, 17(1): 83–92.

Roessler, R. T. and Gottcent, J. (1994) 'The Work Experience Survey: a reasonable accommodation/career development strategy', *Journal of Applied Rehabilitation Counselling*, 25(3): 16–21. This paper is based on the experience of five subjects with MS describing their experience of accommodation based on the administration of the Work Experience Survey.

Russell, D. (2006) 'Employer willingness to consider workplace adjustments for people with mental health problems', *Journal of Occupational Psychology, Employment and Disability*, 8(2): 211–23.

Sandsjo, L., Valtonen, K., Grundell, L. O., Karlsson, A.-K. and Viikura-Juntara, E. (2008) 'Assessment of working conditions and implementation of changes among employees with spinal cord lesion – A case series', *Journal of Vocational Rehabilitation*, 28: 121–8.

Targett, P. S., Wehman, P. H., McKinley, W. O. and Young, C. L. (2004) 'Successful work supports for persons with SCI: focus on job retention', *Journal of Vocational Rehabilitation*, 21: 19–26.

Wehman, P., Kreutzer, J., Sale, P., West, M., Morton, M. V. and Diambra, J. (1989) 'Cognitive impairment and remediation: implications for employment following traumatic brain injury', *Journal of Head Trauma Rehabilitation*, 4(3): 66–75.

Job coaching

Buckley, A. and Buckley, C. (2006) *A guide to coaching and mental health*, Routledge, Taylor and Francis, London.

Carew, D. and Collumb, S. (2008) *Supported employment and job coaching in psychological approaches to rehabilitation after traumatic brain injury*, Tyerman, A. and King, N. S. (eds), Blackwell Publishing, Oxford.

Conyers, L. M. and Ahrens, C. (2003) 'Using the Americans with Disabilities Act to the advantages of persons with severe and persistent mental illness: What rehabilitation counsellors need to know', *Work*, (21): 57–68.

Granger, B., Baron, R. and Robinson, S. (1997) 'Findings from a national survey of job coaches and job developers about job accommodations arranged between employers and people with psychiatric disabilities', *Journal of Vocational Rehabilitation*, 9: 235–51.

McHugh, S. H., Storey, K. and Certo, N. J. (2002) 'Training job coaches to use natural support strategies', Journal of Vocational Rehabilitation, 15: 155–63.

Placements

Fabian, E. S., Luecking, R. G. and Tilson, G. P. (1995) 'Employer and rehabilitation personnel perspectives on hiring persons with disabilities: Implications for job development', *Journal of Rehabilitation*, 61(1): 42–9.

Fraser, R. T. (2008) 'Successfully engaging the business community in the vocational rehabilitation placement process', *Journal of Vocational Rehabilitation*, 28: 115–20.

Johnson, R. and Stoten, S. (1998) *Return to previous employment* in *approaches to rehabilitation after traumatic brain injury*, Tyerman, A. and King, N. S. (eds), Blackwell Publishing, Oxford.

Kluesner, B., Taylor, D. W. and Bordieri, J. (2005) 'An investigation of the job tasks and functions of providers of job placement activities', *Journal of Rehabilitation*, 71(3): 26–35.

Krupa, T. (2004) 'Employment, recovery and schizophrenia: integrating health and disability at work', *Psychiatric Rehabilitation Journal*, 28(1): 8–14.

Mahalik, J., Shigaki, C., Baldwin, D. and Johnstone, B. (2006) 'A review of employability and worksite interventions for persons with rheumatoid arthritis and osteoarthritis', *Work*, 26: 303–11.

Muller, E., Schuler, A., Burton, B. A. and Yates, G. B. (2003) 'Meeting the vocational support needs of individuals with Asperger Syndrome and other autism spectrum disabilities', *Journal of Vocational Rehabilitation*, 18: 163–75.

Parenté, R., Stapleton, M. C. and Wheatley, C. J. (1991) 'Practical strategies for vocational reentry after traumatic brain injury', *Journal of Head Trauma Rehabilitation*, 6(3): 35–45.

Schuster, R. and Marantz, S. (1994) 'Increasing accuracy in job placement for the brain-damaged client', *NeuroRehabilitation*, 4(1): 15–24.

Szymanski, E. M. and Parker, R. M. (2003) *Work and disability: Issues and strategies in career development and job placement*, 2nd edition, Pro-Ed, Austin, TX.

Retention

Mercer, G. (2005) 'Job retention: a new policy priority for disabled people', in Roulstone, A. and Barnes, C. (eds), *Working futures? Disabled people, policy and social inclusion*, The Policy Press, Bristol.

Tsang, H. W. H. and Li, S. M. Y. (2010) 'Work related social skills and job retention', in Lloyd, C. (ed.) *Vocational rehabilitation and mental health*, Wiley-Blackwell, Chichester.

Thomas, T. and Secker, J. (2005) 'Getting off the slippery slope: an example from the UK', in Grove, B., Secker, J. and Seebohm, P. (eds), *New thinking about mental health and employment*, Radcliffe Publishing, Oxford.

Glossary of abbreviations

ABI	Association of British Insurers
ABI	Acquired brain injury
APIL	Association of Personal Injury Lawyers
ASSET	Assistance to Employment and Training
AVEVO	Association of Chief Executives of Voluntary Organisations
BABICM	British Association of Brain Injury Case Managers
BAOT/COT	British Association/ College of Occupational Therapists
BIS	Business, Innovation and Skills (Department of)
BPS	British Psychological Society (www.bps.org.uk)
BSI	British Standards Institute (www.bsigroup.com)
BSRM	British Society for Rehabilitation Medicine
CBI	Confederation of British Industry
CIPD	Chartered Institute of Personnel and Development
CMOP	Canadian Model of Occupational Performance
CMP	Condition Management Programme
CMSUK	Case Management Society UK (www.cmsuk.org)
CPA	Care programme approach
COPM	Canadian Occupational Performance Measure
COTNAB	Chessington Occupational Therapy Neurological Assessment Battery
DDA	Disability Discrimination Act
DEA	Disability employment advisor
DfEE	Department for Education and Employment
DH	Department of Health
DOT	Dictionary of Occupational Titles
DRO	Disablement resettlement officer
DM	Disability management
DWP	Department for Works and Pensions
EAT	Employment Appeal Tribunal
EHRC	Equalities and Human Rights Commission
ELCI	Employers Liability Compulsory Insurance
ERC	Employment Rehabilitation Centre
ERSA	Employment Related Services Association
ESA	Employment and Support Allowance
FCE	Functional capacity evaluation
HPC	Health Professionals Council
HSE	Health and Safety Executive

IB	Incapacity benefits
ICF	International Classification of Functioning, Disability and Health
ILO	International Labour Office
IMF	International Monetary Fund
ICF	International Classification of Functioning, Disability and Health
IRU	Industrial Rehabilitation Centre
JCP	Jobcentre Plus
JIS	Job Introduction Scheme
JRRP	Job Rehabilitation and Retention Programme
MOHO	Model of Human Occupation
MS	Multiple sclerosis
MSC	Manpower Services Commission
MSD	Musculoskeletal disorder(s)
NDDP	New Deal for Disabled People
NHS	National Health Service
NICE	National Institute for Clinical Excellence
NIDMAR	National Institute of Disability Management and Research
OECD	Organisation for European Co-operation and Development
OH(S)	Occupational Health (Service)
OJE	On-the-job evaluation
OT	Occupational therapist
(IB/ESA) PA	(Incapacity Benefit/Employment and Support Allowance) Personal Advisor
PCT	Primary Care Trust
PI	Personal injury
PACT	Placement, Assessment and Counselling Team
RNIB	Royal National Institute for Blind People
RTA	Road traffic accident
RTC	Residential training college
RTW	Return-to-work
SEU	Social Exclusion Unit
SME	Small and medium sized employers
SMI	Severe mental illness
SIG	Sheltered Industrial Group
SPS	Sheltered Placement Scheme
TBI	Traumatic brain injury
UKRC	United Kingdom Rehabilitation Council (www.rehabcouncil.org.uk)
VCWS	Valpar Component Work Samples
WCA	Work Capability Assessment
WEIS	Work Environment Impact Scale
WFHRA	Work-Focused Health-Related Assessment
WHO	World Health Organisation
WIS	Work Instability Scale
WRI	Worker Role Interview
VR	Vocational rehabilitation
VRA	Vocational Rehabilitation Association

Index

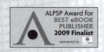
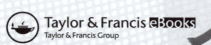